Speech Production and Pei

Other books by Mark Tatham and Katherine Morton

EXPRESSION IN SPEECH: Analysis and Synthesis

DEVELOPMENTS IN SPEECH SYNTHESIS

Speech Production and Perception

Mark Tatham
and
Katherine Morton

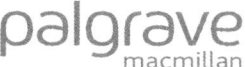

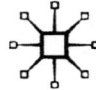

© Mark Tatham and Katherine Morton 2006

All rights reserved. No reproduction, copy or transmission of this publication may be made without written permission.

No paragraph of this publication may be reproduced, copied or transmitted save with written permission or in accordance with the provisions of the Copyright, Designs and Patents Act 1988, or under the terms of any licence permitting limited copying issued by the Copyright Licensing Agency, 90 Tottenham Court Road, London W1T 4LP.

Any person who does any unauthorised act in relation to this publication may be liable to criminal prosecution and civil claims for damages.

The authors have asserted their rights to be identified as the authors of this work in accordance with the Copyright, Designs and Patents Act 1988.

First published in 2006 by
PALGRAVE MACMILLAN
Houndmills, Basingstoke, Hampshire RG21 6XS and
175 Fifth Avenue, New York, N.Y. 10010
Companies and representatives throughout the world.

PALGRAVE MACMILLAN is the global academic imprint of the Palgrave Macmillan division of St. Martin's Press, LLC and of Palgrave Macmillan Ltd. Macmillan® is a registered trademark in the United States, United Kingdom and other countries. Palgrave is a registered trademark in the European Union and other countries.

ISBN-13: 978–1–4039–1732–4   hardback
ISBN-10: 1–4039–1732–9   hardback
ISBN-13: 978–1–4039–1733–1   paperback
ISBN-10: 1–4039–1733–7   paperback

This book is printed on paper suitable for recycling and made from fully managed and sustained forest sources.

A catalogue record for this book is available from the British Library.

Library of Congress Cataloging-in-Publication Data

Tatham, Mark.
  Speech production and perception / Mark Tatham and Katherine Morton.
    p. cm.
  Includes bibliographical references and index.
  ISBN 1–4039–1732–9 (cloth) – ISBN 1–4039–1733–7 (pbk.)
  1. Speech. 2. Phonetics. 3. Speech perception. I. Morton, Katherine.
II. Title.

P95.T32 2006
414'.8—dc22   2005044661

10 9 8 7 6 5 4 3 2 1
15 14 13 12 11 10 09 08 07 06

Printed and bound in Great Britain by
Antony Rowe Ltd, Chippenham and Eastbourne

Dedicated to the memory of Peter Ladefoged, 1925–2006

Contents

List of Figures and Tables — xiv

Introduction — xvi

Part I Speech Production Theory

1 Classical Phonetics — 3
Introduction — 3
Assumptions of Classical Phonetics — 3
The claims of Classical Phonetics — 6
System in Classical Phonetics — 7
Parameters for classifying segments — 9
Combinatorial constraints on phonetic features — 10
Segments 'in' the speech signal — 11
What is a segment? – the speaker focus — 13
What is a segment? – the listener focus — 14
Phonemes — 14
The nature of symbolic representations — 16
Phonetic transcription and linguistically relevant information — 17
Confusion over what speech sounds 'represent' — 18
The domain of speech theory — 19

2 Coarticulation: the Phenomenon — 21
Introduction — 21
What is coarticulation? — 22
Right-to-left coarticulation — 24
Phonetic under-specification — 26
Overlap — 26
Contextual 'accommodation' — 27
Adaptation — 28
Coarticulation and 'phonetic accommodation' — 29
Coarticulation or co-production? — 29
Blocking and coarticulatory spread — 30
The spreading model and linear causation — 31
Target theory — 32
Correlation between the input target specification
  and the articulator target — 35

	Non-variable targets, variable targets and management	36
	The unknown input	38
3	**Coarticulation Theory**	**40**
	Introduction	40
	Characterising the *results* of coarticulation	41
	What must a theory of coarticulation include?	49
	The focus of coarticulation theory	53
	Theories and models of coarticulation	55
	Models of coarticulation – presuppositions	55
	Coarticulation – basic theory	57
	Symbolic representation and linear context	58
	Technical criticism of Wickelgren's approach	59
	Lashley's serial ordering approach	60
	Öhman's vowel carrier model	61
	MacNeilage's three-dimensional spatial targets	61
	Holmes' linearly conjoining model	62
	Lindblom's coarticulation model	64
	Lindblom and Öhman compared	64
	Henke's look-ahead model	67
	Intrinsic and extrinsic allophones	70
	Ladefoged's approach to allophones	71
	Classical Phonetics confuses assimilation and coarticulation	72
	Kim's 'systematic synthesis' model and coarticulation	74
	Daniloff and Hammarberg – coarticulation as feature spreading	75
	Keating's model of coarticulation	76
	Window setting – target constraints and their domains	82
	Coarticulatory resistance and aggression	86
	Revisions of the Window Model	87
	Coarticulatory resistance	89
	Co-production theories	91
	Coarticulation *vs.* co-production	92
	Sources of intrinsic variation	95
	Inter-segment coarticulatory influence	96
4	**Speech Motor Control**	**99**
	Introduction	99
	Two dimensions to speech production theory	100
	The purpose of phonetic descriptions	101
	Speech production models	104
	Levels of abstraction	105
	Articulatory Control	106

	Models of speech production	107
	Serial ordering – the Lashley/MacNeilage legacy	108
	Ordering in Öhman's early model of coarticulation	110
	Rhythm and temporal ordering	111
	Lashley's control mechanism	111
	Action Theory	112
	Task Dynamics	116
	Articulatory Phonology	117
	Speech production theory – changing direction	118
	Unifying the approach	119
	Ruling out explicit segmentation	120
	The Gestural Score	120
5	**Speech Production: Prosody**	**121**
	Introduction	121
	Spanning – an intonation example	122
	Prosodic effects	123
	The correlation between abstract and physical prosody	124
	Linguistic distinctiveness	124
	Syllables	125
	Prosody – focus on segments detracts from good prosody models	129
	Features for prosody *vs.* features for segments	131
	Syllables and stress	133
	Prominence and stress	136
	The metrical organisation of speech	144
	Stressed syllables form the basis of rhythmic structure	145
	Declination	148
	Prosodic Analysis	150
	Prosody and parametric modelling	152
	Prosodic effects on segmental articulation	153
	The basis of intonation modelling	156

Part II Speech Perception Theory

6	**Dynamic Model Building and Expressive Content**	**167**
	Introduction	167
	What levels of representation are necessary?	167
	Modelling and the physical world	168
	Requirements of the model – feedback	169
	The speech production model	171
	Cognition develops models of speech processes	172

Planes	173
Details of the speech production model	174
Supervision	176
Predictive modelling – anticipatory cognitive processing	179
Expressive content in speech production	179
The dynamic nature of the waveform	181
Prosody as information bearing	183
Sources of expressive/emotive content	184
The perception of expressive content	184
The listener is active	187
Some questions that need answering	188
Pragmatics in phonetics	189
Language pathology and clinical neuroscience	192
Language teaching/learning	192
The simulation of speech – speech technology	193

7 Speech Perception and Prosody — 194

Introduction	194
Consonants *vs.* vowels	195
The listener's perceptual goal	196
The principle of sufficient perceptual separation	197
The perceptual task	198
The general problem of speech perception	199
Models of Speech Perception	201
Passive models – template-based models	204
Passive theories – filtering	205
Direct Perception (as opposed to 'mediated perception')	206
The Motor Theory of Speech Perception	207
The Analysis by Synthesis Theory	209
Hybrid models of speech perception	209
Categories	210
Direct Realism	212
Stevens' Quantal Theory	213
The quest for invariance	213
The Associative Store Theory	213
Similarity of production and perception	216

8 Speech Perception: Production for Perception — 218

Introduction	218
Ease of articulation	220
Targets – representations of which level?	221
Adaptive Variability Theory	222

Articulator 'response' and its relevance to perception	223
The basic units for speech – segments again	224
Functional and physical definitions – potential conflict	225
Segments – psychological reality	226
Discrete units in the cognitive world	226
Impossibility of isolating cognitive considerations from physical considerations	227
Segment 'boundaries' and asynchrony	228
Two possible control models	229
Uniqueness of segments as 'targets'	229
Trubetskoy and the continuum of speech	230
'Rule governed' processes?	230
General theory related to phonetic theory	231
A theory of speech production must cover both phonology and phonetics	232
Do phonological or phonetic representations dominate the perceptual processes?	233

Part III Areas of Focus, Modelling and Applications

9 Applications: Cognitive and Physical Modelling — 237

Introduction	237
Duality	238
The phenomenon – what is being modelled	239
Spoken language	239
Speech and hearing/perceiving disorders	240
Language teaching	240
Speech simulations	241
Current modelling	241
An old problem	242
Cognitive and physical modelling	245
Modelling the phenomenon – theory	245
Modelling the phenomenon – the empirical approach	246
Application models within theory	247
Usefulness of empirical work	248
Testing models	249
Theories available for application – linguistically oriented models	250
Cognitive and physical modelling	251
Physical to physical – motor to acoustic	252

		Deficiencies of current theory	252
		When more than one model is needed	254
		Metatheory	254
		Our proposal	255
		A computational approach	255

10 Speech Technology — 256

- Introduction — 256
- Speech synthesis – how natural? — 256
- Naturalness — 256
- Adaptation and simulation — 257
- Speaker expectation — 258
- Intelligibility – state of the art — 258
- Naturalness in human speech — 260
- Variability — 261
- Style — 263
- Data structures — 264
- Automatic speech recognition — 265

11 Second Language Acquisition — 270

- Introduction — 270
- The relationship between production and perception in SLA — 272
- Production unit size and feedback — 273
- Application of an application — 274
- Theoretically motivated pronunciation training techniques — 274
- Accent and dialect studies — 276

12 Speech Disorders — 278

- Introduction — 278
- Neuroscience applications — 280
- The neuropsychology of speech — 280
- An acquisition disorder – deafness as error — 281
- Cognitive approaches to understanding emotive content — 283
- Perception — 283
- Cross-modal linking — 284
- fMRI evidence — 288
- A basic assumption – phonological awareness — 289
- Levels of representation and the metatheory — 290
- Phonetics related to other areas of linguistic description — 291
- Diagnostic applications — 292

Clinical Phonetics – procedures and expert systems: modelling clinical assessment	294
Areas that need further specification	296
Conclusion	299
References	300
Name Index	311
Subject Index	314

List of Figures and Tables

Figures

3.1 Waveform of *I want to go home*. A represents an overlapping coarticulation model: symbols indicate the start of each segment. B represents a LR inertial model: targets 1 and 3 (t1 and t3) are marked, together with the period of coarticulatory inertia (c) between the first three targets. Both models are first approximations, shown for illustrative purposes, as are the degrees of coarticulation and overlap   42

3.2 Waveform and spectrogram of *How are you?* Notice the continuousness of the signal and the constant 'movement' of the formants. There is no indication of any discrete segmentation   43

3.3 Waveform and spectrogram of *It's not that I decided not to go, but that I was told to stay away*. The emphasis is on the second *not* and the word *told*. In both cases there is final plosive release, though this would not have been expected – and in general the emphasised parts of the utterance are rendered slower and with more precision   45

3.4 Waveforms and spectrograms of *null, moll, frond, vans, once, Banff*. In *null* and *moll* LR nasalisation can clearly be seen after the onset of the vowels, and into the final voiced segments of *frond* and *vans* – so long as the vocal cord vibration persists. With *once* and *Banff* there is no obvious LR nasalisation   46

3.5 Waveforms and spectrograms of *man* and *mad*. Note how nasalisation extends throughout the vowel of *man* (LR and RL coarticulation) but only part way into the vowel in *mad* (LR) coarticulation. A stylised estimate of nasal airflow has been superimposed   47

3.6 Waveforms and spectrograms of *i[m]put* and *i[n]put*. Since the lips are involved in both the [m] and the [p] of *i[m]put* we would expect more formant bending throughout the first part of the word, than in *i[n]put* – where the [n] does not involve the lips. There is perhaps more formant bending in *i[m]put*, but certainly not none in *i[n]put*   57

3.7 Waveforms and spectrograms of (A) English *pat, bat* and
(B) French *patte, batte*. Notice the delay in vocal cord
vibration onset following the release of [p] in *pat*, and the
'pre-voicing' preceding the [b] in *batte* 95
5.1 Waveforms and spectrograms of *bad* and *bat*, with the final
plosives unreleased. Note that the greater duration of
vocal cord vibration in *bad* can be assigned to the final
'devoiced' consonant rather than to the 'vowel'. If this is
the case the rule which lengthens vowels before voiced
consonants is too simplistic, since the vowel section of
the vocal cord vibration is approximately the same in
both *bad* and *bat* 141
5.2 Waveforms and spectrograms of *I want to go home*,
rendered fast and slow. Notice the unusual release of the
final [t] of *want* in the slow version, and the way in
which individual 'segments' are rendered differentially in
the two versions 146
6.1 The *planes/wrapper model* in outline. Notice the abstract
exemplar output from static processing and the actual
instantiations output from dynamic processing. Notice how
dynamic processing is constrained from external sources,
and in particular how dynamic phonetic processing is
constrained by the predictions of spatial, acoustic and
perceptual outcomes of dynamic rendering (adapted
from Tatham and Morton 2005) 175
6.2 The emotion space, showing the furious-angry-irritable
and happy-ecstatic vectors (adapted from Tatham and
Morton 2004) 185

Tables

5.1 Classification of various features by segmental or
prosodic domain 132
5.2 Basic queries concerning feature domains, with
appropriate responses 133

Introduction

Until the middle of the 20th century phonetics was largely concerned with recording the sounds of languages and how they are made, together with making comparisons between the sound inventories of languages. We are still with that legacy in many ways. We compare surface events noted in one language with another, or note observations in spoken language and assign symbols with a system that requires interpretation in the act of assignment. This technique is useful, but we cannot see that it is productive in describing what speech *is*, or how it can be most usefully modelled. Our view is that we need to know *what* sounds can be produced, and then incorporate neurophysiological and acoustic modelling into the discipline. Cognitive neuroscience should be able to tell us what is possible in terms of production and perception, and acoustic modelling should be able to characterise the actual sounds made.

As experimental techniques have developed the focus has shifted toward general data gathering, and as a result we now know that there are some significant discrepancies between what phoneticians had thought was going on in speech and what the new experiments are revealing. But even more importantly, in terms of the theory of speech there has been a paradigm shift from theories about the nature of speech toward theories about how it is produced and perceived. The new paradigm attempts speech modelling from high-level cognitive processing through the acoustic signal to its high-level cognitive perception in the listener.

There are some serious problems in speech modelling. For example: there is no serious empirical basis yet for characterising with any degree of certainty the pre-motor stages of speech production. We assume a physical input – something we call the 'utterance plan', and this is a physical copy of the abstract output from prior cognitive or phonological processing. But we have no experimental evidence for the exact nature of this plan – other than that it somehow reflects earlier cognitive processes. In general we are short of coherent underlying principles for uniting the highly abstract modelling of linguistics and the accumulating mass of physical data collected in the last half century.

In this book we outline a possible underlying model, with a view to providing a basis for showing associations between some cognitive and some physical evidence. The model is a sketch, and we are aware of many of its limitations. The intention however is to show that it is possible to realise the accepted goals of science within the theory of speech production and perception. So we have suggested a model that seems to be justified in very general terms, and according to our interpretation of work done in areas *outside* the usual domain of phonetics, such as cognitive neuroscience, which follows scientific procedures developed outside linguistics. It is important that the exchange be two-way, since not only do linguistics and phonetics import data and ideas from other sciences, we also *export* to those sciences: we emphasise the need for a common basis for this exchange. We also suggest that researchers slow down data collection for its own sake, and work more consistently within the overall concept of modelling processes and tasks designed to develop a robust core theory in the light of how it might be used.

It was suggested we discuss some possible applications of phonetic modelling to application areas such as speech disorders, second language acquisition and speech technology. With this in mind we have suggested some areas of application where our model might be useful. If it is *not* seen to be applicable by specialists in these applied areas, then the model can and should be modified.

Part I – dealing with speech production – begins with a discussion of Classical Phonetics – the basic foundation of our science. There are some shortcomings, and we suggest how the subject might develop in line with a paradigm shift away from a linear model toward a true hierarchically based model of speech production and perception. We show how the concept of *explanation* truly improves the credibility and robustness of phonetic theory. Next follows two chapters dealing with coarticulation, arguably the biggest area of research in the last 50 years or so. We discuss the phenomenon itself and give a critical review of the major models which have been developed in the area. We continue with chapters on the theory of speech motor control and prosody.

Part II – dealing with speech perception – develops the idea that perception and production are so interconnected that they have to be modelled together. Indeed much of what we have to say under this heading looks as though it is about speech production – but this is production optimised for perception: a new and important concept which was first introduced along with the 1960s paradigm shift. Prosody figures in this part too, for the same kind of reason, along with modelling expressive content in speech.

Part III – dealing with areas of focus, modelling and applications – is where we introduce the notion that speech theory should perhaps develop with applications in mind. We have discussed just three: clinical application, spoken language acquisition and speech technology. These are intended to be examples only, since there are many areas where our science has potential relevance provided it is made fully compatible. The piecemeal application of small snippets of the theory may even be counterproductive in the long run.

Finally, this book assumes a good deal of the elementary material underlying the subject – there are a number of excellent books that cover the ground. We have, rather, addressed this book to intermediate and postgraduate students and researchers, and have necessarily been selective, designedly so, for the sake of coherence and continuity to theme. Our subject area is coming into maturity as a science, but not all of its accumulated material meets the necessary criteria of commonality of approach and purpose. We have tried to present the material in the light of the kind of thing which is necessary for a truly scientific explanatory approach; but in the end what we propose is no more than a suggestion toward this end.

Note: Throughout the book our own ideas and model are collectively referred to as 'TM'.

Part I
Speech Production Theory

1
Classical Phonetics

Introduction

We begin with a brief discussion of Classical Phonetics as it stood prior to the serious questioning about its status which developed in the 1960s. For examples of Classical Phonetics see, among others, Cruttenden's (2001) *Gimson's Pronunciation of English*, Gimson's (1989) *An Introduction to the Pronunciation of English*, Jones's *An Outline of English Phonetics* (1918), and Wells's *Accents of English* (1982).

Assumptions of Classical Phonetics

Classical Phonetics is a theory just like any other theory in science – though it is a little primitive in some sense because it only characterises observations about speech without *explaining* those observations. For this reason some purists might think of Classical Phonetics more as a kind of 'pre-theory'. Like any theory, though, it rests on a certain number of basic assumptions, and also like any theory in any other science it is bound to be found to be *wrong*, in the sense that it is bound to be felt at some point that it cannot explain some of the data which can be observed. This is the key to what a theory does: it is the means of characterising or describing – and hopefully of also *explaining* – observed facts about a phenomenon. So what were the observed facts that Classical Phonetics incorporated and how did it deal with them?

The clearest, and later the most controversial of the assumptions made by classical phoneticians was that speech consists of strings of discrete sounds, or rather more accurately is appropriately *described* as consisting of strings of such sounds. As a consequence all utterances are to be regarded as linear permutations or rearrangements into strings of a small number of such sounds: around 45–50 is usually taken as the norm for a single language. The *assumption* that speech *is* a string of sounds was made because all speech, in all languages, is clearly perceived to be like this, although the size of the 'chunk' may vary a little between languages. People who know nothing about linguistics or phonetics readily report their feelings that an utterance is a string of sounds, and they can usually quite easily tell you what they are. This is an observation – that people can do this – which needs to be accounted for in the theory. As scientists, phoneticians have shared the observations of the layman, and consequently the 'fact' of the discreteness of the individual sounds which make up speech was not seriously questioned until the mid-20th century.

The *robustness* of the assumption of the existence of individual sounds in an utterance depends, however, *not* on the actual acoustic facts but on how the acoustic signal of speech is either *perceived* by the listener, or *planned* by the speaker. There was no really reliable way of getting at the acoustic facts before around 1950, and phoneticians had to rely on their training in objectively listening to speech to report the acoustic facts. The most they were able to say was that, as trained observers, they could detect that the individual sounds were not exactly abruptly abutted, but that there were *on-glides* and *off-glides* 'into' and 'out of' these sounds respectively. Lay listeners are not normally aware of these glides.

It seems that listeners and speakers process speech cognitively in terms of *categories*, and this may well be the origin of the discreteness idea. People almost certainly have cognitive 'images' or *representations* of discrete sounds, even if the discreteness does not exist in the acoustic signal. We could say that a speaker's cognitive *plan* for speech is worked out using discrete categories, and that the cognitive perception of speech also works in terms of discrete categories. The remarkable thing, we now know, is that speakers and listeners seem unaware that in the physical world of acoustics the discreteness they *wanted* (the plan) and the discreteness they *perceive* is not actually there!

Phoneticians, even with their objective training, came to the wrong conclusion that speech is actually discrete in the physical world. It follows that if they wanted to write down how utterances sound they were bound to use an essentially alphabetic representation system (phonetic transcription) which also assumes speech to be made up of discrete sounds – just as laymen had done in languages where alphabetic writing is used.

Sounds used functionally

Classical phonetics goes beyond this, however. It is not only concerned with the 'sounds' and 'articulations' of speech; it also wants to discuss how these sounds get used functionally in languages. So, on the one hand we are concerned with the sounds, and on the other with how they function. Study of the functionality of sounds was called, in Classical Phonetics, *phonology*. Phonology tried to account for such observations as the restrictions on sound sequencing at the beginning of words and syllables: we cannot, for example, have more than three consonants preceding a vowel at the start of a word in English – and if there are three then the first must be /s/ and the second must be one of /p/, /t/ or /k/ – and the third is likely to be /l/ or /r/. These are obviously phonological constraints on segment sequencing.

Allophonic variation

Phoneticians have also observed that certain allophones, or 'variants of phonemes' in classical terms, occurred predictably in certain contexts. So, for example, at the end of words [b], [d] and [g] which are normally 'voiced' tend to lose their voice, and this phenomenon can be generalised to voiced fricatives. Another example: although [p], [t] and [k] (the 'voiceless' plosives) are normally aspirated in English initially before vowels, in words where they are immediately preceded by [s] they are not: examples are *stop, spit* and *scant*. There are many allophones which occur, phoneticians have observed, like this. Their approach to accounting for these phenomena was to think of all these allophones as being how speech was 'realised' in articulatory and acoustic terms. The allophones could be grouped into sets and these sets could be *labelled*. So all the possible different allophones of /t/ could be grouped together and given a label – /t/. In Classical Phonetics this label is called a 'phoneme'. Transcriptions in terms of phonemes, phonemic transcriptions, or which reflect only the grossest of features of the sound or articulation, 'broad' transcriptions, are given between slashes, those in terms of allophones or intended to reflect the details of sounds or articulations, allophonic or 'narrow' transcription, are given between square brackets. Transcriptions dealing with functionality are normally thought of as phonemic, transcriptions trying to point to the details of the sounds rather than how they function are normally allophonic.

In contemporary speech theory we make a sharp hierarchically based distinction between functionality and detail. Functionality is handled by *phonology* and physical detail is handled by *phonetics*. Functionality is generally considered to be about cognitive processes (phonology is a 'mental component' in modern linguistics), and details are generally considered to be about motor neuro-physiological, anatomical, aerodynamic or acoustic processes (phonetics is a 'physical component').

The claims of Classical Phonetics

Classical Phonetics had been the dominant paradigm in phonetic theory since before the beginning of the 20th century, and it remained so until the 1960s. As in the development of any science researchers eventually raised questions which the theory was unable to answer. Thus began, in the early 60s, the paradigm shift which saw the erosion of the classical theory.

Classical Phonetics was characterised by a number of either explicit or implicit claims, for example:

1. speech is a *linear string of sound objects*, called 'phonetic segments';
2. these segments can be described and classified in terms of their *surface physical properties* at the articulatory and acoustic levels, as perceived by the trained phonetician;
3. they function *linguistically* in particular languages – this defines the 'phonology' of a language;
4. there are some phenomena which span groupings of these segments – these are called 'prosodic features'; they collectively form the *prosody* of a language, and are usually described acoustically.

For the Classical Phonetician speech is a phenomenon which can be characterised in terms of the movement of the organs of speech – articulatory phonetics, or by listening to the actual sounds – auditory phonetics. Phoneticians were concerned with describing what they could see and hear. There was no emphasis on how such articulations or sounds had been *decided* (their underlying phonological structure) or *controlled* (their rendering by the motor control processes). For Classical Phonetics the focus was strictly on the surface phenomena of people's actual utterances. However, despite careful training they maintained a subjective colouration in their observations and descriptions – that is, their science lacked an acceptable level of objectivity.

One of the consequences of subjectivity in phonetics was that researchers felt that speech could be segmented into a sequence of discrete phonetic segments. Such descriptions involved isolating the individual sounds and treating them 'out of context'. The descriptions were always 'static', paying little attention to the dynamics of speech, and were often prescriptive – *This is how the sound should be pronounced.*

An important contribution of Classical Phonetics was that the description of individual speech sounds was formalised within a universal framework. A methodology was set up which could handle the sounds of *any* language. This included a means of classification (the vowel and consonant charts are examples of this) which was parameter based (was about the sound's features), and a means of representing surface sounds symbolically (phonetic transcription). It is important to notice that the term 'sound' is used with systematic ambiguity: it means both a sound segment and how that sound is made in articulatory terms. At the same time phoneticians were keen to show the functional role of these segments within individual languages, and to compare roles between different languages.

System in Classical Phonetics

Phoneticians noticed that it was not enough just to enumerate the properties of these sounds: there was some kind of system behind them.

- Firstly, there seems to be a relationship between the sounds which is to do with how they are made (the same articulators get involved in pronouncing different sounds), and
- secondly, the way sounds sequence in words and utterances, and sometimes 'change' seems to be patterned.

The relationship between individual sounds, or the *system* into which they appear to fall, is for the Classical Phonetician based primarily on which articulators are involved in making the sounds. Phoneticians provide a prose description of the various articulations, but at the same time present the material graphically using the *consonantal chart* and the *vowel chart*. In these matrices the cells formed by the intersection of rows and columns contain symbols representing the various sounds. The symbols, like the term 'sound', simultaneously represent both the sound and how it is made. This is an important idea: the symbols are systematically ambiguous in terms of what it is that they represent.

The consonantal chart

The *blank* chart represents a universal set of coordinates for relating all the consonants of all languages – at least in principle, though this may turn out to be difficult in practice. It becomes 'the chart for English' or 'the chart for Welsh', and so on, when we start putting our symbols on it. In the symbolic representation for sounds that the Classical Phoneticians devised as members of the International Phonetic Association, called the International Phonetic Alphabet or IPA (1999), the idea was 'one symbol for one sound', irrespective of what language was involved. In practice they soon found that this idea could not be sustained, even with the use of diacritics. Hence the consonantal chart is two-dimensional with an x-axis and a y-axis and a top-left origin. The horizontal x-axis, or the rows of the matrix, represent 'places of articulation' beginning on the left with the lips and extending toward the far right, the glottal area. The vertical y-axis, or the rows of the matrix, represent 'manner of articulation'. Manners of articulation are the different ways of actually causing the airstream to produce the different types of sound, for example plosives, affricates, etc.

The vowel chart

Here the chart using a grid of rows and columns represents a mapping of the two-dimensional (vertical) space within the oral cavity through which the tongue can move as it positions itself to provide appropriate resonances for the various vowels in languages. Once again, the grid itself is universal – the extreme coordinates of the map being the universal 'abstract' extremes of the human possibilities for vowel formation. Points are placed on the grid to represent the 'position' of the various vowels of a particular language. Originally thought of as points representing some part of the tongue (sometimes the 'highest part', sometimes the 'significant part') they in fact more likely represent some abstract positioning in a perceptual space, *which can be related to both the physical articulatory space and the acoustic space occupied by vowels.*

There are various theoretical problems with both charts and symbols, even within the classical theory itself, mostly surrounding the two-dimensionality of the graphics and the failure of the symbolic representation to cover all possible details of variation. This latter point is explained quite simply by the mismatch between the subjective use of the IPA – as a symbolic representation – and any attempt to use it to represent objective detail. It works best for representing symbolically abstract or perceived notions about speech (Cruttenden 2001).

The main principles of the mechanics of Classical Phonetics can be summarised as:

- there is a systematic relationship between the way consonants and vowels are made as articulations in the vocal tract, and the way they are symbolised;
- two dimensional matrices can be set up to represent this on a universal basis, that is, which will apply to all languages;
- the matrices can be filled in with symbols relevant to a particular language (or accent of a language); the chart then becomes 'the

consonant chart for Japanese', or 'the vowel chart for Polish', and so on.

As for the IPA symbolic representation, its main features are that it

- adopts a segmental, alphabetic approach, but says almost nothing about how the symbolic objects relate to the actual physical articulatory or acoustic signals which prompt them – in particular how *discrete* objects are derived from *continuous* signals;
- recognises the possibility of marking the boundaries of linguistic units, though does not explain the existence or position of boundaries;
- neglects (in the basic system) prosodic features – but where these are included it is almost as a afterthought, underlining the fundamental notion in Classical Phonetics that prosody is subordinate to segmental phenomena;
- shows nothing of any systematic relationship between segments in the transcription – that is, it shows no linear relationships (except concatenation) nor any underlying non-linear relationship.

The last two negative features are included because it would have been useful, at the very least, to have enabled within the transcription some mechanism for relating prosody and segments, and at the same time used the transcription to reveal phonological relationships between segments, if only relationships arising from their linear context.

Parameters for classifying segments

In Classical Phonetics and its attendant IPA transcription system segments are classified on a parametric basis. This is important because it enables classes of segment to be identified, and then additionally characterised according to their phonological or phonetic behaviour. For example, in English, we can group together all consonants which are voiced, subdividing them into perhaps the stop and fricative subsets – these groupings are made according to the parametric makeup of these segment types. But we can now go on to say that all voiced stops and fricatives share several functional properties: for example, they regularly devoice at the end of words or syllables which are also word final. The use of parameters and the way they enter into phonetic and phonological generalisations is less formal than that found in early Generative Phonology (Chomsky and Halle 1968), but does have similar potential to account for the regularities in the way sounds relate to each other, *and* pattern within a language. Gimson (1989) has a huge collection of such observations. Cross-language and cross-accent accounts can also make use of the classificatory and an functional properties of the model; an archetypal example is Well's *Accents of English* (1982).

Theorist phoneticians differ in how many parameters they want to include for classification and enumerating segmental functioning, and their reasons for including this or that parameter are often quite informal. However, few would disagree with the following representative set:

1. for dealing with the nature of the *airflow source*
   - airstream mechanism,
   - airflow direction;
2. for the *acoustic source*
   - phonation type and location;
3. for detail of the *airflow path*
   - state of the velum,
   - centrality *vs.* laterality;
4. for detail of the *articulation* or *constriction*
   - force (amplitude) of articulation,
   - prolongability (duration);
5. traditional initial *consonantal classification*
   - place of articulation,
   - manner of articulation;
6. traditional initial *vowel classification*
   - vertical positioning (open-close dimension),
   - horizontal position (front-back dimension),
   - lip configuration.

Combinatorial constraints on phonetic features

An important consideration in phonetic theory concerns the combinatorial constraints on these parameters, and in particular how such constraints influence the assignment of values to the parameters. For example the vertical positioning of vowels critically interacts with their horizontal positioning – errors produce morphemic clashes, but in English the duration of a vowel produces only a feeling of error of accent (failure to deliver the right extrinsic allophone), but rarely a morphemic identification problem. In other languages duration of vowels, and indeed of consonants, *is* critical and seriously affects morpheme differentiation. Sometimes it is necessary to introduce only binary values for segment parameters (for example, phonologically vowels are either nasal or not in a language like French), but sometimes scalar values are important (for example a few accents of English have a systematically greater degree of nasalisation of vowels than others). Rather vaguely in the theory, such considerations depend on a number of different factors, among them:

- Are any details to be discussed intrinsically phonetic or phonological?
- Are they dependent on context, and if so is this phonological or phonetic?
- How critical are they for perceptual purposes?

Classical Phonetics focusses on the static description of segments – their articulatory and acoustic properties often enumerated using parameters along the lines of the above set. There is a pervasive acceptance that segments are what they are, both vertically (parameter combination) and horizontally (segment sequencing), but characteristically little attempt at explaining questions such as these:

- Why is this combination of parameters appropriate and this one is not?
- Are the constraints on segment sequencing linearly or hierarchically organised?
- What externally sourced constraints are there on the formation of segments, or how they pattern in the language?

Segments 'in' the speech signal

The notion that speech *is* a string of conjoined articulatory or acoustic units or segments is demonstrably false, and the approach which attempts to characterise it as though it were such a string has proved confusing. Apart from the occasional abrupt change in the articulatory or acoustic flow these physical properties exhibit *continuousness*. Various experimental techniques such as movie or video sequences derived from *x*-ray micro-beam scanning (Westbury 1994), or simple spectrograms of the acoustic signal quickly convince that segmentation working on just the available signal is not possible.

Segmentation
Many researchers working in phonetics begin with an assumption that the near-continuous nature of the acoustic and other signals of speech is

the result of what Laver (1994, p. 101) calls 'the complex interaction of the different elements of the vocal performance'. The argument begs the question, of course. Segments are presupposed in such an approach, and inevitably the next step would be to address what becomes, *because of the approach*, a difficult problem: how to perform segmentation of the continuous signal. As Laver observes, the acoustic signal is 'continuously changing ... with few natural breaks and steady-state stretches', and then goes on to ask 'what analytic approaches could be proposed for phonetic segmentation of the stream of speech'. The problem here is that the question would not even be asked (certainly not in this form) unless it had been presupposed that it was a useful question. Phoneticians rarely adduce a scientific theoretically based attempt to justify the approach.

One possible justification however would be based on the observation that lay users of speech invariably perceive it as strings of segments. If this is the case then the question becomes something like:

- Given that there is some psychological reality to the notion of segmental strings in an utterance, what would be an appropriate way of undertaking the objective analysis of speech? and
- Can our theory justify an attempt at a description which mirrors the perception of segments?

The answers are not simple because the perception of segments may rest on two co-existing underlying sources:

- Segments are the perceived objects because the listener's perceptual system and the speaker's utterance planning system operate on a *symbolic representation* which is constrained to be in terms of sequenced discrete objects – i.e. the *mechanism itself* works in terms of segments;
- Segments are perceived because language operates on layered symbolic representations of discrete objects – i.e. the *use* to which the mechanism is put uses segments.

This is a classical chicken-egg situation:

- Is the planning (in the speaker) and perception (in the listener) segmental because *all* planning and perception is segmental or category-based? or
- Is only speech/language segmentally organised?

The answer to this question will lie within the domain of cognitive psychology. Linguistics notes that both linguistically-naive language users and linguists (as scientists) almost invariably speak of language in terms of organised discrete objects without systematically exploring underlying explanations. Cognitive psychology is perhaps the proper domain of such underlying explanations because the category phenomenon reflected in discrete objects is not confined to language but recurs throughout the processing of sensory data.

Given the reporting of the discreteness of speech in the cognitive planning or perceptual processes there is an assumption that properties of the vocal tract and the way it responds to motor commands transform the discreteness into continuousness. The scientific error here is the idea that a *physical* process can alter something completely *abstract:* of course, it cannot.

It seems quite difficult to persuade some theorists that the fact there is psychological reality to segmentally based symbolic representations does not presuppose a linear correlation with a corresponding neurally based representation. We shall see when we come to discuss coarticulation theory (Chapters 2 and 3) that this idea is the basis of assumptions that the speech output is somehow a degraded version of what is intended – which may be an appropriate explanation, but which, as we have said, is hard to show.

What is a segment? – the speaker focus

Two possibilities for the segment:

1. It is an object which is located in a period of articulation or acoustic signal and which is tied to relatively steady states of the various phonetic parameters – like tongue movement or formant frequency. As such it can be discovered in the soundwave either by a human listener or by an automatic speech recogniser. To get around the a-synchrony of the various features proponents of this theory speak of different 'phases' to the segment, or 'overlapping' segments. This definition is the one adopted by Classical Phonetics.
2. It is an object which is no more than a label assigned to an indistinct portion of a soundwave: '*Somewhere around there is part of the signal which makes me assign this particular label in a sequence with other labels.*' This is a more recent definition and one to which we subscribe.

Definition 1 has the segment as a parametric physical object which can be discovered in the articulatory and acoustic signals. Definition 2 has the segment as an abstract label which is assigned to a portion of signal: the label is not in the signal.

What is a segment? – the listener focus

Models which associate the continuousness of the acoustic signal with their abstract cognitive representation deal with the act of segmentation in two different ways:

1. the listener can identify places in the temporal flow of the signal where boundaries between segments can occur – that is, the segmental boundaries are found or located in the signal, or
2. the listener can construct an overall representation in their mind which has segment boundaries imposed on it – that is, the signal is used only to trigger a segmentalised representation in the listener's mind, which only loosely correlates with the signal itself.

Of these we prefer the second – that the listener imposes the segmentation, rather than the first – that the listener finds the segment boundaries, since, outside the human mind, no reliable way of simulating this particular behaviour has been found. If it were the case that segments exist in the soundwave, then we should be able to find them whether apparent in a segment-by-segment model or an overlapping parametric model. In Chapter 3 we examine the way those researchers who have taken the first option above attempt to model coarticulatory continuousness of whole segments (coarticulation theory) or parameterised segments (co-production theory).

Phonemes

Phonetic theorists have offered many definitions of the phoneme, ranging from 'sets of sounds' (grouped by linguistic function, or articulatory specification) to 'abstract labels' assigned by speaker/listeners to objects which phonologically permit the differentiation of morphemes. In contemporary linguistics we would take the line that, if we wished to retain the concept, a phoneme must be a highly abstract object existing deep in phonology. Its relationship to the soundwaves produced by speakers is complex, though speakers and listeners are able to report about and discuss objects which apparently have phonemic properties. We propose to spend very little space on the concept: it is adequately dealt with in hundreds of articles and books in the literature. We discuss here the general concept of abstraction and how it relates to cognitive processing in general and to speech production and perception in particular.

Defining the phoneme – Trubetskoy and others

Trubetskoy (1939) presents one of the enduring paradoxes of defining the phoneme. His characterisation and arguments are remarkably relevant to contemporary theory. Pointing out that Baudouin de Courtenay (De Courtenay 1875) had defined the phoneme as 'the psychic equivalent of the speech sound' he shows that there could be several speech sounds corresponding to the same phoneme 'each having its own psychic equivalent' – and this *could not be*. Trubetskoy takes an alternative position: when we listen to speech we 'extract individual speech sounds' from the continuum by a process of *matching up corresponding sections of the speech wave to specific phonemes*. In modern terms this means that we use the sound waves to enable us to assign appropriate phoneme labels to an utterance. These labels are known to us as listeners. Since phonemes are abstract it is *not possible* to assign boundaries to the labels. For Trubetskoy, importantly, 'the speech sound can only be defined in terms of its relation to the phoneme' (p. 38). In our terms this means that a stretch of speech audio can only have 'meaning' (be a proper stretch of speech) by reference to its ability to have labels assigned to it. In TM (the Tatham–Morton model) such labels in the initial stages will probably be extrinsic allophonic rather than phonemic – though there is yet little relevant empirical data on the issue.

Trubetskoy (p. 40) speaks of two levels or types of abstraction.

1. abstraction 'on the basis of acoustic-articulatory similarity';
2. abstraction 'on the basis of the relation of the sounds to their environment'.

The first of these is phonetic abstraction and the second phonological abstraction. Trubetskoy criticises Jones (1918) for a phoneme concept related too much to the question of transcription, rather than to linguistics. He is quite clear:

> The phoneme can be defined satisfactorily neither on the basis of its psychological nature nor on the basis of its relation to the phonetic variants, but purely and solely on the basis of its function in the system of language. (p. 40)

Trubetskoy continues to disassociate linguistics from psychology – not necessarily a view we would take today. For us language is a cognitively originating phenomenon and linguistics is the study of that phenomenon. For Trubetskoy linguistics seems to be the description of language without reference to where it happens – in the cognitive world.

Trubetskoy has so clearly exemplified for us what appears to be a commonly assumed property of theoretical linguistics – its relative isolation from major sources of potential explanation. In speech production and perception we have tried to characterise (Chapter 6) a model which is dynamic and which begins to explain actual utterances, rather than confine itself to the static characterisation of exemplar utterances.

The nature of symbolic representations

We have to be careful of how we use words like *vowel* or *consonant*, as well as the symbols we assign to particular sounds. The words are invoked as characterisations of particular acoustic signals, but they *are not* those signals. Vowels and consonants are abstract entities which it suits us to use in our characterisation of speech; this does not mean that they exist as physical entities in the soundwave itself. Similarly with the symbolic representations of the IPA or any other similar representation of speech. [ɑ] is not a sound, it is a symbolic representation of sound. This is why we are able to use a symbolic representation like [kip] or its orthographic equivalent *keep*, to represent *all* instantiated utterances of the word. If the representation were to be the soundwave we would need as many representations as there are different soundwaves associated with this word – technically an infinite number. The use of single symbolic representations [kip] or *keep* for any repetition (complete with all the variability associated with repeated human behaviour) successfully captures part of human cognitive behaviour: namely that for the speaker and the listener all repetitions (within reason) are perceived as the *same*. The symbolic representation of ordinary orthography or typical phonetic or phonological transcriptions have in common therefore with our cognitive processing in planning, uttering and perceiving the soundwave, that there is *identity* where in the signal there is nothing by *variability*. Human speakers and listeners perceive repetitions to be the same and assign them the *same* symbolic representations. It is very important to distinguish, we repeat, between the assigned representation and the physical phenomenon itself. It follows from this that no symbolic representation assigned by the scientist/phonetician or assigned by the speaker/hearer can ever be detailed enough to capture the entire range of variability possible and actual in the physical world. It also follows therefore that if some detail is to be represented it has to be properly defined separately.

Phonetic transcription and linguistically relevant information

Formally IPA symbols are intended to represent only linguistically relevant information (Cruttenden 2001, Ladefoged 2005); that is they exclude the recording of information which does not have a bearing on the linguistics of the utterance. So, for example, a speaker's cough in mid utterance is not generally given a symbolic representation – though there are extensions to the system to permit the kinds of sounds which have to be dealt with in clinical phonetics and any general approach to speech disorders.

But what is and what is not linguistically relevant? It could easily be argued, for example, that intrinsic allophonic (Wang and Fillmore 1961) information is rarely linguistically relevant, but no-one would want to exclude the possibility of indicating some such information. For example, we may want to point out that the place of articulation of [t] immediately preceding [u] is more retracted than it is when followed by [i]. This particular example might be regarded as a minor featural change, but others are more significant. Are all of these linguistically relevant? Or none of them?

In modern times we use our IPA symbolic representations to stand for both linguistically relevant and linguistically non-relevant objects – where the line is drawn between the two is a matter for the particular context of the representation. For example if the representation is actually intended to show intrinsic variability, then of course there must be a way of doing this – even if the variability is not normally perceptible to native speakers and so could not have linguistic significance.

Symbolic representation

In our own model we can recognise three basic levels of transcription which focus on externally motivated symbolic representations. These three levels involve

1. symbols associated with the unique representation of morphemes,
2. the symbolic representation of linguistically determined (extrinsic) allophones, and
3. the symbolic representation of physically determined (intrinsic) allophones.

A fourth level of transcription also involves symbolic representation, but of a less systematic nature and is less linguistically motivated:

4. the symbolic representation of fine acoustic (or articulatory) detail.

Transcriptions of this fourth type do not focus on the utterance's phonology, but try to represent some pre-defined level of detail. Note, though, that sometimes in defining that detail it is not possible to proceed without at least some reference to phonology (and phonetic theory).

Many theorists, in attempting to define different types of transcription, fail to distinguish between variants occurring as the result of phonological processes (2. above) and variants determined by phonetic processes (3. above), though most do make the distinction between systematic transcription and attempts to record fine acoustic or articulatory detail (4. above). The distinction between extrinsic and intrinsic allohones is important because of the direct relationship between the former and the representation of meaning, and the more tenuous relationship between the latter and the representation of meaning.

There are two ways in which intrinsic allophones may relate to the representation of meaning:

- One rests on the hypothesis that coarticulation, which is said to be responsible for their occurrence, is either deliberate or is co-opted by the system to assist listeners in deciding what it is the speaker intends.
- The other rests on the hypothesis that although intrinsic allophones originate in the mechanical or aerodynamic sub-systems which are only incidentally related to the linguistics, they nevertheless constitute candidates for subtle linguistically determined manipulation. The Theory of Cognitive Phonetics (Morton 1986, Tatham 1986a, 1986b) in TM is about this aspect of coarticulation (Chapter 6).

Some researchers have used the term 'allophone' to correspond to what we are calling extrinsic allophones and 'phone' to correspond to what we call intrinsic allophones. However, these researchers do think of phones as being able to be heard, presumably by the phonetician, thus not ruling out some intrinsic allophones which the ordinary native speaker will *not* perceive. However we do have to be careful: intrinsic allophones are allophones *and their labels* derived by intrinsic coarticulatory processes, whereas phones often seem to be acoustic objects.

Confusion over what speech sounds 'represent'

Laver (1994) makes the comment that 'speech-sounds can ... be thought of as representing, or "symbolizing" abstract linguistic units such as consonants and vowels, in a many-to-one relationship' (p. 18). There is a confusion here: it is the abstract linguistic units which are the representations or symbols associated with utterances, not the other way round. The symbolic representation which is the set of consonants and vowels is rendered by the speaker in such a way as to produce an acoustic output signal. Sound could be thought of as an encoding of some underlying cognitive representation by a speaker, with the goal of enabling listeners to assign a similar cognitive representation to the sound they hear. The association between the speaker's utterance (planned as a symbolic representation), the acoustic signal, and the listener's perception of the plan as an assigned symbolic representation is clearly non-linear and imperfectly understood.

Laver introduces into his phonetic theory the notion of 'convenient fiction'. Neither his terminology nor his conclusions are appropriate.

> If one accepts the metaphorical function of convenient fictions in theory-building, then for every fiction postulated, a compensating counter-fiction needs to be invented. (p. 568)

Theory building is not about the assembly of 'convenient fictions' – in fact there is no place at all for such things. Assertions or hypotheses within a theory are not fictions: they are well-motivated pillars of the theory. A hypothesis, or claim formulated as a hypothesis, is not a fiction, if only because it leads quickly and explicitly to further research and must always have a built-in means for its own destruction. 'Metaphorical function' is also a loose and inappropriate turn of phrase. The function of claims and hypotheses is not one of metaphor, but one of coherent and explicit *insight* and *explanation*.

The domain of speech theory

We need to ask ourselves whether the domain of speech theory takes in analysis within the articulatory/acoustic domain, or synthesis of the processes underlying the domain. Classical Phonetics is essentially about the *analysis* of speech in the articulatory and acoustic domains, using various tools including phonetic transcription, trained phonetic perception and some instrumental techniques. What is interesting about the TM model and one or two others is that they focus on *synthesis* – the speech waveform is the end point, not the starting point. A model of speech production for researchers in the Classical Phonetics tradition is a coherent account of some piece of speech or perhaps speech in general. For us a model of speech production is an account of how acoustic signals are assigned to otherwise unspoken sentences. This includes, of course, high level phonological planning.

In such an approach, the synthesis of phonetics and phonology is an account of hierarchical processes which explain all speech soundwaves, and therefore any *one* soundwave. It is true, though, that earlier and *off-line*, such accounts must be based in part on analysis of what is possible in actual speech output – the observations potentially described in Classical Phonetics. This is why, in TM, we set up static and dynamic areas of the model (Chapter 6): static areas characterise a generalised set of processes which can be accessed by dynamic areas to produce specific acoustic instantiations of utterances.

For us *perception* is the assigning of some meaningful symbolic representation to input sensory data. The assignment is based on a characterisation of possible symbolic representations held in the listener's mind. Thus perception is essentially an act of interpretation since it is clear that there is no linear correlation or 'direct path' between the acoustic signal and the assigned symbolic representation. What perceivers do *not* do is discover or register the linguistic objects of what they hear – this would imply that these objects and their labels are in the soundwave. What they do is interpret what is heard in a complex process of assignment, from what they already know, of symbolic representations.

2
Coarticulation: the Phenomenon

Introduction

Coarticulation Theory was developed in the late 1960s and early 1970s explicitly to overcome a serious problem in Classical Phonetics (CP), the descriptive theory dealt with in Chapter 1.

In CP the model is based essentially on how phoneticians *perceive* speech, rather than on explicit knowledge of how speech is *produced:*

- the *phonetic* descriptions of CP involve isolating individual sounds and treating them as discrete sounds out of context (for example, '[p, b, t, d, k, g] comprise the set of stop consonants in English');
- there is detailed description of speech sounds on articulatory and acoustic (for example, 'this vowel sound is made with the tongue high in the front of the mouth and involves vocal cord vibration');
- the *phonological* descriptions of CP treat the functioning of these discrete sounds in linear context (for example, 'palatalised $[l_j]$ is used before vowels in English, but velarised $[l_w]$ is used at the end of words or before other consonants at the end of words');
- the descriptions are almost always static, paying little attention to the dynamics of speech (for example, exceptionally: '[k] is fronted before front vowels, as in *key*, but retracted before back vowels, as in *car*');
- an actual utterance is thought of as a linear concatenation of sound segments, or 'phones'.

From the early 1960s researchers began to move toward a new hierarchical approach, with phonology preceding phonetics as a *planning* component operating at an abstract or cognitive level. This change was symptomatic of the paradigm shift from a linear account essentially based on how speech is perceived to a hierarchical account based on speech production. The move was from a surface descriptive model to a hierarchical production model.

With improved experimental techniques:

- the 1950s sees advances in the development of the technology for objective investigation of speech, particularly of the acoustic signal;
- it quickly becomes very apparent that far from being a sequence of discrete sounds speech is characterised by its dynamic continuity;
- physical segmentation of an utterance's acoustic signal is observed to be rarely possible with any degree of certainty;
- researchers begin to seek an *explanation* for the fact that in dynamic acoustic data, focussing on time, it is rarely possible to be sure that sounds actually have a beginning and ending;
- hence the research focus shifts from a characterisation of the idealised isolated segment to a characterisation of dynamic or connected speech.

Work initially sought to explain how the discrete segments had become continuous in both the articulation and the soundwave. Importantly the idea persisted that discrete segments had *become* continuous. No theory was put forward at the time which completely abandoned the idea of discrete segments. The first influential theories in modern times dealing with *phonetics* and using an asynchronous (and therefore non-discrete) approach was the co-production idea in Fowler's (1980) Action Theory and Browman and Goldstein's (1986) Articulatory Phonology. The formal treatment of an asynchronous *phonology* had been proposed earlier by Firth (1948). But prior to Fowler's proposals the main theory proposed to explain the continuousness of speech persisted with the idea of an underlying segmented level which becomes continuous during the phonetic rendering process. We shall see later that researchers were at pains to discover just at what stage in the overall speech production process (from underlying abstraction to acoustic signal) the switch from discrete to continuousness takes place. This very approach perpetuates the idea that there *are*, at some level, discrete objects. The main theory became known as Coarticulation Theory.

What is coarticulation?

Coarticulation is traditionally roughly defined as the effect of the influence of an articulatory segment on adjacent segments. Two subdivisions of coarticulatory effects are generally made:

- left-to-right (LR), perseverative or carry-over effects, in which properties of a segment carry over to influence those of following segments;
- right-to-left (RL), or anticipatory effects, in which properties of a segment influence those of earlier segments.

Coarticulation is universal in the sense that in all languages neighbouring segments interact phonetically with one another, but the extent of the effect and the balance of the two possible directions of the effect vary from language to language. There are many coarticulatory effects observable in English, with RL effects usually said to be commoner than LR effects.

Some researchers have linked coarticulation with the so-called *Principle of Least Effort*. The idea here is that speech production at the phonetic level need be only as accurate as is necessary to communicate the required segmental, and hence morphemic, contrasts to enable meaning to be transferred. This idea assumes that the most accurate realisation of a phonological string would involve the precise rendering of the articulatory and acoustic features which make up individual segments: they would not blend with each other and each would be fully realised. Because phonological segments and their phonetic correlates are generally over-specified and contain redundancy the information they encode can be communicated even if phonetically segments fall short of full realisation. Since, from the point of view of the motor control of speech, accuracy and precision are therefore less than completely necessary, the Principle of Least Effort holds that they will be relaxed as far as possible whilst maintaining a good level of communication. Relaxation of the precision of motor control results in segments running into one another, and target positioning of the articulator sometimes being missed. We might say that a balance is struck between using the least effort possible to render the articulation and the need to render the articulation sufficiently accurately to prevent loss of communication.

An earlier term, *assimilation*, was used for the phenomenon, now called coarticulation, at both the phonological and phonetic levels. In general the modern usage is to reserve assimilation to refer to influences of one phonological segment on another, and coarticulation to refer to influences of adjacent or near phonetic segments on one another. Phonological assimilation may reflect the phonetic tendencies of coarticulation, but is *voluntary* or *optional*. Phonetic coarticulation describes effects which are not under voluntary control – though the degree of the effect can often be manipulated (Chapter 6).

From the theoretical point of view the notions of assimilation and coarticulation are interesting because they rely heavily on the idea that speech at both the phonological and phonetic levels is made up of a string of discrete segments, blended together to produce a relatively continuous articulation and soundwave. In fact there is little evidence of an experimental nature to support the idea that speech *is* made up of a string of discrete segments which have become blurred together. The main piece of evidence we have is that when questioned about speech people usually refer to it as though they *feel* it to be made up of individual sounds: those who know nothing of linguistics or phonetics will readily, for example, refer to the three sounds in the word *dog* or state that the last two sounds of *dog* are the same as the last two in *fog*. At the cognitive level of speech production and perception the segment appears to have reality. It is not necessarily the case, though, that the segment has reality at the physical level.

The usual traditional model of speech production at the phonetic level does however *assume* the physical reality of the segment (Chapter 1). Speech is said to consist of strings of gestures of the vocal organs which are realisations of canonical targets. In the articulation of isolated, steady state segments these targets are said to be fully realised. When the segments are strung together execution of the targets is less than full: targets get missed as phonological assimilatory and phonetic coarticulatory effects are introduced. The effects are progressive in the sense that the more we depart from the ideal of isolated steady state segments the more the effects occur.

In coarticulation the predominant influence on the extent to which ideal targets are missed in running speech is *time*. The greater the rate of utterance the greater the degree of coarticulation. This suggests that the effects are mainly mechanical, since mechanical systems are particularly sensitive to constraints such as inertia and friction which tend to smooth out and blur the 'precision' of rapid or finely detailed movements. The accuracy of motor control is heavily influenced by rate of utterance. Motor control failure at a *higher* level than the control of the mechanical system results in the slurring of speech, for example under the effects of alcohol or other drugs which might affect the central nervous system or the response of the musculature to neural impulses.

Right-to-left coarticulation

Some researchers have tried to explain RL anticipatory coarticulation in terms of a *weighting* on an articulator or area of the vocal tract, relating its 'position' to how that position is specified in the current target and the next target. Ladefoged (1993) summarises this as:

> Coarticulation between sounds will result in the positions of some parts of the vocal tract being influenced largely by the one target, and others by the other. The extent to which anticipatory coarticulation occurs depends on the extent to which the position of that part of the vocal tract is specified in the two targets. (p. 57)

The 'extent to which a target is specified' seems to refer either to the precision of the specification or a 'don't care' factor. This is not unlike Bladon and Al-Bamerni's (1976) sketched coarticulatory resistance model or Keating's (1990) window model (Chapter 3). The approach taken in Cognitive Phonetics (Tatham 1985, 1986a) is rather different in that the weighting is a variable which is linguistically dependant, as well as physically dependant.

This anticipatory coarticulation is due to the 'warming up' factor. In an utterance like [əku] the lip rounding associated with [u] is begun earlier than the apparent beginning of the segment because of anticipated articulator inertia and because it is necessary to achieve simultaneity of the acoustic signal at a pre-determined point. Knowledge of inertial and other motor properties determines the start point of the warm up. Notice, though, that the output effect (visible lip rounding, though not muscular contraction) is altered if the articulator is required to do something different during that warm up phase. Thus, if the sequence is [iku] the lip rounding does not visibly (or audibly) begin till part way through the [k] – spreading and rounding compete for articulator participation (the lips are completely involved in both spreading and rounding, and since these are opposites something has to give). The underlying musculature though is different, and spreading might well continue well into the rounding; and rounding might well have begun, muscle-wise, well before spreading has apparently 'given way' in the positioning of the lips. This means that to speak of target positioning of the lips is too simple. What has to be involved is the target position and, importantly, timing of the gestural parameters. This is the co-production approach of Fowler and others.

Researchers point out that the relationship between phonological segments and motor or articulatory targets is not linear, and often not obvious. But most conclude that there is *some* relationship of some kind – there must be – which can be modelled. This is where the hierarchical approach scores since the known factors in the development of the utterance plan and its rendering or realisation can be assigned to different processes in the hierarchy:

- *overall cognitive specification* (the utterance plan) to one level,
- *plain and inevitable inertial factors* can be assigned to another,
- *cognitive intervention* for local modification of rendering to yet another perhaps.

Different factors associated with cognitive intervention (Chapter 6) are given their own sub-tiers depending on the relationship between the different factors involved: emotion, attitude, style, phonological precision, semantic and syntactic predictability, etc. It is the total of these interacting tiers in the hierarchy which provides the visible or audible output. To try to model the observed 'coarticulation' on a single level results in the observation that the relationship between this and the underlying plan is complex. Even co-production as it stands has a problem here: co-production really only models the actual motor and articulator movement events, it does not reach behind them to tease out the various factors which go up to making them.

Our recent XML *wrapper paradigm* (Tatham and Morton 2004) moves someway to laying out the format of the model and exposing the layers which might be separately investigated before their relationships become clear to us.

Phonetic under-specification

Many theorists have been worried by the fact that phonological units are aoristic by definition; that is, they have no time. And since, among other things, they have no boundaries they *cannot* overlap. In fact the notion of overlapping segments so often referred to in early coarticulation theory could not exist without modifying any theory which seeks to relate phonology and phonetics in an integrated production model. Keating (1988) reasoned from this that coarticulation must be sourced other than in the phonology, since it reflects 'graded changes' and 'pliant boundaries'. For her it is phonetic *under-specification* which allows coarticulation to take place: the phonetic gesture is insufficiently robustly specified, so can vary.

Overlap

It is worth pointing out, though, that attempts to explain apparent segmental overlap beg the question. Segments could only overlap temporally and consequently interact with one another if they had a temporal existence. Alternative models which do *not* focus on segments of the traditional kind are possible.

- A very simple example – already present in several theories – could specify the unit as the *syllable;* anything internal to this unit could be regarded as 'part' of the *whole* unit rather than as a string of segments in its own right; though eventually of course the syllable has to be assigned a time dimension (that is, make the transition from phonological object to phonetic object).
- In another example, *gestures* could be the focus. Here time would be the most important consideration since gestures are by definition dynamic objects.

The problem exists because of the assumption that there is a linear relationship between representation in the mind, which is probably in terms of discrete segments of some 'size' (allophones, syllables, etc.), and physical representation – perhaps just *assumed* to be in terms of discrete segments. It is this *latter* assumption which causes the dilemma, rather than the assumption of discrete segment representation in the mind. The hypothesis of discrete segments represented in the mind is fine, and has been demonstrated many times. But this only works if it is not assumed that there is a linear correlation with *anything at all* at the input level in the physical description of the hierarchical rendering processes.

Contextual 'accommodation'

Some researchers have gone beyond the hypothesis that contextually determined coarticulatory adjustments occur passively in phonetic rendering, and assumed that these processes might be a property of the motor control system or of the way in which the motor control system is used in speech. Most though would favour the hypothesis that coarticulation (rather than co-production) probably has nothing to do with active neuromuscular control, but is entirely mechanical or aerodynamic in origin. This view easily accommodates the possibility that even the neuromuscular system has *passive* 'inertia' – though this is probably insignificant compared with mechanical and aerodynamic inertia.

In our view some researchers (for example, Laver 1994) assume too much of the dynamics of speech to be under direct motor control, in the sense that events result directly from the speaker's intentions, whether or not the speaker is themself aware of these intentions. There is no reason to assume that *all* movement of the articulators is directly under neuromuscular control – clearly it is not, and could not be.

However, it is clear that anticipatory (RL) coarticulation presents a serious problem to the inertial model, as does the observed spread of coarticulatory effects over several segments in either direction. This spanning of multiple segments by a coarticulatory phenomenon is even more difficult to explain when it is observed that unexpectedly some segments do not 'succumb', and the phenomenon appears to 'jump' these segments to affect one or two beyond them. This situation is more likely as a candidate for an explanation calling on active neuromuscular control. It should not be too difficult to devise experiments which show the limits of passive coarticulation, but we do not know of any which effectively cast light on the problem.

Adaptation

Adaptation is the process invoked by some researchers when modelling coarticulation; it is a more detailed attempt to model LR coarticulation. That is, adaptation occurs when articulatory movement to a given target is changed because of the detail of the previous target. One or two researchers have however suggested that the process can be bi-directional. Certainly in our own early electromyographic data (1969) there was some evidence that the signal from *m. orbicularis oris* associated with lip closure for [b] varied depending on whether the previous vowel was rounded. Here is the argument:

- If a target segment *S* shares relevant properties with the previous segment *S-1*, then movement toward *S* is altered, since the articulator is either already closer to the target or further from it than it would have been if segment *S-1* had been completely neutral with respect to this feature. What in this context constitutes a 'feature' has to be defined, but since the movement of articulators is in the end down to the degree of contraction of individual muscles then 'feature' would have to mean *muscle* here, rather than *articulator position*. One immediate problem is that articulator position is determined by the differential contractions within a set of muscles – modelled either on an *ad hoc* basis, or in terms of coordinative structures. So, we could say that it is the configuration of a group of muscles which might be best characterised by an abstract cover term, like *articulator position*.

Thus it would be how the entire configuration shifts toward the entire new configuration, and for a set of 6 muscles, say, each with perhaps

10 distinct levels of contraction, the calculation of the change would be considerable. There is something wrong with the argument: the computation is getting to be too large.

However, the computation only looks too large when viewed as a complete process being re-computed on a moment by moment basis by some central processor. For the musculature we can introduce a sub-model, the coordinative structure (Fowler 1980), which passes on a continuous basis through various 'configurations' against which we might put some abstract label – a 'segment'. The calculation only looks complex when viewed as a set of independent sub-calculations. But if the set is viewed as internally interactive and *self-organising* (in the manner of a complex spread sheet) then it is possible to see that local low-level 'arrangements' could take care of ongoing sub-calculations.

Put another way, we can say that some observed phenomena might be modelled as either *centrally* organised in terms of motor control, or *locally* organised. Central organisation would involve a great deal of moment-by-moment re-computation of 'targets' to explain adaptation phenomena. However, simple central organisation followed by fast local *self-organisation* will equally explain such phenomena – but this time without any massive loading on the central (cerebral/mental) system. This is the very essence of Fowler's Action Theory and subsequent extensions to the theory (Chapter 3).

Coarticulation and 'phonetic accommodation'

The idea of 'phonetic accommodation' in the phonetics literature is similar to, if not identical with, the notion of phonetic adaptation (see above). Sometimes accommodation is involuntary, sometimes voluntary though which is rarely discussed. However, coarticulation is not a phenomenon which we can switch on or off at will; it is a phenomenon brought about by unavoidable constraints external to the linguistic domain of speech production. Coarticulation shares with many somatic processes the fact that cognition can be brought to bear on its operation, so as to more or less limit or enhance the *necessary* constraints it introduces. In no way does this mean that coarticulation is a voluntary process. At most it means that coarticulation is an *involuntary* process which, like many others, can be *voluntarily* influenced.

Coarticulation or co-production?

Co-production is the telescoping of the parameter values of adjacent gestures during the rendering process; these in their turn may relate to identifiable segments of the utterance plan. Most researchers are clear that LR coarticulation can result from co-production but they are less clear that co-production might introduce a RL effect. We shall see later than RL effects are very often classified as voluntary, and therefore programmed as part of motor control. But the 'anticipation' (in the sense 'deliberately anticipated') of RL effects is perhaps more apparent than actual. Thus in the English sequence [ku] lip rounding is evident even before closure for the stop phase associated with [k], and in the sequence [ki] lip spreading can be observed to behave similarly. The rounding and spreading are only 'anticipated' in the sense that the spreading or rounding parameters (of the gestural programming of whatever coordinative structures are involved) begin before the velar closure associated with [k]. However the use of the term *anticipate* still needlessly adheres to the earlier unrealistic segments-and-boundaries model we associate with Classical Phonetics, and if it does not imply active control introduces a curious sentient anthropomorphic characteristic to articulators.

The effect of co-production *clashes* in telescoping LR and RL processes can be seen in the sequences [iku] and [uki] where there is an apparent change from rounding to spreading or *vice versa* during the stop phase of the [k]. In fact, of course, there is *no* change over from one to the other – the overlap and the final observed *lip distortion* aggregates the underlying gestures, obscuring the timing of the onsets and offsets taking place below the surface. This is the kind of reason we adduce for adopting wherever possible a hierarchical approach to modelling speech production: it is *impossible* to model gestural effects with a linear model which takes in only 'articulators' as its objects. A technique like electromyography reveals how independent gestures overlap to produce an apparent dependence when viewed simply from the surface.

Blocking and coarticulatory spread

At its simplest the blocking model (Chapter 3) proposes that segments selected either on an absolute or relative basis can be blocked with respect to certain coarticulatory effects. Put another way: coarticulation spreads out from a given segment to influence adjacent segments, but the spread from time to time encounters a blocked segment. That is, selected segments do not succumb to the coarticulatory spread. The problem here is that the blocking model has to allow for *variable* blocking. So, for example, it is hard to see how blocking could account for the [iku]/[uki] data introduced above.

What makes it hard to work out a good blocking model are the many variables which need to be accounted for. For example, Daniloff et al. (1980) speak of 'facilitated' when it comes to coarticulatory spreading, but this characterisation is insufficiently neutral; we do not *know* that coarticulatory spreading is something which can be facilitated, or what the mechanism to accomplish this might be. In contrast, Cognitive Phonetics focusses more on the idea that inherent coarticulation deriving from co-production is open to manipulation by the Cognitive Phonetics Agent – but explicitly *not* open to cognitive *initiation*. Daniloff et al. hypothesise that coarticulatory facilitating is positively initiated at will. It seems to us that the use of a hierarchical model with a lower tier of inherent physical constraints (due to whatever source) and the possibility of cognitive intervention is much less complex. We shall see as we proceed that this separation between voluntary and involuntary in a tiered model enables us to show a gamut of underlying sources for such cognitive intervention – all feeding into the active processing power of the Agent (Chapter 6).

The spreading model and linear causation

One flaw detectable in many writers on coarticulation is the presumption that speech sounds are 'influenced' or 'altered' by adjacent sounds (Borden and Harris 1980). What such writers must really mean is that from time to time we can observe at the surface regular alternations which enable us to set up a model in terms of targets and target departures. But it must be going too far to suggest that neighbouring sounds *cause* these alternations in some linear 'spreading' way, as though error (as a kind of living entity) were *seeping* across the surface fabric of speech. The characteristics of the surface signal might well, for some researchers, point to a model (among several possible) suggesting that there are targets and that the targets have regular alternations – that is they are regularly seen to vary in rendering. A weak explanation of these alternations, based on their apparent regularity, is that they are *caused* by the juxtaposition of the targets. The idea comes simply from the observation that the alternations are present when the targets are linearly juxtaposed: but this is *correlation*, not cause and effect. The causation model suggests an *active role* for targets – that they can, of themselves, distort their neighbours. Some researchers go so far as to suggest that they 'enhance' rather than distort, but this introduces a perceptually-based role for *motivation* of the cause – rather far fetched unless the entire process is quite literally under some higher control. There *is* place for enhancement which is perception oriented, but it is as a cognitive overlay layer rather than an overriding explanation of coarticulation.

- The worst possible formulation of the causation model hypothesises that a *segment* (an abstract linguistic unit) causes a physical coarticulatory effect – this is absurd. What causes observed coarticulatory effects is the rendering process: it is inherent in phonetic rendering that its surface outcome does not linearly reflect its apparent segmental input. If we are obliged to speak of cause, we might say that phonetic rendering causes surface articulations or acoustic signals which do not of themselves reveal the sources or processes involved in their own derivation.

Target theory

Central to Target Theory (see MacNeilage 1970) is that in speech production there exist strings of underlying discrete objects characterised as articulatory or acoustic specifications or 'targets'. These composite objects are what the system is to aim for or execute as part of the speech production process. The targets are represented at some stage as a *physical* specification of the chain, though the representation itself may be cognitive, of course.

In general areas of behaviour, invoking the concept of targets is felt by some researchers to be necessary to link surface observations with underlying abstractions which are almost invariably in terms of sequences of goals, and in the case of language (if not other modalities) in terms of strings of symbolic representations. It has made sense in target theory to have the output of the abstract system underlying the physical system as a string representation of required targets which 'translate' more or less linearly into a string of similar targets for physical rendering. The match is not quite linear because of things like time which has to take quite different forms in the two worlds.

Sequenced targets

Sequential target theory focusses on strings of discrete objects, cutting the linear cake, so to speak, in notional and later physical time, and lending to these objects the idea of boundaries. It is these boundaries which have to be 'removed' by coarticulation since they fail to materialise at the surface. Discrete segmental representation, however, is not a *sine qua non* below the phonological level, and it might be possible to abandon the sequential object notion even before the conclusion of the cognitive phase of the system. The replacement involves re-orienting the focus through 90 degrees to produce a parallel and continuous featural representation in a *prosodic* manner. A major problem introduced by this non-discrete approach, though, is the squaring of *cognitive parameters* with the subsequent *physical parameters* needed for rendering. It is simplest and perhaps most scientifically expected that the parameters at the cognitive level should be those found to be most useful in the linguistics of speech, and those at the physical level to be those found most useful in the area of the motor control of speech: the problem is finding an equivalence. The reason for the problem is that what is cognitively best is not necessarily physically best. Thus

cognitive parameters ⟶ cognitive/physical interface ⟶ *physical parameters*

It is easy to diagram the progression, but difficult to actually provide any argument for the equivalence, particularly in the light of a serious lack of empirical evidence. For example, take tongue height. In the abstract we might speak simply of, say, high-front or low-back vowels. The *vowel, high, low, front* and *back* features are quite meaningful in linguistic theory and hopefully have some psychological reality. But how this translates into motor control is difficult. Are we to keep the commonly found notion of the *articulatory unit* – in which case *high, front, low* and *back* need some kind of less specific specification more able describe overall tongue *shape* rather than apparently refer to some single point on the tongue surface? But perhaps they should be specified in terms of target contractile states of the tongue musculature to be achieved by the appropriate coordinative structure? Or both, with an equivalence table provided? Or both with a linking set of association rules provided?

We would ourselves prefer a physical representation here which makes sense to the speaker/listener in *cognitive terms;* and for this reason we prefer some kind of reference to articulators. The motor control system with its reliance on the knowledge stored within the low level muscular structural system's network could then take over the process which would be and remain completely opaque to cognitive awareness. We need something like this to explain why it is that speaker/listeners cannot discuss this aspect of motor control: they cannot discuss it because they do not know about it, or even know that it is there to discuss. But they *can* discuss the cognitively real objects and they can discuss 'abstract' physical objects or concepts like 'the tongue as articulator'. The physical object here is paradoxically abstract because it is not necessarily *per se* involved in the motor control of itself! A good parallel would be the way in which individual grass plants collaborate to give us a *lawn*: there is a strikingly true sense in which there is no such thing as a physical lawn, just an abstract lawn.

Reconciling abstract representations with physical representations

In the TM model we contribute to the problem of reconciling abstract representations with physical representations in this way. We extend the earlier more traditional view of speech to include the concept of *abstract physical objects* which can be related 'directly' to non-abstract physical objects, but are also transparent in their apparent relationship to abstract cognitive objects.

In a linear sequential model this is exactly the dilemma. There are as many different objects to combine as there are occasions to combine them, because every context for their occurrence is by definition different. Hence researchers sometimes refer to a 'physical path through articulatory inner space', which while predictable cannot be specified in terms of constantly changing motor control. Hence the need for coarticulation theory to account for the apparent surface uniqueness of every event.

There are two choices: compute everything every time at the higher level and set up the motor control for each unique event, or compute a detail-free or idealised (that is, abstract) sequence of abstract events, and allow the lower level rendering process to supply the uniqueness of the event. Put another way:

- *surface events are unique to a single event* (because of their variability which makes them members of an infinite open set);
- *underlying events cannot be unique to a single event* (because they are not variable, but members of a closed set);
- *transformation must take place* between the two in a one-to-many mapping.

There are at least two possible places for the transformation:

1. before the cognitive/physical interface – this gives rise to an impossibly large number of permutations of control specifications to explain the subsequent uniqueness;
2. after the interface – this throws the burden of supplying the uniqueness onto the rendering process.

These positions have been adopted as follows:

a. coarticulationists who believe the effects to be an *active process* reflecting deliberate distortion of targets favour the first approach;
b. coarticulationists who believe the effects to be largely *passively derived*, reflecting inertia based merging or blending of segments, favour the second approach;
c. co-productionists opt for a mixture of the two, and this also goes for the Cognitive Phonetics approach – though in a different way.

Correlation between the input target specification and the articulator target

Following MacNeilage (1970), we are saying that there is a direct correlation between the input specification (the target) and the final 'spatial target', but that the means of getting to the final target is variable. Using MacNeilage's own words in a diagram:

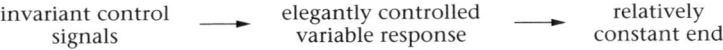

invariant control signals ⟶ elegantly controlled variable response ⟶ relatively constant end

There are several problems with the MacNeilage model, one of which is that the 'central signals' are not actually *known* to be invariant: this is no more than an assumption deriving either from a intuition or from the way they are modelled in Classical Phonetics and most speech production models. The variable response formulation is useful, but 'elegantly controlled' probably means no more than 'complex'. What the 'constant' end could be is not quite plain, either, because of coarticulation variability depending on timing and other mainly prosodic factors. Basically MacNeilage's model (Chapter 3) makes sense however because it avoids the problem of specifying variability and its causes too early in the derivation.

Size of targets

Most speech production models before Action Theory have targets which are equated in size to the domain of an extrinsic allophone. Since an extrinsic allophone is an abstraction it cannot have a duration, but it can have scope or domain. The relationship with an acoustic signal is that its domain covers the duration of an acoustic signal which can be assigned the allophone as a label. In the hierarchy the extrinsic allophonic domain covers an associated stretch of acoustic signal.

Returning to MacNeilage, his spatial targets are not abstract phonological segments, but *are* segment sized. As neural representations they exist in the physical world and are also rendered in the physical world: they cover a coherent set of articulator positions within the vocal tract space. The space is emphasised as three-dimensional, presumably to dissociate it from the two-dimensional geometrics so common in the writings of the Classical Phoneticians. The sharply focussed edges of these segments are subsequently blurred by inertial constraints and, interestingly, by deliberate overlapping – thus foreshadowing two types of coarticulation: voluntary and involuntary. The time-governed overlapping processes can distort the target timings.

- Note that neural representations are abstractions because they are just that: *representations*. This notion here of abstraction is not the same as the abstraction of the phonological segments which eventually comprise the utterance plan. Neural representations are descriptions of something which exists in the physical world; the utterance plan is a description which does *not* exist in the physical world. These distinctions are not niceties: they are *fundamental* to the theory of phonetics.

It is not entirely clear whether MacNeilage's set of articulator positions is the range of positions for each parameter, or the set of parameters itself. A representation could be

- a set of positional parameters within the three-dimensional space of the vocal tract, or
- a set of values for each position in the space.

If the set of positions is a set of values for *each* target then MacNeilage is moving toward Keating's window model within the TM model (Chapter 3).

Non-variable targets, variable targets and management

Before Action Theory it was felt unlikely that target specifications comprised unique values for sets of muscle parameters because of the ability of the system to compensate when interfered with. Several researchers have shown (for example Lubker and Parris 1970) that external interference in articulation does not impede speaker success in achieving spatial targets. There are two possible reasons for this

1. there are related sets of targets and the appropriate one is chosen to take care of external interference – this is an adequate model if the interference is long-term or gradual;
2. there is no more than a narrow range of targets, but this is coupled with the ability of the musculature involved to compensate rapidly within its own 'system' – this is a powerful model if the interference is sudden or short term.

Fowler's Action Theory calls for the second solution – the system within the musculature referred to as a *coordinative structure*. Coordinative structures are self-organising intra-communicating groupings of muscles specifically designed to maintain the *status quo* of a target as a constant. The structure's internal communicating system operates by calling on the readily available and comparatively fast gamma arc feedback mechanism (Matthews 1964).

Thus a set of *generalised* abstract commands is indeed possible, provided there is a low level mechanism to interpret the commands and organise compensation when necessary. This extension of the MacNeilage model moves toward Action Theory, but is not quite there because it still supposes detailed programming from above – not detailed enough to be more than a generalisation, but still more detailed than Action Theory or Cognitive Phonetics. These latter relegate a great deal of the detail in the end result to the low level structures themselves, which have *learned* how to take care of simple goal instructions from above.

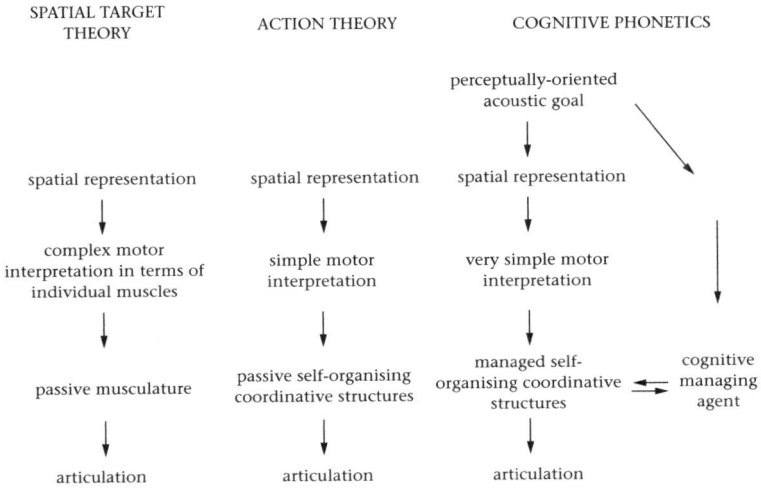

The diagram compares the basic properties of spatial target theory, Action Theory and Cognitive Phonetics. The essential property of Action Theory and Cognitive Phonetics is that they remove a great deal of the detail of articulation from the higher level planning and interpretation stages of speech production, and place it within low level physical structures of the musculature. These models rely heavily on the self-organising properties of coordinative structures. Cognitive Phonetics reduces the reliance on self-organisation by introducing the Cognitive Phonetics Agent to manage its operation. We shall see that the gain here is that local detailed and rapid adjustments are possible by using the CPA to supervise not just the linguistic features but also extra-linguistic features associated with expression (Chapter 6).

The unknown input

There is one major and quite simply expressed problem with all approaches to modelling speech production. The modelling technique is quite standard: a model is developed which derives a known output from a known input. The problem is that we do not know the input. Hence

input (unknown) ⟶ production process (unknown) ⟶ output (known)

If we do not know what we are processing to achieve the measured output we cannot work out what the processes are. Those researchers in speech production theory who are aware of the problem explicitly discuss and evaluate hypothesised plausible inputs to try to gain entry into how the production process might work. So what precisely do we not know? We do *not* know how

- speech is represented in the mind and brain
- speech is processed in the mind and brain
- anything to do with the brain correlates with anything to do with the mind

We need to know about mental representation in speech *production* because we draw on the mental representations of speech and other linguistic processes characterised by contemporary linguistics. But at the same time we need to understand how this cognitive processing 'interfaces' with physical neural and motor processes to derive the physics of speech. The task is near impossible, but awareness of the problem and the dangers of proceeding ignorant of the scientific consequences of cascading 'unknowns' have led to some useful insights about speech production.

3
Coarticulation Theory

Introduction

That coarticulation has occurred is taken as being signalled by the occurrence of a segment whose features vary from those specified in its target. A coarticulated segment is one whose features and/or feature values are not those predicted from its target. This idea assumes that we know the 'correct' or intended identity of the segment and have its target specification. Thus, in the word *width* we predict an alveolar plosive after the vowel, but we observed that in fact the plosive turns out to be dental. So, coarticulation has occurred.

Diagnosing the occurrence of coarticulation in this way presupposes that we had ruled out *assimilation* – which is often defined similarly. The difference is that assimilation is phonological, voluntary and the result of phonological processes operating on phonological objects *prior to* the full characterisation of the utterance plan. Coarticulation is phonetic, at first glance involuntary, and the result of phonetic processes operating on phonetic objects *during* the rendering process; it arises both logically and temporally *after* the utterance plan.

The idea of coarticulation rests on the assumption that there is an invariant or target phonetic specification for each segment. That is, that there is a representation of segments characterising their unique specifications. This representation is stored, and exists prior to the utterance; it is consequently independent of the planned utterance. Note that this would be equivalent to a 'table' of target phonetic values for extrinsic allophones (the units of the utterance plans) not phonemes (the units underlying the planning process). Such tables are abstract – the nearest they can become to physical rendering is when an individual extrinsic allophone is planned in isolation; this does occur in real life, though rarely. Time is an important parameter for the coarticulatory process since the inertial processes are time-governed. The inertial effect increases as time decreases. In sharp contrast phonological assimilation cannot have time as a parameter since there is strictly no time in phonology due to its wholly abstract nature.

Characterising the *results* of coarticulation

Almost paradoxically there are two ways of looking at the results of coarticulation, and there is some dispute in the literature. The segment rendering left by coarticulatory processes is

- a *degraded* version of the intended segment, or
- an *enhanced* version of the intended segment.

The segment can be thought of as having been degraded in the sense that, all things being equal, the parameter values have been altered such that there is a less than perfect match with the target specification. In terms of time the revised specification may have some temporal portion matching the original specification, but this will be less than the total duration of the segment. In the worst cases there is no time in which the target specification is hit.

The segment can be thought of as having been enhanced in the sense that it now contains information at its boundaries which reveals something of the adjacent segment(s). At the start of the segment this means that there is a 'reminder' of the previous segment's specification, and at the end it means that there is a 'preview' of the next segment. Provided there is sufficient time allocated to an approximation to the segment's own specification, a few researchers argue that this additional information could potentially enhance the perceptual process.

Mathematically, a first approximation model of left-to-right (LR) coarticulation would characterise the effect as a low pass filtering or smoothing process. As such the sharp edges at segment parameter boundaries would have their 90° angles increased. Figure 3.1 illustrates the point. Notice that it is the individual parameters of the segment that are differentially subject to this filtering, not the segment itself. Earlier researchers spoke of whole segments being coarticulated, but this is clearly not the case. In the *width* example above it is only the tongue positioning parameter which has coarticulated – in this case the smoothing is between the more alveolar positioning of the tongue tip associated with the [t/d] plosive and its more dental positioning associated with

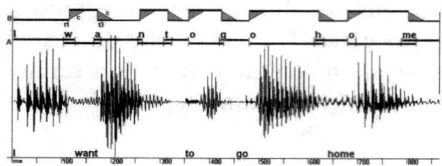

Figure 3.1 Waveform of *I want to go home*. A represents an overlapping coarticulation model: symbols indicate the start of each segment. B represents a LR inertial model: targets 1 and 3 (t1 and t3) are marked, together with the period of coarticulatory inertia (c) between the first three targets. Both models are first approximations, shown for illustrative purposes, as are the degrees of coarticulation and overlap.

the [θ] fricative. Most early researchers into coarticulatory effects would have spoken of the way the [θ] 'influences' the [t/d], though with little regard to an accurate explanatory modelling of just how or why this process might be accomplished.

The initially widely accepted smoothing model, once the details are filled out, in effect distributes information across adjacent segments. It is this idea of the distribution of information which has influenced those researchers who feel that the perceptual process has thereby been assisted: the unique information afforded to segment *S* is now distributed into segment $S - 1$ and $S + 1$ (at least) – thereby improving perception's chances of spotting it. The error here is to forget that segment $S - 1$'s information has now been distributed into segment *S* along with a part of the information relating to segment $S + 1$, as can be quite readily seen by observing the formant trajectories of the phrase *How are you?* in Figure 3.2. It could easily be argued that the resultant multiple and multi-directional distribution gives rise to nothing less than a very confusing continuousness to the flow of information, to which the perceptual process has a hard time assigning a copy of the speaker's original *discrete* specification.

That coarticulation assists perception is to us a counter-intuitive assertion – the assignment process is surely hindered. We have not yet come across any convincing experiments showing that perception degrades as coarticulation is reduced, and there are a great many examples of deliberate speaker *reduction* of coarticulation ostensibly to try to *improve* the listener's chances of assigning the correct interpretation to a signal. Figure 3.3 shows the result of a speaker trying to make sure that the listener understands correctly the phrase *It's not that I decided not to go, but that I was told to stay away*. In the first *not* we find

Coarticulation Theory 43

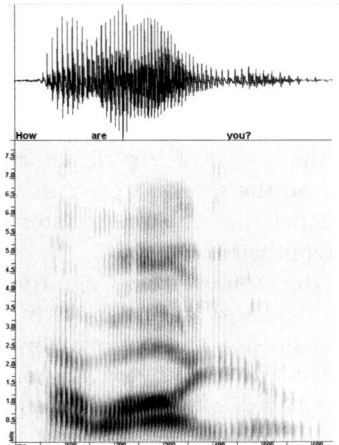

Figure 3.2 Waveform and spectrogram of *How are you?* Notice the continuousness of the signal and the constant 'movement' of the formants. There is no indication of any discrete segmentation.

an unreleased dental [t], but in the second a fully released alveolar version – where normally we might have expected the [t] to coalesce with the [t] at the beginning of *to*. Similarly the [d] at the end of *told* is fully released. These are examples of increased precision of articulation to assist perception. It would be hard to argue that perception is assisted by *decreased* precision of articulation.

Some researchers have even gone so far as to suggest that perception might be the 'reason' for coarticulation. That is, perception might *explain* coarticulation. There are two factors here:

- inertia (predominantly mechanical or aerodynamic) – including the parameter overlap effects focussed on by Action Theory and Cognitive Phonetics (Tatham 1986a, Morton 1986);
- speech perception itself and whether it can work independently of speech production.

The occurrence of inertia and parameter overlap is in principle *not* optional. It is arises from factors *outside* speech production, and a characterisation of those factors constitutes a true scientific explanation of the coarticulatory phenomenon. Perception, on the other hand, is not outside the system: we are concerned with the perception of *speech*, and both production and perception are within the same system and inextricably linked. This makes it difficult to invoke perception as a true explanation of the phenomenon (Chapter 8).

If the inertial factor might be optional, the perceptual factor would also be optional – a speaker could decide whether or *not* to include coarticulatory phenomena: but is this really the case? Is the coarticulatory content of speech ever optional dependent on the speaker's perceptual goal? Almost certainly not: all things being equal, the basic coarticulatory content will always be present, we might hypothesise.

This argument does not disagree with the proposals of Cognitive Phonetics (see below). Here we model coarticulatory effects as having two components arranged hierarchically: the one is a non-optional low-level biological or mechanical rendering effect and the other is a cognitively sourced *intervention* in this process (Chapter 6). This is a far cry from those that believe that coarticulation can be switched on or off at will, depending on perceptual needs.

- Inertial effects in the mechanics and aerodynamics of speech are, let us be clear, unassailable and *must* therefore figure in a model of speech production. That they are unassailable has nothing to do with speech production, and *cannot* therefore be denied from within a theory of speech production. At the same time cognitive intervention in biological and hence mechanical and aerodynamic processes is equally unassailable from within the theory of speech production for precisely the same kind of reason.

Left-to-right and right-to-left effects

In coarticulation both LR and RL effects have been observed by researchers sometimes in the movement of the articulators and sometimes in the resultant acoustic signal (MacNeilage and Declerk 1969). LR effects are those most usually cited as reflecting inertia in articulator movement or in aerodynamic processes. Taking just nasality as our focus: examples of LR effects occur in words like *null* [nʌl] and *moll* [mɒl] where nasality bleeds from the nasal stop into the phonologically specified [−nasal] vowels. Another way of saying this is that the utterance plan does not specify nasality for these vowels; the nasality is introduced during the rendering process applied to the plan. Staying with nasality we can also find the effect at the end of syllables when segments following the nasals are phonologically [+voice], as in *frond* [frɒnd] and *vans* [vænz] – provided there is sufficient periodic signal in the [d] and [z]. These effects can be found in the

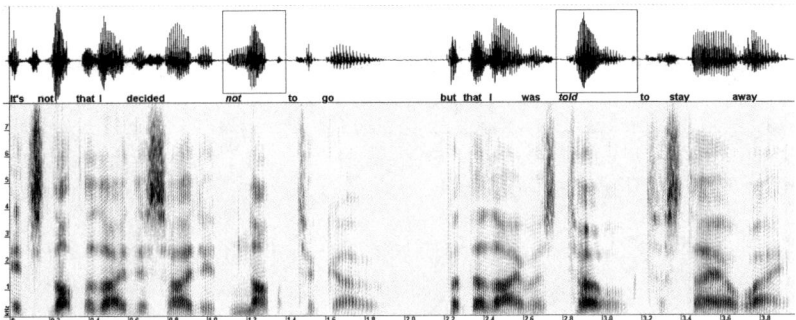

Figure 3.3 Waveform and spectrogram of *It's not that I decided not to go, but that I was told to stay away*. The emphasis is on the second *not* and the word *told*. In both cases there is final plosive release, though this would not have been expected – and in general the emphasised parts of the utterance are rendered slower and with more precision.

acoustics, and are shown in the spectrograms in Figure 3.4. Note that nasality would not be apparent in the post-nasal segments in spectrograms of words like *once* [wʌns] or *Banff* [bænf] – not because there has been no nasal leakage, but because it is not manifested in formant structure. It can, however, be measured as nasal airflow.

Two factors outside the domain of speech production play a role in such inertial effects:

- the biological, mechanical and aerodynamic properties of the articulators, their underlying control mechanisms and the way they interfere with or 'modulate' the air stream system;
- utterance timing – both linguistically global (rate of articulation) and local (segmental timing), as well as global and local effects explicitly related to expressive rather than 'core' linguistic content.

Inertia is a time-governed set of processes applying to the parameters of articulator movement and aerodynamics. These processes and their timing are *initiated* by linguistic and expressive factors, *but they are not the explanation of the processes*. Speech uses mechanisms which are governed by laws which have nothing to do with speech *per se*, but by which speech, because it uses these mechanisms, finds itself constrained.

46 Speech Production Theory

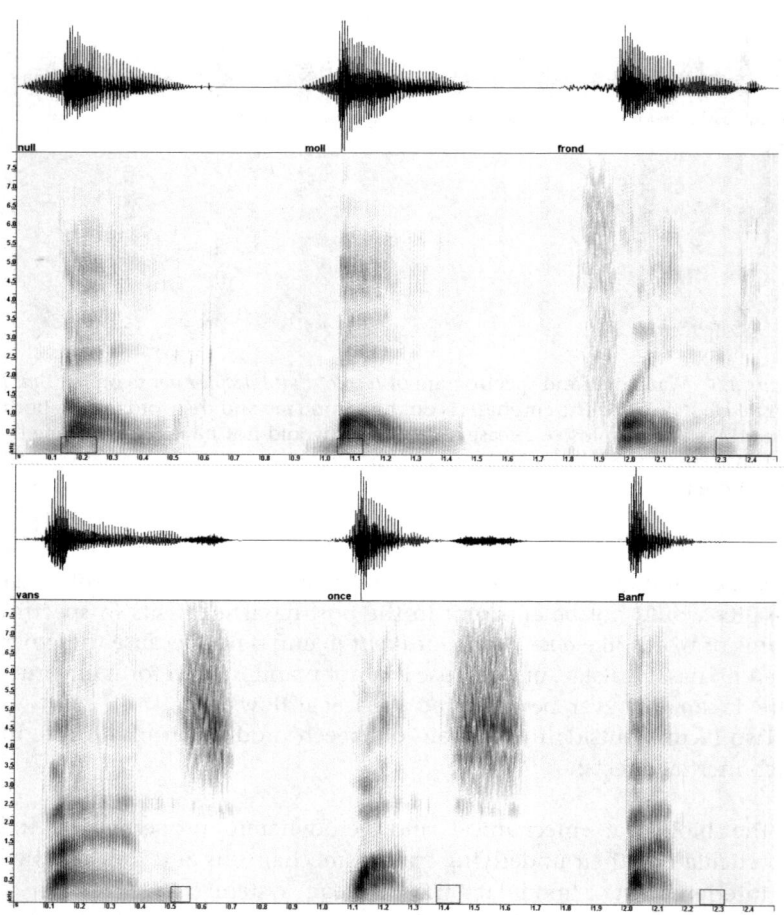

Figure 3.4 Waveforms and spectrograms of *null, moll, frond, vans, once, Banff*. In *null* and *moll* LR nasalisation can clearly be seen after the onset of the vowels, and into the final voiced segments of *frond* and *vans* – so long as the vocal cord vibration persists. With *once* and *Banff* there is no obvious LR nasalisation.

There is one other factor which enters into the results of inertial processes:

- cognitively sourced neuromuscular intervention designed to constrain these processes.

Constraint here is implied in its neutral gloss: the processes are differentially curtailed or enhanced along a continuously variable scale, but never negated by this intervention process alone. Cognitive intervention in biological and biomechanical processes is the basis of Cognitive Phonetic theory, and is used to explain such observations as the systematic variation in nasality of the vowels in words like *man* in various different accents of English, and in tongue positioning for [s] in words like Spanish *sí* and Italian *sì*, both meaning *yes* ([s] in Spanish has greater variability than [s] in Italian).

RL effects are considered to be more difficult to explain. There are a number of factors which could be involved:

- inertial effects of an 'anticipatory' nature were often cited in the early literature.

So, for example, the nasalisation of the [−nasal] vowel in *man* often runs throughout, but in *mad* does not. That the nasalisation continues beyond the start of the vowel can be modelled as anticipatory of the syllable concluding nasal consonant. If we examine the nasal airflow during the vowel we see that it reduces from the vowel's onset to some 'central' portion of the vowel, only to begin increasing as the vowel continues toward the nasal consonant (see Figure 3.5). In our view this is

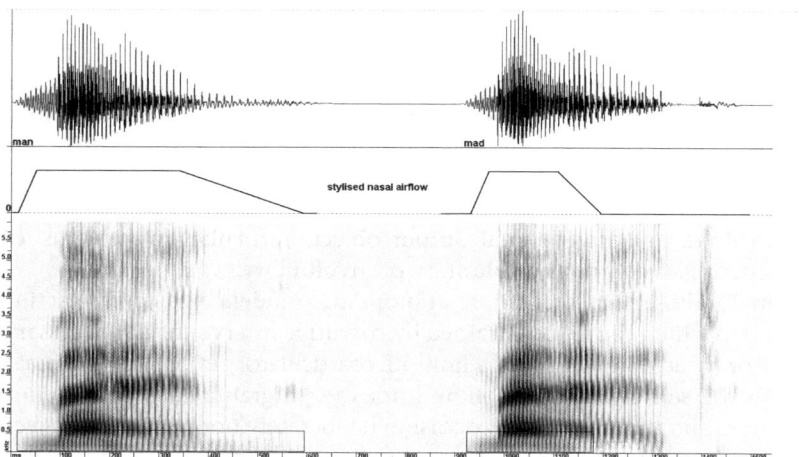

Figure 3.5 Waveforms and spectrograms of *man* and *mad*. Note how nasalisation extends throughout the vowel of *man* (LR and RL coarticulation) but only part way into the vowel in *mad* (LR) coarticulation. A stylised estimate of nasal airflow has been superimposed.

not true inertia, and is much better modelled as parameter overlap. The nasal parameter of the final consonant has to begin while the overall acoustic is still associated with the syllable's vowel nucleus – and it is this which can be attributed to inertia: the velum has mass enough to require an early start in its trajectory from near closed to fully open. However, note that at the start of the vowel the velum is being raised against gravity, but toward the end of the vowel it is being lowered with gravity. We do not support the model which allows gravity to drop the velum because speakers produce very similar effects when gravity works in the opposite direction – when they are standing on their heads. This example serves to underline just how complicated it is to model effects such as inertia in speech production and how they relate to 'intended' effects.

The difficulty of providing a true inertia-based explanation for RL effects leads to the possibility that

- RL effects are deliberate and 'programmed into' the articulation.

Such effects are unlikely, though, to be phonological in origin. That is, they are not part of the phonologically derived utterance plan. There is a great difference between saying that systematically distributed variant like $[l_j]$ and $[l_w]$ ('clear' and 'dark' [l] respectively) are 'programmed' and that the variant nasalisation of the vowel [æ] in *can* (nasalised) and *cad* (not nasalised) is programmed. In a descriptive phonetics we would call the [l] variants 'extrinsic allophones' and the [æ] variants 'intrinsic allophones'. Extrinsic allophones originate during the production phonology to contribute to deriving objects in the abstract utterance plan, whereas intrinsic allophones arise during phonetic rendering to contribute to deriving final output objects (articulatory or acoustic). Rendering effects can be voluntary or involuntary.

In TM RL effects are, where appropriate, modelled as co-production overlap which can be constrained by cognitive intervention if necessary. The only sense in which TM admits RL coarticulatory effects as 'deliberate' is in the sense that they follow from the programmed co-production process and that they are on occasion deliberately not constrained, even if they could be. Examples of co-production induced anticipatory coarticulation might be the more palate-central (here 'fronted') positioning of the constriction associated with [k] in a word like *keep* [kip] in English, or the more palate-central (here 'retracted') positioning of the constriction associated with [t] in a word like *tarp* [tɑ(r)p].

What must a theory of coarticulation include?

If we follow the above definitions we are obliged to include certain properties in a theory of coarticulation. A model of coarticulation must

1. accept the notion of *underlying discrete segment objects* which at some level are contextually invariant (the deepest phonemic level) – these are symbolic units of representation;
   - The reason for this is that by definition a theory of coarticulation only exists if it presupposes that there are discrete segments to coarticulate. It must, however, trace the origin and development of these segments so that any inherited properties which might influence the coarticulation can be taken into account.
2. accept that logically posterior phonological processes, which include assimilation, derive *equally discrete objects* selected from a language specific set of extrinsic allophonic segments – these are also symbolic units of representation;
   - Phonological processes derive further levels of representation from the deepest level. The final output comprises a string of extrinsic allophonic segments which on the one hand retains some of its derivational history, and on the other hand points toward the utterance plan. Assimilatory processes transform their *entire* segment-sized domain (though not their entire parametric representation) – there are none of the graduated or progressive effects of physical coarticulatory processes, because of the aoristic nature of phonological segments.
3. accept that not only do these underlying discrete objects exist in the phonological structure as symbolic entities, but also that they have no temporal feature other than simple sequencing;
   - Coarticulation occurs during phonetic rendering *after* a clock time dimension has been assigned. Prior to this sequencing is the only time-like feature the phonological segments underlying the utterance plan can possess.
4. hypothesise that these or at least some equivalent and correlating objects exist also logically simultaneously at the deepest *physical* level – they have been 'copied across' between the cognitive and physical worlds;
   - There are two worlds to be included in the theory: the cognitive and the physical. The scientific metatheory does not provide us with any clear route to automatically correlating the two. However, the correlation cannot be avoided in speech production theory.

A first approximation hypothesises that abstract objects can be copied across from the abstract world to the parallel physical world. Quite simply this means that the theory should be able to account for the co-existence of both types of object and their worlds (abstract and physical), if only by explaining the *necessity* for their coexistence.

5. assign these deep physical objects with some primitive temporal feature;
   – Classical Phoneticians and in particular early Generative Phonologists characterise abstract representations of *exemplar* utterances, which in a speech production model is equivalent to the characterisation of specific utterances. These characterisations are completely abstract, and in the production model equate to the results of the cognitive stages of processing. TM calls them utterance plans. In the 1960s and 1970s coarticulation literature the starting point of the phonetic rendering process is a target representation of the utterance – itself a sequence of *segmental* target representations. These targets have a 'primitive temporal parameter' which goes beyond the utterance plan's abstract time, making provision for the development of clock time. Primitive time involves phenomena such as normative intrinsic segmental durations or normative prosodic rhythmic structures (Tatham and Morton 2002). The rendering processes transform these primitive temporal structures into actual structures which are bound by prosody and potential pragmatic and general expressive content (Tatham and Morton 2004).

6. attempt to explain the nature of any physical processes which might transform the discontinuities of discrete objects into a continuous flow – the explanation must be truly *external* and must not therefore derive from language or from the perception of speech;
   – Since the basis of coarticulation theory is that otherwise discrete objects in a linear string are *smoothed*, the smoothing processes must be explained in terms of the independent mechanics and aerodynamics of the vocal tract. There may also be motor control effects which contribute to the smoothing, though these would need to be unravelled from *intended* motor control. The theory will need to distinguish between overall smoothing effects which are intended and those which are not – and in a more advanced model, distinguish between linguistically constrained or enhanced smoothing processes and those which are 'allowed' to operate unconstrained.

7. in terms of the articulators involved in the smoothing process, list and account for constraints on the physical transformational processes in terms of their own *intrinsic structures* – the processes must constitute a system which is *internally* constrained, that is, they interrelate in a non-random way;
   - There is every reason to suppose that the smoothing effects are not independent of each other. Thus inertia in tongue movement is not independent of inertia in jaw movement when it comes to spatial parameters such as tongue 'height'. The relationship and consequent *interaction* between the various sources of inertia needs to be characterised.
8. in terms of the physical structures outside the articulators involved, characterise any constraints there are which derive from or provide for *externally sourced interventions*;
   - It is not hard to imagine that there are external constraints on movement. The most obvious one is gravity, but there are others of a more mechanical nature. The inertia 'holding back' an articulator's potential movement may be augmented by an opposite resistance of some kind. The intended movement of an articulatory gesture may be impeded by the fact that it begins its movement from a position unexpectedly beyond its normal resting place. There are significant possibilities for articulatory movement which do *not* stem from the intrinsic mechanical properties of the articulator itself.
9. account for any *specific functions* assigned to coarticulation by the speaker and detail the mechanism enabling the speaker to do this;
   - Those researchers who attribute a linguistic motive to coarticulation or to some coarticulatory phenomena need to include a characterisation of the mechanism by which coarticulation is taken into account in speech production as an *active* linguistically dominated property. They need to explain how a speaker knows of the effects in a way enabling firstly prediction and secondly control. Remember that such models explicitly claim that speakers *use* coarticulation to assist perception; they less frequently take the weaker position that speakers count themselves lucky that coarticulation occurs and that perceivers know enough about the phenomenon to inversely filter its effects to gain insight into the underlying segments that it had smoothed.
10. account for how listeners can distinguish between 'unwanted' and 'wanted' coarticulation, and in addition how they distinguish between assimilation and coarticulation since these effects are often

confused even by researchers in the area;
- If coarticulation plays a role in speech perception, either because it accidentally cues aspects of underlying production or because it is intended actively by the speaker, or because it has been manipulated in a rendering management process (Tatham 1995), then it falls to a theory of coarticulation to explain how perception can do all this. But importantly, how do perceivers distinguish between coarticulation which is linguistically relevant and that which is not?
11. account for any *use* made of the results of coarticulation and any constraints by the listener's perceptual system which might limit the use of coarticulatory results;
    - The perceptual processes which can use coarticulation to assist assignment of symbolic representations to heard acoustic signals cannot be infinitely able in this respect – there must be limitations. What are these, and how does a speaker know them? What are the differential limitations on decoding the 'meaning' of coarticulatory effects? – some will be easier to unravel than others. For example, coarticulation is clearly a variable, and if listeners can make use of it, then the theory must explain how listeners are able to take this variability into account.
12. point explicitly and in detail toward a *simulation* or a *computational model* able to predict all observed coarticulatory phenomena.
    - The theory of coarticulation has been so central to elucidating speech production that it must be detailed and fully explicit. Not only must the model be properly and fully explanatory, it also needs to be *predictive*. These days the most appropriate and productive route to prediction is *via* a fully computational model: one which will simulate the human-based outcome and explain how it arises.

The above presupposes that a model of coarticulation accepts as input a string of discrete objects and outputs a continuous articulation or a continuous waveform. It also supposes that there is a close relationship between speaking and perceiving. Listeners do assign appropriate symbolic representations for continuous waveforms, and most models of perception would attribute this to an active process which brings knowledge to the perceptual process, rather than a more passive process which discovers the representation *in* the signal. However, for those models of direct speech perception which take the latter and attempt to 'recover' information from the acoustic signal, the model must explain how this is possible – since what appears to be recovered is equivalent to the segmental representation in the speaker prior to coarticulatory effects. The diagram below illustrates the two ways of modelling the decoding process: in either case a detailed account of the perceptual processes is necessary (Chapter 7), and in the case of the direct models an account of *how* the underlying segments are present in the acoustic signal.

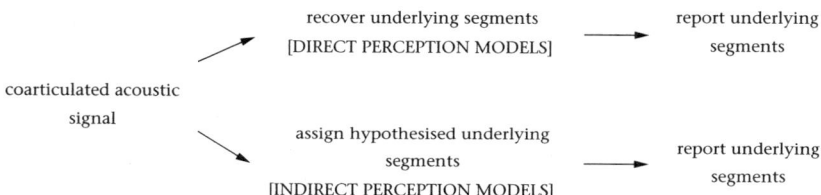

The focus of coarticulation theory

Research into coarticulation has focussed on a number of different levels in the system hierarchy in an attempt to establish at what point(s) plans and targets transform – and why. These are the main levels of attention:

1. the nature of the units of utterance planning – these units and how they are used to represent the putative utterance are not known but *hypothesised*, although they constitute the model's input;
2. the relationship between planning units and the deepest level of physical representation of the utterance – the planning units are cognitively sourced as part of a production phonology, but at the same time they relate to the input to the physical processes of speech;
3. the representation of the physical units as targets – at some stage target or idealised specifications for speech production must be accessible, either as target 'segments' (static focus) or as targets for temporally ill-defined stages of articulatory gestures (dynamic focus);
4. the hierarchical system of motor control – from motor cortex through direct muscular innervation, intermediate muscle response, feedback systems and indirect ('pure' reflex and coordinative structure 'managed' reflex), to final muscle response;
5. the physical (mechanical) behaviour of muscles – their interaction and the way in which their contractile behaviour results in the desired articulatory configuration;
6. the aerodynamic system – how this responds to dynamic articulatory configuration to produce a final acoustic signal;

7. possible perceptual models which are sensitive to coarticulation – either in that they are able to 'recover' the intended utterance by inversely filtering the signal, or able to use coarticulatory information to assist (rather than hinder) the perceptual process.

At the deepest planning levels we can see that assimilation, as an optional phonological process, results in the transformation of the featural specification of a phonological object or unit. The assimilatory transformation is predictable in the sense that only particular features change in line with the marking of such features in adjacent segments. Thus in the word *input* the underlying object /n/ is transformed for utterance planning into a derived /m/ in accord with the bilabiality feature of the following object /p/. It is optional in that although speakers of English would almost always use the assimilation, they sometimes do not – as when for example, they may wish to stress that they are speaking of *in*-put rather than *out*-put. This implies, importantly, that they know they do not have to assimilate; and so they also know *when* and *when not* to assimilate.

Because phonological units are abstract and clock time ostensibly plays no role in phonology the units are considered to be individually simultaneous – that is, they have no beginning and no end in the physical sense. The nature of phonology (itself constrained by general cognitive processes) is such that assimilation applies to the whole of the simultaneous object, and cannot, by definition, arise or decline gradually 'during' the object – there cannot be a 'during' for such abstract objects. So, to misuse phonetic transcription for the moment, but to make the point:

- underlying / ɪ n̠ p ʊ t / derives
  1. / ɪ m̠ p ʊ t / (where /m/ is a bilabial extrinsic allophone of /n/), but cannot derive
  2. /ɪ-ɪ-ɪ n-n-n-m p-p-p ʊ-ʊ-ʊ t-t-t /, nor
  3. /ɪ-ɪ-ɪ n-m-m p-p-p ʊ-ʊ-ʊ t-t-t /.
  (where the triplets are intended to be a symbolic representation of a temporally prolonged segment).

The second and third representations are not possible because simultaneous segment objects *cannot* be prolonged since they have no temporal dimension. However, having asserted this, we note that in transcription systems such as the International Phonetic Alphabet there is a representational problem with diphthongs and affricates and with the representation of palatalisation, affrication and the like. This does not materially affect the simultaneous nature of phonological objects: diphthongs and affricates do not temporally change within the object in any clock time sense. Thus the representations of the single segments /oʊ/ and /ʧ/ should not imply a temporally based change 'during' the segment any more than /p/ implies a temporally based change from 'stop phase' to 'release phase'; the changes are *logical* not temporal. Misconceptions of this kind are the result of using a phonetically-based transcription phonologically, and alternative representations like the matrices of distinctive feature theory (Jakobson *et al.* 1952) do not fall into this trap.

The *input* example is open to experiment to determine whether there is any attempt during physical rendering to produce a dental. Can a lay speaker feel tongue contact with the alveolar ridge? Can we show in the laboratory that the 'segment' in the articulatory or acoustic signal begins with a dental and ends with a bilabial? In Figure 3.6 we show two spectrograms, the first of the acoustic signal from planned /ɪmpʊt/ and the second from planned /ɪnpʊt/. /ɪmpʊt/ should show no movement of the second or first formants, but there should be movement of these formants with /ɪnpʊt/. If there is movement with /ɪmpʊt/ then the assertion that the entire extrinsic allophone has been substituted in incorrect. We agree with Keating (1990) that assimilation is about aoristic phonological segments – she sees them as whole or indivisible – whereas coarticulation has a more gradual, time-related effect on temporally governed phonetic segments.

Theories and models of coarticulation

Coarticulation is a phonetic phenomenon and not something to do with phonology. In our TM model there are cognitive phonetic processes which could be regarded as spanning phonology and phonetics – they are *not* phonological, but they are not physical in the way ordinary phonetic processes are (Chapter 6).

Models of coarticulation – presuppositions

Models of coarticulation invariably presuppose that there exists at some point in the hierarchical description of how an acoustic signal is produced objects which are timeless and discrete. In such a model lexemes (objects retrieved from the lexicon with full underlying phonological specification) have a phonological representation consisting of linear strings of symbolic objects. In such models the function of coarticulation theory is to explain how such a representation becomes the continuous soundwave. One reason for having phoneme sized objects is to capture the apparent psychological reality of these objects for speaker/listeners.

Speakers and listeners are able to talk about objects of this size, and give an account of their role in making up syllables and words.

The symbol–object model is a pre-supposition of coarticulation. If there are no objects like this there is nothing to coarticulate and the model is superfluous. Early writers in coarticulation theory were quite explicit about this – they usually introduce their writings with a statement of the problem of 'reconciling' the discrete objects of phonological descriptions with the continuousness of the physical speech signal (articulatory or acoustic). They ask questions like: *At what point in the production hierarchy does the discrete representation give way to a continuous signal (or sometimes a continuous representation)?*

The *theoretical* problem is that the discontinuous representation is symbolic and abstract, whereas the continuous one is physical, and that it is too simplistic to speak of the discrete *giving way* to the continuous. In a sense the abstract representation is less secure or robust because it could take many different forms (which would have to be justified on a 'purpose' basis – *Why does it have to be like this?*) whereas the acoustic signal *is* just that: the acoustic signal. Any graphical re-representations we can 'inspect' are trivial: waveforms, spectrograms etc. as they appear on a computer screen. Without independent justification, necessarily external to the linguistic domain, the abstract representations could be many, each perhaps equally justified. Thus we could have a system which consists of processes characterised as sets of productions, or artificial neural networks or as an expert system, or as a hidden Markov model, and so on. It could be procedural (a putative 'speech production model') or it could be declarative (a descriptive model characterising the knowledge needed to generate exemplar utterances) or a mixture of the two (a knowledge-based production simulation).

One property of our TM model is that we 'copy' the phonological surface representation to the deepest entry representation in the phonetics. That is, we get around the levels of abstraction problem literally, by jumping the two levels. In effect what we are saying is that the *plan object*, conceived cognitively and represented abstractly at the exit point of the phonology is *copied* to the phonetics entry point, including whatever abstraction adjustment is necessary between the two levels. Thus the *phonological plan object* is not exactly the same (in terms of level of abstraction) as the *phonetic plan object*. This is not a question of transformation between the two objects, it is a question of re-interpretation of the object in new terms (terms which are less abstract) and its *transfer* to a parallel world – a world of different constraints and conditions.

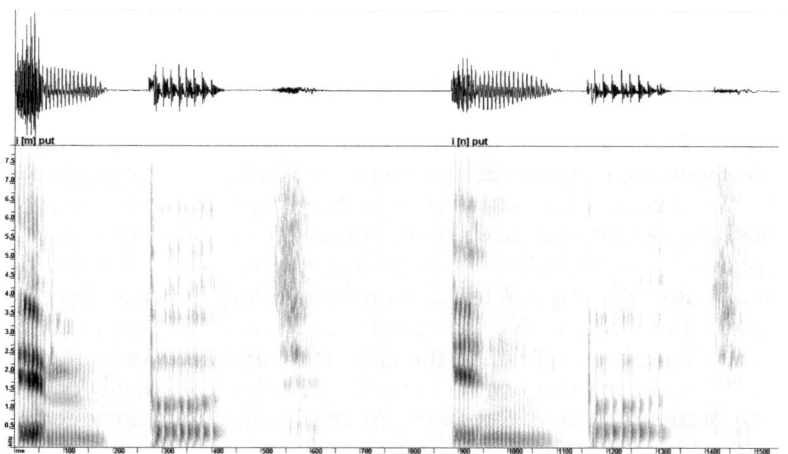

Figure 3.6 Waveforms and spectrograms of *i[m]put* and *i[n]put*. Since the lips are involved in both the [m] and the [p] of *i[m]put* we would expect more formant bending throughout the first part of the word, than in *i[n]put* – where the [n] does not involve the lips. There is perhaps more formant bending in *i[m]put*, but certainly not none in *i[n]put*.

Coarticulation – basic theory

Hardcastle and Hewlett (1999) describe coarticulatory effects and the discrete units involved as 'the result of the integration of those units in the continuously flowing activity of the vocal mechanism' (p. 29). This is saying that the vocal mechanism is predominantly a device of 'continuously flowing activity' – irrespective of language. That is, the continuousness is scientifically correctly explained by reference to physical phenomena outside the domain of language. However, for Hardcastle and Hewlett this continuousness interacts with the discreteness of the *phonological* units. But this cannot be right because those phonological units are abstract, and the *physical* constraints of the vocal mechanism cannot logically interact with *abstract* objects. What we might say is that there exists at some underlying physical level a representation of the cognitively planned utterance which is itself discrete in correlation with the psychologically real discreteness of the plan units. In a neuro-motor model we would perhaps be obliged to say that the cognitive plan is transferred to a neural plan (in the motor cortex?) which looks just like the cognitive plan except that it is physical and not abstract. This, of course, is the mind-body problem whose detailed discussion is well beyond the scope of this book. All coarticulation theories presuppose the existence of utterance plans which are physically represented at the deepest level of motor control, and they all presuppose that these plans relate (hopefully on a linear basis) to yet deeper cognitively represented plans.

There seems little escape from this situation. Human beings can introspect about their utterances and when they do so they report their thinking to be in terms of discrete and identifiable objects – which we choose to call in our science of phonology: phonemes, extrinsic allophones – or some such name. At the cognitive level this is hard to deny.

But what of the physical level? Do human beings report or discuss a parallel set of physical objects? We call them parallel because to us the only useful pro-tem solution to the mind-body problem (which may be a pseudo-problem, of course) is to speak of related and parallel objects which cannot be directly correlated. We think not. When someone says *The sound I just made was a [t]*, for example, they mean *The sound I just made was one which I identify* [a cognitive activity either on the part of the speaker or the listener] *as a [t]* [an abstract symbolic representation in their mind]. They do not report how the sound is physically made on any level of the production hierarchy (neuro-motor, articulatory, aerodynamic or acoustic), unless they have trained as phoneticians or introspected unusually about how speech is produced.

Symbolic representation and linear context

Wickelgren (1969) proposed a descriptive model (*not* a speech production model) in which he uses a symbolic notation to capture the immediate phonological context of linearly concatenated utterance plan objects. Many researchers have been perplexed by this model, and many have misinterpreted it as a phonetic rendering model.

Wickelgren's model hypothesises that the *basic units* of speech are context sensitive, rather than context free in the way proposed by other models. Thus the units which correspond to our extrinsic allophones are units which differ depending on their context. In many models a unique utterance plan comprises extrinsic allophones drawn from an inventory where they exist in a context-free state: their context is supplied by the hierarchically organised derivational history of the plan. In Wickelgren the allophones are inserted into the plan as already context-sensitive: a linear model whose final outcome is the *same* utterance plan. Wickelgren was trying to characterise the psychology of the utterance plan (and, to a certain extent its recovery in the listener), not the physical detail of its rendering.

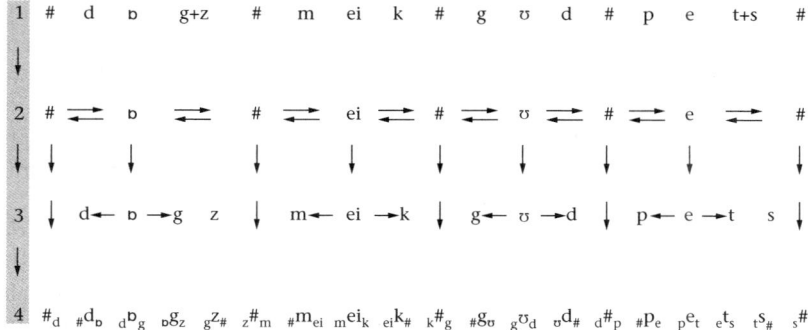

The diagram represents a revised version of Wickelgren's contextualised model, arranged hierarchically. Tier 1 is the phonologically derived utterance plan, expressed as extrinsic allophones; tiers 2 and 3 show a two-stage rendering process with 2 developing an Öhman-style coarticulated vowel 'carrier', and 3 showing the consonantal sequence to be 'dropped' onto the vowel carrier – with the vowel's 'influence' indicated by horizontal arrows. Tier 4 is the resultant fully coarticulated output, represented symbolically in Wickelgren's subscript notation – note that the notation does not allow for separate vowel-vowel and vowel-consonant coarticulatory effects to be shown. If fully developed the model would be able to indicate pre-rendering cognitive assimilatory effects and effects such as the cross-boundary suppression of the initial plosive release in the pairs [$_k\#_g$] and [$_d\#_p$].

Technical criticism of Wickelgren's approach

Even though we believe that much of the criticism of Wickelgren's model has been misguided there are one or two technical problems of basic model building procedure:

- The model requires an inventory of large numbers of extrinsic allophones capable of characterising linearly all assimilatory processes. The counter-approach is to have a small finite number of objects and a finite set of rules to derive the exhaustive output – this is the classical Chomsky (1957) approach to modelling syntactically the infinite set of sentences which comprise a language.
- Wickelgren's model of adjacent segment influences is linguistically naïve since there are several phonological processes which spread beyond adjacent segments. To take just one simple type, consider the normal pronunciation of the Russian word *хорошо! (Good!):* [χəra'ʃo].

The underlying phonological representation will have the three vowels as identical /o/, but the derived representation (equivalent to our utterance plan) will be /χəraˈʃo/. The linear sequence is not 'responsible' for the variants in the derivation, but presumably Wickelgren could only index his objects according to their immediate linear context: #χ₀ χOr ₀rₒ rO ʃ₀ʃ₀ʃO#. This will not do because the variants must be derived *before* the representation not after it.

- Additionally any processes which are cognitively derived and which participate in the TM-style *management* of coarticulation also occur after Wickelgren's representations so are left completely unaccounted for in his model, since he has no means of controlling subsequent coarticulation other than by contextual specification within the plan.

The main fault ascribed erroneously we believe by some researchers to Wickelgren's model is that it misses important 'normal' coarticulatory generalisations, such as the fact that vowels nasalise before nasal consonants. But Wickelgren's representation is intended to be *subject* to the later coarticulatory processes, not account for them. Similarly, some of the criticisms that Wickelgren fails to capture some of the detail of variants (as, for example, when a speaker restricts coarticulation by deliberately increased precision of articulation) are met by introducing a *third* level similar to that introduced by Lindblom (1990) or TM.

Finally, the entire argument surrounding Wickelgren's approach rests on precisely what his contextual objects correspond to in the traditional models. If they embody a derivational history covering only assimilatory effects, as we believe, then there is no significant reason to criticise, other than the fact that Wickelgren does not give us a true hierarchically based approach. But if they represent segments which are supposed to have already undergone coarticulatory processes, then the model fails on several fronts.

Lashley's serial ordering approach

Lashley's account of serial ordering (Lashley 1951) is not as parametric as, say, that adopted in Articulatory Phonology (see below), and does not therefore easily enable gestural overlapping. However, events, whether segmentally delimited, or gesturally limited (and therefore overlapping) are still serially ordered within the gestural parametrically parallel framework. This is not a contradiction. For the psychologist Lashley, as for most linguists and most lay speaker/listeners, speech is a serially ordered chain of events, and remains so despite the complex rendering of 'serial' at the phonetic level. Gestural models do not contradict the serial approach; they merely make it more complex, and indeed are potentially more productive.

Öhman's vowel carrier model

Öhman's model (Öhman 1966, 1967) is pre-Action Theory, and as such relies on the notion of *independent* controllability of phonetic features. The articulatory structures (lips, jaw, tongue) enumerated by Öhman are what he hypothesised must be independent because of their differential roles in the articulation of vowel and consonantal sounds as characterised in Classical Phonetics. Öhman hypothesises that coarticulated vowels form a continuous carrier onto which consonants are 'dropped' on demand by the utterance plan.

Öhman's coarticulation model belongs to the 'missed target' genre. There are target shapes – necessarily idealised because they are potentially never fully rendered, even when segments are rendered in isolation. Öhman, like so many other coarticulationists, makes a technically weak case for associating abstract plans based on sequenced discrete phonological objects (extrinsic allophones) with abstract targets for corresponding physical objects, expressed as parameter sets. In the tongue control model we have three parameters:

- the apical – associated with the primary constriction of consonants toward the front of the vocal tract,
- the dorsal – associated with the primary constriction for mid/back consonants (palatal and velar), and
- the tongue body – associated with setting up the primary constriction for vowels.

The consonant/vowel dichotomy is cognitive in origin since it is essentially a phonological concept; even in Classical Phonetics, despite attempts to give different physical definitions to consonants and vowels, the distinction is functionally descriptive – that is, phonological. Öhman extends the separation of vowels and consonants to the possibility of physical control, and structural differences, affording vowels the dominant 'carrier' role.

MacNeilage's three-dimensional spatial targets

The basic unit for speech production in MacNeilage's model (MacNeilage 1970) is the 'phoneme'. This is equivalent to 'extrinsic allophone' in later models and in TM. Extrinsic allophonic segments are stored in a three-dimensional psychological space as a 'map' – a representation – of articulator positions within the vocal tract. Since in the production of some sounds more than two dimensions are involved the representation has to be in terms of a three-dimensional mental map of the articulatory space.

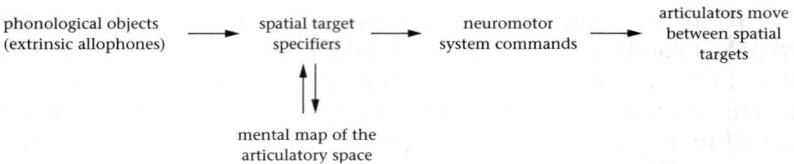

The command system in the MacNeilage model is *open loop*. That is, there is no reliance on feedback to influence the nature of the commands. The motor commands incorporate *deliberate* coarticulation. One reason why such a system would have to take in whole utterances would be to account for coarticulation beyond the immediate segmental context. This implies a high-level mental image of chunks of utterance as potentially executed – including the detail of coarticulation, thus explaining coarticulatory 'spanning' as an *intended* phenomenon, rather than as a low-level segment by segment inertial effect.

MacNeilage does however include a closed-loop stage, presumably for its stabilising effects. MacNeilage himself invokes the 'gamma motor system' (Matthews 1964), with its ability to 'tune' the musculature and to react quickly to stretch forces. But he is writing without the benefit of the low-level coordinative structure network model introduced later into speech production theory. MacNeilage seems to anticipate the coordinative structure's essential property of being able to self-organise by constant messaging around the network. It may well be that since the coordinative network involves the gamma system MacNeilage is foreshadowing Fowler's Action Theory (Fowler 1980) and subsequent similar models.

Holmes' linearly conjoining model

Although essentially a model developed for the Holmes text-to-speech synthesis system (Holmes *et al.* 1964, Holmes 1988) this model is important because it foreshadows later models, and may well have provided the inspiration for some of them.

Essentially a table-driven system, the model takes segments from a table, and modifies them according to phonetic context. These segments are called 'phonetic elements', and are expressed as sets of acoustic parameters corresponding to those used in the Holmes parallel formant synthesiser. Each parameter is specified in the abstract with a target value. This target comprises

1. an underlying generalisation from which actual values will be derived – a 'target specification which might often not be reached, but which can be regarded as an ideal that would be aimed for in long isolated utterances' (Holmes 1988, p. 84);
2. two important accompanying indices:
    a. indicating the intrinsic duration of the segment – an abstract, idealised timing,
    b. a weighting factor attached to the segment which expresses its degree of influence on adjacent segments when it comes to conjoining or coarticulation – or, conversely, its degree of resistance to the coarticulatory influence of adjacent segments.

Holmes had observed that segments do not all exert the same 'strength' of influence on their neighbours, nor do they all succumb equally to similar coarticulatory pressures from neighbours. Additionally, the *consonant* determines the transition between a consonant and a vowel:

> For example, nasal consonants have acoustic properties that change only slightly during the oral occlusion, but cause rapid changes at the boundary between consonant and vowel, and fairly rapid but smooth formant transitions during the vowel. Fricative-vowel boundaries, on the other hand, can also have quite clearly discernable formant transitions during the frication. Types of transition are largely independent of what vowel is involved, although the actual numerical parameter values in each transition obviously depend on the associated vowel target value. (Holmes 1988, p. 85)

Notice importantly that the model begins by considering the type of transition between *classes* of segments, not between individual segments. A generalisation is involved here which hinges on the *manner of articulation* of the segment. This recognises that the transition effects are down to articulator properties rather than linguistic properties.

Lindblom's coarticulation model

Lindblom's (1963) formulation of coarticulation theory is very basic and cannot explain extended temporal influences spanning multiple segments. Here, as with many other theorists, the 'principle of economy' is what underlies coarticulation. What is economical, for example, requires some kind of value judgement, and may itself be a variable, changing with different contexts. Introducing the term 'economy' does, however, go beyond a simple reporting and characterisation of the observed data – that is, moves towards explanatory adequacy.

The principle of economy shows up in two dimensions:

- vertically (focusses on the segment): the actual targets (for example, undershoot dependent on duration),
- horizontally (focusses on utterance timings): movements between the targets.

Lindblom has the speaker's goal as the acoustic signal *which is to be perceived*, not just the acoustic signal. And this goal is dominant in determining many of the features of the way the sound is itself produced. This notion accords well with the TM goal of producing a signal which optimally triggers the correct perceptual assignment of a copy of the underlying representation. Lindblom is similarly able to incorporate the notion of constrained coarticulation and timing to allow for speaker style (see Lindblom 1990).

Lindblom and Öhman compared

Lindblom's (1963) coarticulation model matched phonological invariance to physical target invariance, as does Öhman (1967). For both, observed variations in the utterance arise after the motor command level, so are essentially properties of the mechanism receiving the motor commands. This is archetypal coarticulation theory, and forms the basis of almost all subsequent models – those which espouse the same theory, and those which evoke it for the purpose of illustrating improved theories. In Lindblom articulatory economy smoothes the 'joins' between segments on a *parametric* basis.

Lindblom's coarticulatory phenomenon is almost entirely one of mechanical inertia modelled linearly in terms of the sequence of targets and the inertial and temporal constraints which smooth the transitions between targets. Öhman, however, puts forward a model of a hierarchically organised system involving, in effect, the articulatory transformation of motor commands as consonants *collide* with vowels. The tongue body parameter moves independently and smoothly from target to target (or under certain conditions, from missed target to missed target) while consonant targets drop into the system from time to time to distort this smooth movement to give an output in which both LR and RL coarticulatory effects are observed.

The diagrams compare Lindblom's linear model with Öhman's more hierarchical model. In Lindblom the coarticulation is between adjacent segments; in Öhman the dominant coarticulation is between vowels in the vowel carrier, with consonants dropping onto this carrier. Optionality of consonants is indicated by bracketing them, and inter-segmental effects are indicated by double arrows.

Lindblom ... $(C_a) \leftrightarrow V_1 \leftrightarrow (C_b) \leftrightarrow V_2 \leftrightarrow (C_c) \leftrightarrow V_3$ ...

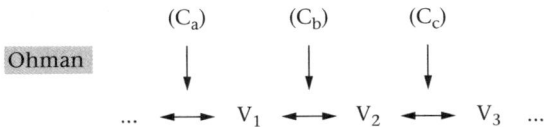

Ohman

We can re-interpret these ideas from a modern perspective. The underlying phonological plan is a sequence of syllable objects, each of which begins with an optional consonant cluster and ends with an optional consonant cluster, but which must contain a vowel nucleus between the consonant clusters; the whole is organised as in hierarchical system. In the general case for English the surface phonological sequence is:

$$\$ \ C^{0-3} + V_1 + C^{0-4} \ \$ \ C^{0-3} + V_2 + C^{0-4} \ \$ \ C^{0-3} + V_3 + C^{0-4} \ \$$$

where $\$$ is a syllable boundary, superscripts on C indicate the number of consonants which can occur in this syllabic position, and subscripts on C indicate the sequencing of vowels.

The underlying plan above *gives rise to* an appropriate sequence of phonetic targets where in Lindblom these remain in the planned surface sequence. But Öhman hypothesises that these targets are re-organised in a way corresponding to constraints of motor control which dictate that vowel targets are the primary initiators of a smooth and continuous articulator displacement, and where the smoothing results from constraints imposed by the inertial properties of the tongue body. In Öhman the consonant targets then displace the vowel trajectory according to regular coarticulatory constraints.

One problem with Öhman's model as he formulates it is that although we can in the abstract conceive of it as a hierarchical model, in terms of actual physical motor control there still needs to be a linear system – unless the motor commands for vowels and consonants comprise separate channels of access to the musculature. Separate channels would be possible on single innervator nerves if the control information were multiplexed.

One source of difficulty in Öhman's model arises because the concepts *vowel* and *consonant* are concepts from phonology where they relate to the functional properties of objects which are sufficiently distinct to the classified into two subsets. The functional property usually involved is their role in the structure of syllables noted above. Öhman carries over this abstract notion into the physical domain of articulator control. Ostensibly this is a productive way of modelling what is observed at the surface, but it does not necessarily reflect what actually goes on in the speaker: the formalism used for phonology may have had too much influence on the way the physical phonetics is modelled. If this is a criticism it is one which has to be levelled at *almost all* proponents of speech production models.

Öhman's data, he argued, is consistent with a model in which the control of vowels and the control of consonants are separate, with a continuous vowel control and spot consonantal control. It is important to remember that this is only one possible way of explaining the data which Öhman had gathered – and in any case constitutes a model, not of course a characterisation of fact. How vowels interact to form the carrier, especially when their mutual influence clearly varies depending on their individual durations and weightings (see the Holmes model above). So far there has been little discussion of weightings between vowels or between consonants, and most researchers have assumed that Öhman is not proposing coarticulation between consonants. But there clearly *is* coarticulation between consonants, as in the occurrence of a nasalised [z] in the word *bronze* in English, and many other examples.

The conclusion of Öhman's hypotheses is that vowels form a basic *bias* and within their vocalic domain mutually coarticulate to produce a smooth flow of articulation and therefore of acoustic output. Consonants are spot dropped onto this vocalic flow. The coarticulatory effects of consonants distort the vocalic flow, leaving inertially determined traces in their wake. We have not done the necessary analysis of the signal, but it should not be impossible to subtract such consonantal overlays if the hypothesis is tenable.

In modern terms it would be better to speak of coarticulation between syllables and perhaps primarily between syllable nuclei. The concept of the syllable and its nucleus is essentially a concept within phonology – but there is scope for extending a similar concept into phonetics (notwithstanding the pulse, etc. ideas for defining syllables – see Abercrombie 1967).

Henke's look-ahead model

Henke (1966) proposes a look-ahead model in an effort to explain some aspects of anticipatory RL coarticulation. Speakers look ahead to see whether there are any motor actions which could be taken up in advance of their local requirement for a particular segment. The idea is that if there is nothing between now and the time for this segment which might require some other specification for these particular motor actions then it is possible to get on with the articulation early. This would particularly apply if the articulator to be moved involved high mass or the distance to be covered was large.

Thus the look ahead model predicts correctly the lip rounding observed during (even earlier than) the articulation associated with the first vowel and the consonant in the sequence: [ə'ku], and also predicts lip rounding onset at some point during the period associated with the consonant in the sequence [i'ku] – that is, the lip rounding seems delayed because the lip articulatory parameter is 'in use' for the [i] in a different mode (spreading), thus preventing an early start for the [u] rounding.

A difficulty with Henke's look-ahead model is the mechanism which prompts look-ahead. How does the system know what is coming up? The look-ahead mechanism could be cognitive – scanning ahead in the utterance plan – or it could be physical – all articulatory parameters proceed with a lead time unless there is mechanical inhibition (as with [i'ku] above).

In psychology, cognitively sourced intervention in somatic processes is modelled overall as a two-tier process: the basic process is physical, but is amenable to a dominant tier which permits *cognitive intervention*. Notice that cognitive intervention does not imply some decision to switch on or off at will the appropriate physical process – the on/off process *per se* is not under cognitive control. On this basis, and adopting the modelling approach of psychology, it would be a gross exaggeration to claim that coarticulatory effects are cognitive in *origin*.

The original approach adopted by the Theory of Cognitive Phonetics in the 1980s was borrowed from the psychologists' approach:

- there are somatic processes (in this case constraints on articulator movement in time), and
- these can be interfered with once they have been identified by the cognitive system.

These processes are amenable to constraint in both positive and negative directions. The amount of constraint which can be applied is not the same for all processes, nor is the degree of application along a *positive* ← *zero* → *negative* vector symmetrical. Positive constraint involves no less than an enhancement of the inherent physical constraint, and negative constraint involves a limiting of the effects of the inherent physical constraint. Over the years many examples of constraints applied to mechanical and aerodynamic effects have been adduced, ranging from the control of 'areas' within the articulatory and acoustic spaces for segment target rendering, through to systematic adjustment of the timing of aerodynamic effects for promotion to phonemic level. An often used example is the systematic exaggeration of voice onset time for the phonemic use of, say, four degrees of VOT (negative, zero, positive and enhanced positive) to provide the potential for four contrasting plosive types.

Cognitive Phonetics has a cognitively organised look-ahead mechanism which tries to account for some of the difficulties with Henke's model and others of a similar type. In the Cognitive Phonetics model – which is listener goal oriented – there is a continuously running prediction of the results, both articulatory/acoustic and perceptual/acoustic, of plan rendering. This look-ahead mechanism forms the basis of rending management – a system which takes charge of how physical rendering unfolds. This mechanism in predictive mode clearly has access to what is about to happen (in motor, articulatory and acoustic, as well as perceptual terms), and can adjust articulation accordingly. If there is a least effort component in rendering, or simply a practical component which gets things going early so as to optimise rendering, then this will be known to the manager – the Cognitive Phonetics Agent (Chapter 6).

Coarticulation Theory 69

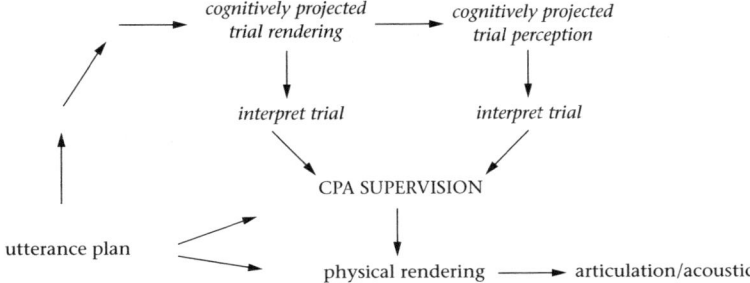

In the CPA model the Agent has access to the original utterance plan, and also to cognitively organised trial renderings and trial perceptions of the plan. On the basis of running these predictive models the CPA can supervise the actual physical rendering of the utterance plan, thus optimising the rendering.

Henke's model is segmentally based, which is why it includes abrupt discontinuities at segment boundaries. This is the consequence (as with most other coarticulation models) of mapping the abstract phonological segmental object directly into a physical phonetic object and consequently having to introduce the notions of boundary and duration (which are not possible parameters for the abstract phonological object). The model is also *linear*, and it is the linear context which purports to explain both RL and LR coarticulation.

Henke's look-ahead model has the important and significant asset of being computational. His units are phonemes-sized segments, and these are specified parametrically in terms of a set of articulatory targets. Thus an utterance is specified as a matrix in which the columns are the segment targets and the rows are the articulatory specification for these targets. Movement between targets occurs instantaneously at the boundaries between columns. The comparative non-abruptness of the observed movement of the articulators or the acoustic signal results from

- the past linear phonetic history of parameter values as we move from target to target – this is RL coarticulation, and
- from inertial and neuromotor constraints – this is LR coarticulation.

The key property of the model is that phonemic segments are implemented as articulatory commands. The target matrix therefore itself embodies the conversion from an abstract whole target specification to a physical featural detail specification. The matrix itself *is* the converter between the symbolic representation and the physical representation or interpretation. Much more simply: what we have, of course, is a lookup table, exactly paralleled by Holmes' (Holmes *et al.* 1964) acoustic parameter lookup table. The Henke and Holmes models share a lot of properties, not least that they rely on linear context and that they are both computational.

Intrinsic and extrinsic allophones

Wang and Fillmore's (1961) original distinction between extrinsic and intrinsic allophones (p. 130) speaks of 'secondary cues' and divides these into two types, reflecting

1. the speech habits of a particular community – in our terms characterised as *phonologically derived* extrinsic allophones, and
2. the structure of the speech mechanism in general – in our terms characterised as *phonetically derived* intrinsic allophones.

In practice this means broadly and as a first approximation that extrinsic allophones are those variants produced in the phonology by language specific processes, and intrinsic allophones are those variants produced in the phonetics by universal processes. Wang and Fillmore are unravelling the term 'allophone', rather than providing it with a formal definition. Later we see that Kim (1966) invokes Ladefoged for a more formal definition which introduces an element of explanation.

In TM terms (and in those of many other researchers interested in speech production models), and assuming a segmental rather than a gestural model of speech production, intrinsic allophones are objects derived in the rendering process: they are rendered extrinsic allophones and reflect processes intrinsic to the speech production mechanism and the way it is controlled. Processes which are intrinsic to the speech production mechanism are, by definition, universal and are *explained* by reference to domains *outside* the domain of linguistics. For example mechanically and aerodynamically determined constraints influence the way in which mechanical and aerodynamic rendering proceeds. To a certain extent we can say that rendering is *explained* by invoking the mechanical and aerodynamic constraints involved. These limit the freedom of the rendering process, such that the articulatory and acoustic goals of rendering might themselves be ultimately constrained by them.

Ladefoged's approach to allophones

Ladefoged's (1965) definition of the two types of allophone is clearer than Wang and Fillmore's, and at the same time moves toward explanation. Intrinsic allophones are those which are caused by the way 'articulations of adjacent phonemes' *partially overlap*. We have to be careful of the terminology here: in TM terms we would speak of the overlapping during the rendering process of parameters of the extrinsic allophones (phonemes are too abstract and too unitary) to be found in the underlying utterance plan (as output from the phonology and input to the phonetics). Extrinsic allophones are not simultaneous once they move into the phonetic rendering domain: they are already time-constrained and for rendering purposes the onsets and offsets of their component parameters are not precisely synchronised. An intrinsic allophone occurs when the offset of a particular parameter for segment S ends later than the onset of the same parameter in segment $S+1$. The result is what we might call 'edge distortion' of the parameter (and perhaps, if it is significant in the whole segment, of the segment itself). This is co-production, a parametric view of the way observed coarticulatory effects occur. It is the variants which arise from these *overlapping effects* which are called intrinsic allophones. This is not to say, of course, that all intrinsic allophones derive from co-production and overlapping parameters. There is no denying that the earlier idea of articulator inertia results in coarticulation – it is simply not the only source of the phenomenon.

- In speaking of intrinsic allophones, we have to be careful to distinguish between a physical event, and its description. Ladefoged and many others (including ourselves at the time) regularly make no apparent distinction between the event or object (the allophone) and its symbolic representation (the allophone). This ambiguity is all-pervasive, yet clearly it is productive to distinguish between an object and its representation.

For Ladefoged, extrinsic allophones are the result of phonological processes operating on deep objects. Extrinsic allophones in TM are wholly abstract objects (or their symbolic representations), are timeless and therefore simultaneous: there is no possibility of a graduated effect spread over time *during* an extrinsic allophone. Intrinsic allophones are wholly physical objects (or their symbolic representations) and must, of course, have time. It follows that they can have effects graduated during their lifespans (the time from their beginning to their end). Extrinsic allophones change in their entirety therefore, *because* they have no durations, but intrinsic allophones can show partial changes, where 'partial' means spanning only part of their durations. Loss of the voice parameter in a phonological segment means that [+voice] changes to [−voice]. Loss of the vocal cord vibration parameter on the other hand in a phonetic segment means that we need to specify that this means an amplitude reduction which may be progressive over a given period of time, or over a specified portion of the duration of this segment. Thus there would be a major difference in the meaning of a phonological rule which assigned [−voice] to an underlying [+voice] segment, and a phonetic rule describing a loss of vocal cord vibration in the rendering of an underlying [+voice] extrinsic allophone.

Classical Phonetics confuses assimilation and coarticulation

Some writers in the Classical Phonetics surface-descriptive tradition confuse assimilation and coarticulation, as defined from a more modern perspective. Thus we sometimes find the observation that *nasal assimilation* and *voicing assimilation* are partial because they are due to co-production processes, making them (to use Ladefoged's terminology) 'intrinsic features'. The problem is deciding whether these processes and others like them are cognitive and phonological, or physical and phonetic. These processes are clearly determined by constraints on phonetic rendering which are physical in origin, and in most cases are caused either by inherent inertia or by parameter overlap (as discussed above). The 'partial' outcome of the processes is enough to show that they have operated in time, and must therefore be phonetic. This is not to say that all phonetic processes are temporally partial, but it is to say that *no phonological processes can be temporally partial*.

It is the case that that these intrinsic processes sometimes vary beyond the variability introduced by the physical structures themselves (cognitively adjusted coarticulation). The variation is often systematic, and it is for this reason that some theorists have felt obliged to classify them as phonological. The TM model prefers other criteria: a process is phonological if the objects it operates on are themselves phonological, and a process is phonetic if it operates on phonetic objects. All phonological processes will be cognitively sourced, therefore. But some phonetic processes, despite their physical source, will be cognitively adjusted – this is the process of cognitive intervention characterised in biopsychology, and adopted into Cognitive Phonetics.

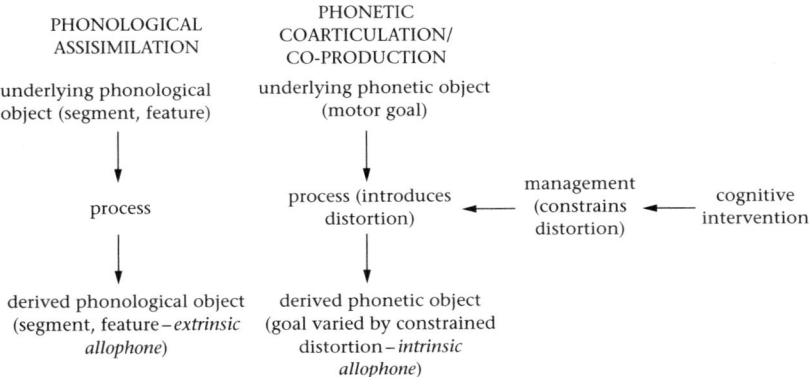

The diagram shows how the processes of assimilation and coarticulation or co-production are kept distinct. What would be unacceptable theoretically is the idea that a phonological object could be varied by a phonetic process. We can see that there is obviously no need to constrain a phonological process by cognitive intervention, since all such processes are themselves cognitive. The only exception here would be the existence of some phonological processes which were deliberately varied as to the extent (not temporal, of course) of their application. Phonetic processes, on the other hand, are less robust and seem to be *supervised*. Since the supervision involves choice and decision it is of cognitive origin, as opposed to the intrinsic physical processes themselves which are entirely of physical origin. This model extends the original Wang and Fillmore definitions of their allophone types, and refines the Ladefoged definition to account for details of the observed properties of coarticulated speech.

- *Assimilatory processes* are phonological and operate on abstract objects (that is, segments which are timeless and whose parameters or features are therefore *simultaneous* or *boundless*);
- *Coarticulatory (including co-production) processes* are phonetic and operate on physical objects which exist in time – the processes themselves are time dependent (so cannot be phonological);

- Separating processes into a hierarchical arrangement which introduces tiers and which differentiates types of process, seems to us to be a *sine qua non*.

Kim's 'systematic synthesis' model and coarticulation

Kim (1969) uses the term 'systematic synthesis' to describe an approach to modelling roughly equivalent to our computational approach. He introduces *conjoining rules* which are in effect rules characterising coarticulatory processes. His approach is to start with a table of values of extrinsic allophones, and from these derive intrinsic allophones by means of conjoining rules. Kim observes that intrinsic allophones vary systematically with their language or dialect. This observation has been made by many researchers, though modelling the effect varies, as we have seen, considerably.

However, Kim wants 'intrinsic allophonic *features*' to be universal rather than language specific. We notice repeatedly, though, that he observes that it is the intrinsic allophones which are language specific. He cites Lindblom (1964) and Öhman (1966) and their conjoining rules – which are really in terms of universal effects. What he says is that if the targets are the same then the intrinsic effects will be the same, even across languages. This is because, following Lindblom and Öhman, the processes arise from the 'structure and potential behaviour of the human vocal tract mechanism' – and these are virtually the same for all human beings. The apparent contradiction is solved by postulating sets of universal rules whose effects shift in a language specific way – as though by the addition of a weighting factor. It is the *set* of rules which has the weighting factor applied to it, thus ensuring a coherent shift from some norm or idealised system in which there is no weighting nor language specific element.

Kim solves the problem of the apparent perception of underlying extrinsic allophones rather than of surface intrinsic allophones by introducing the idea that perception involves the 'projection of the listener's internal knowledge about this language' onto the 'acoustic substance' of what is heard. In effect the listener's judgement is based on his projected grammar – this *becomes* the perception. Kim's innovation was in trying to model speech production and perception as active processes drawing on Chomsky-style 'knowledge' (Chapter 6 for how this idea is incorporated into TM).

Daniloff and Hammarberg – coarticulation as feature spreading

Daniloff and Hammarberg (1973) and Hammarberg (1976) set out their theory of Feature Spreading as a way of explaining coarticulation. They observe that previous coarticulation theories have been obliged to distinguish sharply between an intended physical target (an object ultimately deriving from some cognitive target) and physical processes which distort the target. They point out the implication that any necessary prior *cognitive* phonological processes would appear to proceed without any predictive model of the subsequent *physical* processes and how they might distort the intended target. That is, the system would proceed, even if motor commands were strictly adhered to, to produce an end result at variance with what was apparently intended. This is a classical dualist approach with representations and processes sharply divided between those which are cognitively based and those which are physically based. They try to get around this dualism by assigning coarticulation to the *phonological* component in the speech production process, with features phonologically spreading across and between segments *before* the motor commands are issued.

- This class of model sees the burden of explanation of the observed output phenomena (the coarticulation) as resting within linguistic cognitive processing, and contrasts sharply with the Lindblom–Öhman–MacNeilage class of model which sees the burden as resting with universal *a*-linguistic physical processing. The Cognitive Phonetic and Co-production models see the burden as *shared* between cognitive and physical processes. The problem for these last two models is how to approportion the processes and how to reconcile them with the linguistic descriptions of speech.

Most other proponents of a cognitive element in coarticulation see LR effects as universal and physical, and RL effects as feature spreading 'assimilatory' rules. This still does not deal with an essential difference we have already noted between abstract phonology and physical phonetics: the phonological segment cannot have partial or gradual effects, whereas the physical segment can. So we have to ask whether all the proposed RL effects in these models are all-or-non. The answer, of course, is no – they too are often gradual.

In fact one of the diagnostics for deciding between assimilation and coarticulation is the property of phonolgoical processes that they apply to the whole segment object and not to part of it. *Whole segment* here means 'vertically' whole, features notwithstanding, and *part* means not this or that subset of features, but 'temporally part'; that is, having in practice temporally gradual onset or offset.

So, in the Daniloff and Hammarberg model RL coarticulation should be in the phonology as phonological 'feature-spreading rules', that is, assimilation rules. LR processes are true coarticulatory effects, phonetic rules based on inertia in the articulatory system. In speaking of what they call the 'graded nature' of coarticulation, they do however recognise that the problem with associating this with phonology is that the characterisation of such grading is not possible with a system based on binary values for features. We ourselves would add, importantly, that since phonological segments are abstract not only must the entire feature be all-or-none in its specification, but there *cannot* be a grading within a segment based on time. So gradual spread across several segments is not possible, and also gradual spread within a segment is not possible if we stay with a phonology based on a binary valued feature system.

Keating's model of coarticulation

Keating (1990) suggests that coarticulation can be phonological or phonetic. We summarise the position:

- *Phonological coarticulation* (that is, assimilation in other models) derives from feature spreading rules (Goldsmith 1990), and causes successive segments to share one or more attributes. The attribute spreads between segments, and the feature values either change or they do not. When they change they do so for the segment, and since segments are a-temporal they do so for the *entire* segment, though the word 'entire' is not really appropriate for what is an abstract object. To this extent phonological assimilation could be said to be 'abrupt' in the sense that it has no gradual onset or offset. This is obvious because 'gradual' implies a time function which cannot exist in abstract phonological representations. The nature of phonological feature spreading is interesting because it must be *motivated*; what causes the effects and what the constraints are need investigating.

– Phonological rules are to be thought of as language specific.

- *Phonetic coarticulation* is less abstract, and because phonetic segments are more physically oriented than phonological segments they exist in clock time. This means that they have in principle temporal, rather than simply logical, beginnings and ends, and the concept of 'gradual' for the onset or offset of a coarticulatory effect has important meaning. Indeed we often find that coarticulatory effects are gradual, by contrast with phonological assimilatory effects which are, by definition, abrupt, as are the 'boundaries' between phonological objects in general.

  – Each language can apply a different phonetic interpretation to any unspecified features in the output of the phonology. So phonetic processes are universal, but their application may be language specific.

For Keating it is necessary to think of coarticulation as occurring on two different levels since, she asserts,

- binary features and phonological rules cannot account for the *gradation* observable in coarticulation
- the observed graded variation should not be characterised in terms of phonetic *universals* deriving simply from the speech production mechanism, but presumably in the provision for their application to be language specific.

The process, as we understand it, is shown in the following diagram:

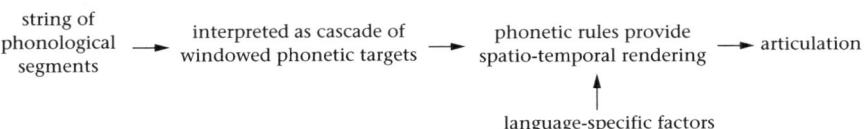

The diagram illustrates Keating's basic model, showing the insertion of windowed phonetic targets as part of the general spatio-temporal interpretation of phonological strings. However, Keating is uneasy about earlier rigid distinctions between phonological all-or-none binarity – arising, of course, from its abstract timeless nature, and about the observations which have troubled a number of researchers, that observed coarticulation is not entirely predictable from any universal mechanical properties of the rendering system.

Hence, Keating's model begins with the assumption that the process of phonetic rendering involves initially converting phonological features (or combinations of features) into phonetic targets: these have both spatial and temporal elements. Importantly, these targets are not invariant in the way earlier models proposed (for example, those of MacNeilage 1970 or Lindblom 1990). In sharp contrast we find that in Keating's model segmental features are associated with value *ranges*, which she calls 'windows', and which represent the overall variability possibility, or coarticulatory possibility for *these* features (or feature combinations) in *this* segment. Wide ranges or windows go along with a segment's greater coarticulatory possibilities.

Keating intends that window *width* should

- either describe the actual coarticulation that results,
- or be what constrains the coarticulatory possibilities.

Any ambiguity here rests on whether this is simply a descriptive model or a predictive procedural model. We assume that Keating favours the latter, since she goes on to talk about variable width windows adjusting the coarticulation. This is an important distinction: Keating clearly has in mind that these windows enter into the actual speech production process, rather than simply characterise the results of that process. The windows have both duration and 'width', and together these characterise the range of possible values for a particular target in the language. That is, the exact *width* of each window is language specific, with all values between the available maximum and minimum possible. Window width can be varied to account for *coarticulatory resistance*. It is unlikely that any language would select a window width at the maximally humanly possible level. In effect the maximum possible width for language (rather than a particular language) is the maximum possible in terms of articulatory control.

In this model if the window is, say, the sum total of all possible coarticulatory variations for the segment (or for the feature), then for any one item there may be a 'bias' to the window: it is not necessarily symmetrical, and any a-symmetry may be important. Note that the set of coarticulatory contexts presumably varies from language to language. It would be useful here to specify some kind of 'universal' window for a segment which may be constrained by its articulatory-place type or articulatory-manner type (or both), and further constrained down by specific language usage. Examples of the kind of question arising here might be:

- Are plosives *more likely* to coarticulate (or coarticulate 'wider') than fricatives?
- Similarly, what about vowels? Are front vowels *more likely* to coarticulate than back vowels, or high vowels than low vowels?
- Can a segment's degree of *coarticulatory freedom* be constrained by context?
- What about those languages with *consonant clusters* as opposed to those which tend to favour more the CV+CV ... pattern? – how are consonant clusters to participate in the cascading window scenario?

As we have pointed out, the window could be said to express coarticulatory resistance, in that the extent of coarticulation or its restraint is defined by window width. Although not made much of by Keating, it would also be possible to set up a system with *variable* windows. For example, window width could be determined for any one utterance by a pragmatically derived prompt such as 'with anger'. In angry speech there is a tendency to increase articulatory precision (or restrict coarticulation), and this could in principle be accomplished by a window narrowing process. Once again though the window concept implies either a linear distribution of coarticulatory possibilities across the window, or a normal distribution of possibilities, and whether this is or is not the case would have to be determined empirically. In such a refinement of Keating's basic approach there could be a whole cascade of constraints applied to the window width, some widening the window, some narrowing it. What such constraints might be and what there sources are would have to be determined, as would be their hierarchical interaction – can they cancel each other out? or are the effects additive or related in some other way? and so on.

Keating's model is within the class of coarticulation models. Offset to this idea is the class of co-production models. Coarticulation models presuppose

- underlying invariance (for example, of units used utterance plans),
- surface variability (for example, of articulation and the resultant acoustic signal).

Co-production models, on the other hand rework the notion of units in the utterance plan as being dynamically specified – functionally defined phonologically derived units called 'gestures'. The term phonological is used to indicate that they are functionally systematic, though the concept of gesture often confusingly spans phonology and phonetics.

Elaborating Keating's model

One reason why Keating felt the need to elaborate on the traditional account of coarticulation as a universal a-linguistic phenomenon is the way in which it appears to apply differently in different languages. A number of other researchers had noted this fact, and it follows that a language-specific characterisation is more appropriate. We shall see, however, that there is more than one way of incorporating the language specific element, and indeed dialectal and expressive, pragmatically derived, elements (see Tatham and Morton 2004). Keating sees traditional phonological 'under-specification' as serious, since it fails to specify some allophonic variation.

Keating has *two* levels in her phonetics; these accommodate

1. effects earlier characterised as belonging within phonology, and
2. effects earlier felt to be universal and physically determined.

In contrast, the TM Cognitive Phonetics account handles the language-specific and universal effects using *three* levels:

1. effects of assimilation characterised in the phonology,
2. effects of universal coarticulation characterised in the phonetics,
3. cognitive phonetic effects characterised in the phonetics – these effects are language/accent specific and often dependent on expressive content.

At first glance it seems that Keating collapses TM's 2 and 3 into her second phonetic level. For her phonetics has the task of 'interpreting in space and time' the output of the phonological rules. This output is, in TM terms, the utterance plan; so the job of phonetics is to interpret or render the plan from its wholly abstract representation as a phonological object into a spacio-temporal articulatory characterisation. Keating is clear in specifying an articulatory rather than acoustic goal.

Keating is attempting in her general model to integrate phonology and phonetics, and her solution is not unlike that of Browman and Goldstein's (1986) Articulatory Phonology in conceptual terms (though not in detail). Time and space are the real problems, and Browman and

Goldstein bring these in by giving their phonology notional versions of these otherwise very physical properties of speaking. These abstract concepts pass into physical representation as speaking moves to the phonetic actualisation stages. In Keating, space and time are assigned to phonological representations through the medium of phonetic rendering of windowed phonetic targets matching phonological objects; these phonological objects are, in a sense, 'spatio-time *ready*'. For us, she shares with TM the highly abstract notion that a phonological object is an object designed not independently of its phonetic rendering, but with its possible range of phonetic renderings in mind. One of the purposes of our accounts of the various models of speech production is to attempt to bring out commonalities of approach. We believe that Keating's solution to more integration of phonology and phonetics, whilst recognising their different approaches, is partly an expression of a two-way interaction: phonological objects and their manipulation have an important and fundamental phonetic underpinning.

Keating's model – summary

Keating's Window Model has phonetic implementation rules whose output is a time-focussed representation derived from an input sourced in the phonology. The model is parametric, and proposes that parameter values for objects be specified in terms of ranges rather than absolute values. Ranges are *windows*, though some researchers have found the term a little misleading in the sense that windows are often associated with stretches of *time*, or views of sections of complex processes. Windows are

- undifferentiated and are used to specify the extent of phonetic coarticulatory variability for any one segment;
- defined in terms of maxima and minima;
- can be very wide where there is extreme contextual variation or narrow where only slight contextual variation arises;
- have their precise limits determined within a given language or accent, and are therefore language-specific.

One criticism of Keating's model is that the explanation for a given range does not explicitly take into account the notion that range may be the manifestation of a complex hierarchically organised system. We are thinking here of the idea where observed coarticulatory variation is the product of actual physically induced ranges overlaid on which are *range modifiers* in the form of constraints and enhancements to the basic physical system; these constraints and enhancements are ultimately sourced in aspects of the linguistics of the system.

At its simplest Keating's model, though parametric, does not develop the idea of a hierarchy of parameters or some system of inter-dependence between parameters. One or two researchers have criticised this aspect of the Window Model. But in principle it can be developed in this way without undermining Keating's original idea. The TM constraint and enhancement overlays are also stated in principle in terms of a block of parameters, but implicitly there is application of constraints by varying the internal system within the parameter set itself. We interpret Keating to intend to model an idealised, error free and expression free speech. In this case the significant constraints are indeed linguistic in origin. But the model is eminently extensible into the domains of expression, in which case the 'core' linguistic constraints would assume a more balanced role in determining the final output.

Although Keating provides the theoretical mechanism for predicting assimilation and coarticulation and how extra-linguistic constraints may impinge on this, it is not made entirely explicit how windows are 'set'. Setting a window is the process of establishing its initial target width and then adjusting that width to take account of linguistic and other (in the extended model) proposed external constraints. Fowler's Action Theory model has tuning to set target parameter ranges, as does the TM model which adopts this concept. The physical mechanism which makes this possible is the coordinative structure. The nature of the coordinative structure is also used in these two models to simplify the complexity of the target signal by introducing a self-organising element at this lowest of levels in the motor system. Although neither tuning nor self-organisation are addressed, clearly both could be added.

Window setting – target constraints and their domains

We might imagine that for each target parameter window there is an intrinsic width. We might further imagine that this width is constrained on linguistic grounds, and by extension, on grounds external to linguistics, such as expression and style. The focus here is on the origin of the constraints. But there is also the domain of such constraints. Are, for example, constraints to apply to each single segment and its linear context leading to a cascade of more or less constrained window widths? These would relate to each other only by reason of their overall domain – the syntactic phase or sentence, or perhaps the phonological utterance – and their one-on-one sequencing.

Or are constraints to depend on some overall prosody? Where there is a general prosodic domain for such constraints the focus would be on the overall utterance and how its prosodic structure influences its segmental rendering. Thus, the coarticulatory resistance claimed by some researchers would be dependent not on linear context but on prosodic context. There have been several attempts to link coarticulatory resistance to prosody, but the most comprehensive study so far has been Cho's (2002). Here we find an attempt to explain much coarticulatory resistance in terms of the prosodic environment, in his terminology 'prosodically-driven coarticulatory resistance'.

Few contemporary researchers have gone so far as to place all coarticulatory effects in a prosodic hierarchy in the way developed in TM. But it is clear that much of the detail of coarticulation is directly linked to an utterance's prosodic structure – including, and perhaps especially, the detail which is due to expressive content.

The prosodic dominance of coarticulatory resistance seen as itself a time-governed whole-utterance variable gives valuable insights into the way coarticulation effects seem to vary as prosody unfolds. But at the same time the nature of the class and individual identity of segments within the prosody also provides us with important insights about coarticulatory resistance. For example we can see that the *rallentando* toward the end of major prosodic domains promotes a progressive reduction in coarticulatory effect, but that some classes of segment are more likely to be affected than others (Cho 2002). As an example of expressive effects we can see that the somatic tensioning associated with anger promotes an increased rate of utterance with, at the same time and (perhaps for researchers in coarticulation theory, a counter-intuitive) *decrease* in coarticulation. Some speakers experiencing these biological effects during irritation or anger may well additionally increase the duration, precision, and acoustic amplitude of voiceless plosives and sibilants in general: *He hissed his anger at me!*

As we have pointed out elsewhere, simply using empirical observation of instances of this kind of effect does not guarantee a complete generalisation either across a language or across human speech in general – accuracy would only come if all possible occurrences (which is impossible) had been observed and measured. The alternative is to examine the mechanism on which the effect depends, and using theory *distinct* from linguistics or phonetics, predict its properties and hence all possible constraints. This approach rests on the idea that the constraints are externally derived (that is, do not have a linguistic origin), and that the external constraints operate truly irrespective of linguistic context. From our point of view it is important to decouple linguistic constraint and selection from properties of the mechanism which derive from sources external to linguistics. It is in this way that we try to ensure *explanatory adequacy* for our approach.

We can propose some modifications to the window concept:

- what Keating calls 'a window' might be in fact be better modelled as a *collection* of windows, where part of putting an utterance together is to select an appropriate window from a set; there is also the possibility of a whole cline of windows in some kind of continuously variable arrangement;
- the width of a window might be better modelled as *variable* – that is, the maximum and minimum settings might be alterable for particular utterances – say, for a particular tone of voice, or a particular rate of utterance delivery;
- the distribution of values across a window should be specified – perhaps for any one utterance, or expression, or style, etc.; the distribution is probably not normal: that is, it is probably skewed, and this might be important.

For a dynamic model, the window needs expressing *parametrically*, and the window's individual parameters need to be specified and set. If they are to be set, then the *conditions* for this or that setting need to be specified, and the setting *limits* need to be specified.

Cho has proposed that window width signals how resistant a segment is to coarticulation. But initially this could only mean for the *basic intrinsic target specification* of a segment. The questions which need now to be addressed are

1. What is the *mechanism for altering window width?* – that is, changing the segment's original resistance/vulnerability setting. The point is that resistance seems to vary.
2. What are the *rules which govern altering window width*? – that is, the basis of the decisions to invoke the width altering mechanism.

We feel that perhaps a useful way of putting these points together in Keating's model might be to characterise the window in terms of a set of parameters, for example

- width – a quantifiable variable for constraining the extent to which this segment 'succumbs' to coarticulation; a vector able to express a range from *maximum resistance* (maximum precision) through *'don't-care'*, to *enhancement* of coarticulation; the width indicates what we'd like to achieve in terms of coarticulation for this segment;
- maximum amplitude – a quantifiable variable indicating the maximum weight that can be put on the width variable: how much do we want to achieve the value given for the width parameter;
- minimum amplitude – as with maximum amplitude, the value here indicates the minimum weight that can be put on the width variable: the system will not work unless width has at least this weight;
- mean amplitude – indicates a longer term (links to adjacent segments) value for weighting how much the coarticulatory constraints are wanted – useful for expressive content;
- linearity – the 'amplitude' parameter is not constant over its width; that is, how much amplitude we can apply to the width parameter varies with where we are along the width vector; this is clearly non-linear with any one segment and can vary from segment to segment.

There are certainly other possibilities as well, but we have chosen here to indicate that windows have width which is quantifiable, reflecting perhaps

- both intrinsic (a property of the segment, irrespective of what the speaker wants) and extrinsic ('desired') resistance to coarticulation, and
- how critically the speaker regards constraining or enhancing coarticulation (width 'amplitude'), and in addition
- the linearity of the system's ability to influence this segment's role in the coarticulatory processes.

We offer these ideas to indicate possible enhancements to Keating's model: we have not ourselves worked through them in any detail. However, we do feel from our own work in Cognitive Phonetics that coarticulatory processes are for the most part universal and outside the domain of linguistics – this is covered by the window and its width, but that these processes are also differentially open to cognitively controlled constraint or enhancement: parameterising the windows and allowing some cognitive control over setting the parameter variables will enable Keating's model to be extended into the notions of *precision control* and *cognitive intervention*. Windows could more accurately reflect coarticulatory resistance (constraint) and 'aggression' (enhancement).

Coarticulatory resistance and aggression

There are three external factors which cause segmental rendering to appear to vary the hypothesised effect of coarticulation on phonetic targets: *contrast, coarticulatory resistance* and *coarticulatory aggression*. Resistance and aggression act as opposites. In TM we have used *constraint* and *enhancement*, where constraint results in a rendering result closer to the abstract target value, and enhancement results in a result further from the abstract target value. In Cognitive Phonetics constraint and enhancement exist on a single vector, and this could be the case, we believe, for the Keating model if the two are regarded as mutually exclusive (that is, you cannot have both played off against each other simultaneously). If necessary, the two could, in both models, be overlapping simultaneous parameters operating in much the same was as agonistic and antagonistic musculature works to stabilise movement.

- It might be interesting to consider whether in fact we can have both resistance and aggression simultaneously. The application of a constraint would arise from a cognitive decision to increase articulatory precision. This is where we have to bring in the idea of a parameterised target, where each parameter has multiple dimensions (according to the target list above). So, for example, it may be possible for a segment to be specified with increased precision of tongue position, but a 'don't-care' or relaxed precision for vocal cord vibration. This brings up yet another dimension. Tongue position precision is a spatial parameter, but precision of vocal cord vibration may involve a time element: *Keep the vocal cords vibrating throughout the segment*. Perhaps *each* has a time element: *Hold the tongue position tightly for at least 80% of the duration of the segment before relaxing to enable smooth transition to the next segment*. And so on; there are a great many permutations possible here.

Although we have argued above against the idea of *constant* width widows, it is an important aspect of Keating's original formulation of the model that window widths should be empirically determined on the basis of context, but are then kept as constants. That is, a set of contextual scores sequentially alter the value of a window until its maximum (and minimum) width(s) are set. This means that the data set must be quite exhaustive (a theoretical impossibility), or at least large and representative, though it is hard to see how we would determine the representative power of any piece of data, except perhaps on a statistical basis. Because 'all' possibilities are used to set up the window, then all possibilities are already covered in the window, and its *boundaries* become its focal point, rather than any points within it. That is, the empirically determined physical window now assumes an abstract status.

Revisions of the Window Model

Guenther's (1995) revision to the window model allows for the variation of articulatory positions dependent on various input factors both linguistic and extra-linguistic (such as utterance rate, 'stress', and so on) in origin. Keating (1996) agrees that this modification is useful because resizing enables her model to depart from the rather abstract exemplar output notion. If the resizing can be dynamic (not obvious in Guenther) then many sources of variability can be accommodated. As we have said, we reserve judgement on such a 'flat' approach, preferring a transparent tiered approach, with individual tiers reflecting contributions from different external domains. The tiered approach not only makes the model more transparent, but it enables ordering of the various influences to be established.

We assume that in the Keating model, the target specifications for utterances appear at the plan level – that is, at the entry point to the phonetic rendering process. It is suggested that this is the point where the window size is to be modified. What this means is that the original plan is thought of as being put together as an idealisation, because in principle *all* renderings are going to be modified from some norm or idealisation by some factor(s). The proposals are that the target should be modified at this point and then not modified subsequently. In sharp contrast, in TM we make provision for varying the rendering process itself, rather than the input plan. The plan remains constant and the Cognitive Phonetics Agent guides the rendering process in the light of, or 'wrapped' by, these external constraints. There are a number of reasons

88 Speech Production Theory

for taking entry points for the sources of variability into the rendering process itself, and variability can of course vary sometimes on a global, sometimes on a local, and sometimes on a continuous basis.

Guenther proposes fixed modifications to the window to reduce the range to some active area. But there is a problem with this: the kind of variability we can observe for both expression (Guenther) and prosodics (Cho) is variable! This is a principal reason why in TM the wrapper *is* a message to the CPA, *within which* the plan is to be rendered. The CPA is sensitive to varying external requirements and knows how to adjust speech production (that is, the rendering of plans) on a continuous, supervised basis, which can take account of this variability.

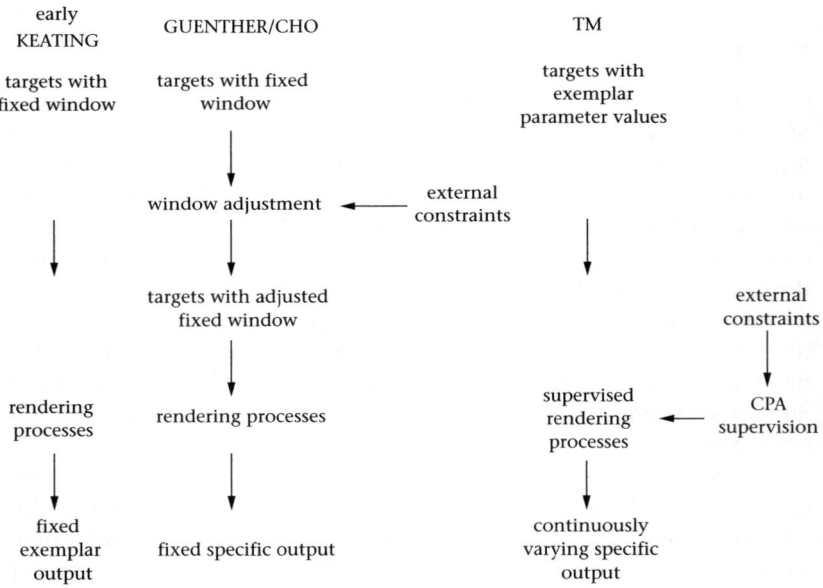

The diagram compares the three models: basic Keating, Guenther/Cho and TM. All begin with targets. Keating's model does not allow for externally derived constraints such as prosody or expression, whereas the other two do. The Guenther/Cho solution is to modify the parameters of the window which indexes the planned segment targets in line with the incoming constraints: this produces an output varied from Keating's exemplar or generic output, but still fixed. TM leaves the target specification unaltered, but varies its rendering by allowing the Cognitive Phonetics agent, sensitive to the externally derived constraints, to supervise the rendering process itself. The result is a *continuously varying* output.

One problem here is that the basic window model is in principle *segment* bound. But we may well want a *group* of segments to have their windows varied in a linked way, and perhaps on a continuously variable basis. The group of segments may well be internally structured (for example, a phonological syllable or a syntactic sentence or a semantic 'paragraph'). Graduated or controlled supervision of the rendering processes seems a good way to do this, particularly as the supervisor is needed for other purposes too. In the TM model the rendering process *cannot* proceed automatically; it is *always* a supervised process – even if the supervision gets sometimes set to zero or 'don't-care'. Multiple channels feed the supervision process: prosodic, expressive, general pragmatic, etc.

We have devoted much space to the Keating model because it incorporates a number of important features. It is potentially dynamic and computational since it is structured in such a way that it can be 'run' in both a static mode (producing exemplar output) and a dynamic mode (producing genuine output instantiations). In principle the entire model is computational and therefore potentially eminently explicit, predictive and testable.

Coarticulatory resistance

There are several early sources for the idea of coarticulatory resistance, based on the observation that sometimes segments seem to resist coarticulation where we might expect it ordinarily to occur. Sometimes the resistance is almost complete, sometimes it is partial. The Holmes computational model (Holmes *et al.* 1964, Holmes 1988) introduces weightings on segments based on their articulatory or linguistic classes (vowel *vs.* fricative, *vs.* plosive, etc.). Coming just one year after Lindblom's (1963) characterisation of the coarticulatory phenomenon, Holmes' insight provides for segment weightings which are indices giving the level of resistance a segment has to coarticulation. In principle these weightings can be varied to respond to calls for resistance. It should be noted that in the majority of models the operation of coarticulation resistance is on a linear contextual basis – that is, the resistance itself and its description in speech production theory is seen as heavily dependent on linear context. The Holmes model is archetypal in this respect.

Tatham (1969 and 1971) introduces the notion that coarticulatory effects are able to be constrained depending on a number of different contexts (see also Tatham and Morton 2004, 2005). This early model is hierarchical rather than linear, and allows not just for coarticulatory resistance but also coarticulatory *enhancement* to explain the frequent observation that both occur. This approach invokes the notion of *cognitive intervention* in biological processes as the *mechanism* for constraint.

Bladon and Al-Bamerni (1976) develop the idea using the notion of inhibition, with 'coarticulation resistance' becoming an index on segments inhibiting the spread of coarticulation in either direction: both LR and RL. The idea of the index is the same as that in Holmes, but for Holmes the index is segment-target focussed, whereas for Bladon and Al-Bamerni the index is context focussed. In Holmes the index is about the segment's resistance, but in Bladon and Al-Bamerni the index is as much about the segment's spreading influence on adjacent segments. The input to their model takes the form of a phonological binary target featural representation, but allows for *scalar* coarticulatory resistance, during phonetic rendering. Most theorists in the area of coarticulation have a phonological-style input representation which either is or becomes the phonetic target from which is derived a scalar output.

Bladon and Al-Barnerni's model incorporates a number of points:

- all *coarticulation* is characterised by *phonological* processes – this is a rather fundamental conceptualisation error;
- assimilatory rules are the basis of coarticulation – another fundamental error because it attempts to conflate into a single domain both the voluntary (assimilatory, cognitive) aspect of coarticulation with its involuntary (coarticulatory, physical) basis; the *origin* of coarticulation is assuredly *not* cognitive;
- assignment rules provide each 'allophone' target with a coarticulatory resistance coefficient or target;
- subsequently the segment's general coarticulation resistance is *transferred* to each boundary condition – this is to cover the notion of coarticulatory spreading and resistance to the phenomenon.

In general the idea of coarticulatory resistance focuses on a segment's articulatory class – resistance being greatest when the area of contact between the tongue and palate is large (Farnetani and Recasens 1999). This is not generally explained other than in terms of the area of contact, but it may, of course, be down not to the *area* but to the *force* exerted (in turn at least partially responsible for the area).

- Note that the domain of resistance can be very local – featural or segmental, local – syllabic or phrasal, or more global – sentential or wider. An example of global resistance might come from expressive content: in angry speech or precise speech the degree of coarticulation is reduced, because, in our view, these modes introduce an extra degree of tenseness which might be manifest in greater force of contact between articulators (for example in plosives) – resulting in minimising the tendency to coarticulate. In fact deliberately precise speech might be characterised by increased tension, designed to *stabilise* the system response to the ideal target values for any particular segment. In the example of angry speech the reduction in coarticulation is *somatic* in origin, but in the case of over-precision the reduction is *cognitive* in origin.

Co-production theories

Theories of co-production, embedded originally in Fowler's (1980) Action Theory, emphasise the articulatory overlap of segments. The action required for a segment S initiates before the conclusion of segment $S-1$, which itself ends less precisely than might be predicted from a simplistic concatenated segment model in the manner of Classical Phonetics or implied in some contemporary accounts of phonology. In effect, the original idea emphasised the way in which *articulatory parameters* spread their actions on either side beyond the resultant *acoustic signal*. Thus the lip rounding associated with [u] in the English sequence [ku] can begin even before the stop phase of the plosive, though its contribution to the utterance is not apparent until much later in the acoustic signal – where, in fact, it becomes periodic in nature (correlating with the 'onset' of the linguistic vowel).

Co-production theories enhance coarticulation theories rather than detract from them. The enhancement takes the form of providing a specific explanation of the otherwise rather vague reference to the effects of articulator inertia. Because of parameter overlapping, *segments* at the output level may appear to have changed, but have only done so because of the interactional effects of the underlying co-production overlaps. Thus the controllable rendering process has not, of itself, altered the output: the effect is a by-product of the way the system works rather than of any underlying target specification. In the TM model we explicitly allow for the effects of the overlap to be enhanced or constrained differentially as part of the supervised rendering process. In Fowler's original model there is no explicit review of how co-production can be productive linguistically; implicitly there could be the means of adjusting the overlap, and therefore its acoustic effects.

Coarticulation *vs.* co-production

Coarticulation theories inherit their viewpoint from Classical Phonetics and its derivatives – a descriptive perspective based essentially on perceived data. Coarticulationists attempt to add explanation to Classical Phonetics by firstly giving the model a dynamic speech production perspective and secondly trying to explain the processes involved in matching the underlying discrete segment 'input' with the smooth non-discrete output. The diagram shows the classic 'black box' approach taken:

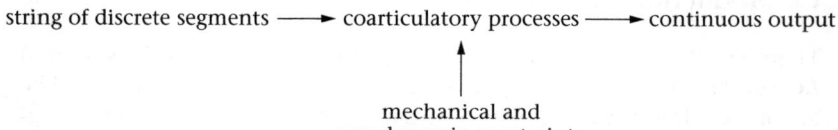

The basic model is properly explanatory in that the constraints on the coarticulatory processes are external to linguistics/phonetics, and to that extent is a useful advance on Classical Phonetics. The most serious theoretical problem with the model is that it attempts to apply physical processes to underlying *abstract* objects. Coarticulation theorists attempted to patch the model by introducing articulatory (or sometimes acoustic) targets at the critical point:

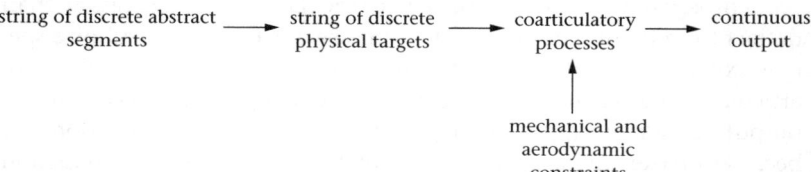

In fact, all this does is push the abstract/physical mismatch problem one stage up in the hierarchy. In practice, even the targets themselves have to be abstract representations of physical objects because they have to be based on generalisations. How precisely abstract phonological objects get converted to physical phonetic objects is rarely mentioned. Fowler's Action Theory is an attempt to tackle this problem, effectively ascribing much of the earlier phonology to dynamic physical processes.

It so happens that gestures – dynamic complexes of motor parameters – have onsets and offsets which *must* overlap in order to achieve acoustic simultaneity for a segment (in segmentally based models) because this is the way the system has to work. Take a simplistic example: for a 'heavy' articulator to arrive at its destination simultaneously with the arrival of a 'light' articulator at *its* destination, the heavy one must begin its movement earlier. The linguistically relevant acoustic signal starts when both reach their destinations. It is easy to imagine that with so many articulators of varying mass and their underlying musculature involved, overlap of parameter movement is going to be the rule rather than the exception. Hard-to-move articulators or muscle groups will cause gestural spreading away from any underlying abstract 'simultaneity' rather more than less hard-to-move articulators. This is the basis of co-production theory. We will see later when we consider perception (Chapter 7) that listeners 're-discover' the underlying simultaneity: how they do this is one of the main areas of perceptual theory.

Thus, for example, we might predict that tongue-root gestures would spread more than tongue-tip gestures because of the greater mass and greater inertia involved with the tongue-root. But we do not *know* this to be the case: it is an empirical question. There has been inconclusive work in this area and quite insufficient to make any authoritative statement yet: the problem is the extreme difficulty in collecting large quantities of appropriate data.

This explanation of observed coarticulation does not imply a cognitively determined option. Co-production of gestures underlying observed surface coarticulatory effects continues to explain those effects in terms of the intrinsic workings of the articulatory mechanism – not in terms of the way it is *linguistically* controlled. Whatever the linguistics – the underlying phonology and its utterance plans – the actual production of a soundwave has to proceed in a particular way. The motor control system constrains how the acoustic signal will turn out. The obvious question now is to what extent these constraints can be influenced.

We need to be careful in attempting to say what is deliberate and what is not when it comes to speech production and the characteristics of the waveform. We know that segments and their combinations in to syllables have 'psychological reality', they are units that speakers and listeners can report on and discuss. So we can say that it makes sense to say that speakers attempt simultaneity of articulation because they know that simultaneity will make sense to listeners. But we also know that there is parameter overlap in the actual physical process, and we know *why* there is parameter overlap. What we should not conclude is that we *cause* parameter overlap because we know speakers can use this to detect simultaneity. Coarticulation, however produced, is *tolerated* by speaker linguistics rather than caused by it; we are able to tolerate it because the perceptual system can deal with it. Speech is about getting across an acoustically encoded message using the available means.

In general it is best to think of assimilatory processes as changing the segmental specification *before* the finalisation of the utterance plan toward the end of a production (rather than descriptive) phonology, whereas co-production processes occur *after* the finalisation of the plan.

Just as segments can assume different status in different languages, so can processes. For example Metropolitan French has only 'clear' [l] as a rendering of a single underlying phonological /l/. However, English has both the clear /l/ and the 'dark' /l/ – as required extrinsic allophones. But Russian uses the clear and dark /l/s to contrast morphemes – a example of status raising or promotion. This is an example of segments fulfilling different functions in different languages, but the same goes for processes. So, the aerodynamic inertial process which causes delayed onset of vocal cord vibration in vowels following plosive release is 'used' contrastively in English to distinguish between phonologically [±voice] stops: in *pat* [pʰæt] *vs. bat* [bæt] the acoustic distinction is only on the delayed periodic waveform. This is illustrated in Figure 3.7A. We have to be cautious about the term 'used', though. This does not mean that the delay itself is deliberate: it means that, given that we have it, it can be used to signal contrast. Notice that in Metropolitan French (though not in most Canadian speakers) and other languages the p/b contrast is not signalled this way (Figure 3.7B). In French the underlying [+voice] segment is rendered with pre-release vocal cord vibration, and the underlying [−voice] segment similarly to the /b/ in English. In TM the co-production process has been interfered with (not caused) by cognitively controlled intervention.

So, although it is unlikely that co-production and other coarticulatory processes are deliberately controlled, it is possible to predict that overlap will occur and what its results will be – thus permitting the possibility of deliberately attempting to constrain or enhance the effect. This is Cognitive Phonetics.

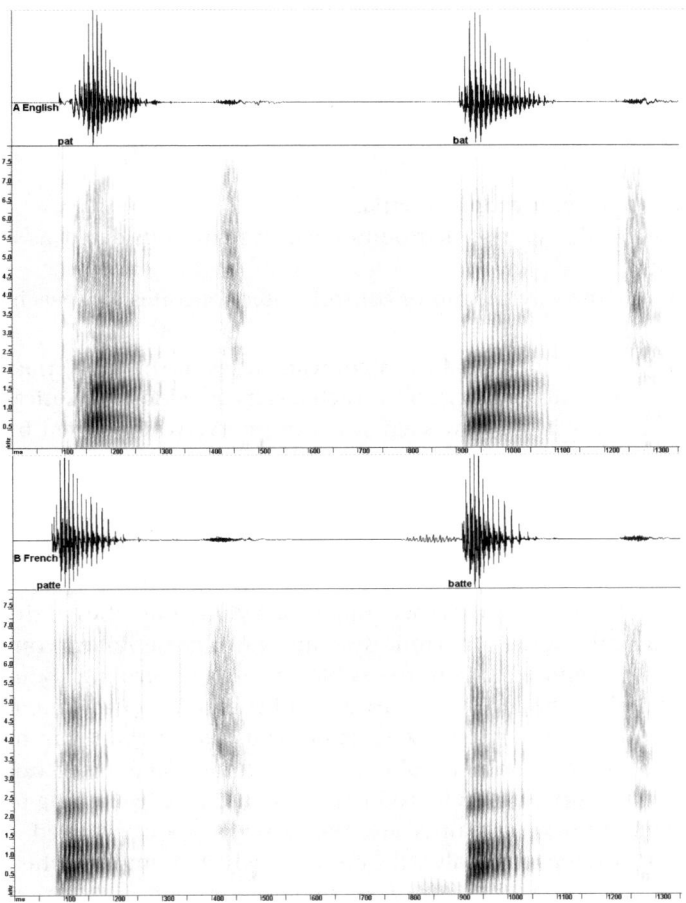

Figure 3.7 Waveforms and spectrograms of (A) English *pat, bat* and (B) French *patte, batte*. Notice the delay in vocal cord vibration onset following the release of [p] in *pat*, and the 'pre-voicing' preceding the [b] in *batte*.

Sources of intrinsic variation

Intrinsic allophonic variations – those that result from co-production and other coarticulatory effects correlate with

- the immediate phonetic context – as specified in the utterance plan;
- global utterance rate – the speed of the entire utterance, taken on average;

- local utterance rate – the speed of parts of the utterance which depart from the global rate.

Underlying these variations on the surface there are a number of constraints we can identify as

- mechanical and aerodynamic inertia,
- limiting properties of the neuro-muscular system considered as a mechanism,
- constraints on the way the motor control system operates for speech.

We have traditionally identified the significant parts of the vocal tract from the speech production viewpoint. Each has its own bio-mechanical properties which constrain how such structures move when driven by their internal (structures like the tongue, lips, etc.) or external (bony structures like the jaw, etc.) musculature.

We can think of a body's inertial properties as an index of how it resists acceleration or deceleration. What makes the situation so complex with speech is that articulatory structures are not mechanically independent. When the vocal tract is used linguistically the properties of the motor, mechanical and aerodynamic systems will impose linked constraints on what is and what is not possible. What is interesting about this situation is that the combined processes of speech production and perception are able to tolerate these constraints up to a certain threshold. Obviously if no constraints could be tolerated the system could not be used, but the theory of speech production should have something to say about what these constraints are and *how* they are tolerated – explaining how the system deals with errors which they impose when 'overdriven'. We shall see that one of the major assisting factors here is the collaboration which exists between the production and perception systems (Chapter 8): they each know about the constraints imposed, and can conceptually, if not actually, reverse them. Thus coarticulatory processes in rapid speech which may totally 'obliterate' a segment from the soundwave, often do not phase the perceptual system's ability to repair the error.

Inter-segment coarticulatory influence

Despite Öhman's early hierarchical model of coarticulatory influence, one or two researchers have attempted a more linear model trying to establish which types of segment are more likely to influence their neighbours.

Several researchers have come up with the following observations, or variants of these:

- vowels influence consonants more than consonants influence vowels,
- consonants influence consonants as much as vowels do.

This implies that coarticulatory influence spreads out from the syllable nucleus. The difficulty is answering the question: How could a mechanical system know about syllable nuclei? What the system might know about is that there are different types of control demands to be made on the system. And *we* know that these correlate with linguistic phenomena.

The syllable nucleus is, of course, a phonological vowel or something vowel-like. In phonology there is a sense in which syllabic nuclei are dominant: there is no such thing as a syllable without one, for example, and consequently if a syllable has just one element this must be a vowel. These are things which speakers know about how their phonology works. With vowels in such a dominant position it is unlikely that they will allow themselves to be influenced more than they influence their surrounding consonants – the anthropomorphic argument. Öhman, of course, has it round the other way: the control mechanism of speech is such that it works with some carrier mechanism which can tolerate spot interruptions. The carrier mechanism has been adopted by the linguistic system to provide what a linguist would describe as a sequence of vowels, and the spot interruptions as various consonants.

Taking a linguistic focus, therefore, on this physical world, we could observe that the *results* of coarticulation appear to *correlate* with the (C)V(C) structure of syllables – this structure does not *cause* the physical results! And we might hypothesise an explanation in the terms used above – the linguistics adapts to whatever mechanism it has available for its message encoding. Let us give an easy example of this: We would predict from the empirical observations available about consonant-vowel coarticulatory interaction that the effects (whatever their source) spread out from a syllable's vowel nucleus to its surrounding consonants. So we can hypothesise that in an initial CC the effect would probably be RL and that in a final CC the effect would be LR. It might be possible to say in phonological terms that the direction of influence accords with the sonority rule (Spencer 1996) in the makeup of phonological syllables. The sonority rule predicts an increase in sonority in consonants in syllable onsets and a decrease in sonority in consonants in syllable codas, though there are times when the rule is violated. It might be the case that the spread of coarticulation is out from the syllable vowel nucleus, deceasing in line with decreasing sonority. Clearly, to support or refute the prediction experiments focussing on inter-segmental influence would need to be carefully conducted.

4
Speech Motor Control

Introduction

Writing about general phonetic theory Laver (1994, p. 95) believes that success will show in 'the ability to describe and explain ... the *phonetic basis* [our italics] for the differentiation of words and other linguistic units in every known human language'. Differentiating words this way is actually a *phonological* task, but this could importantly be elaborated in terms of the phonetics. The way we would elaborate the task is to develop the idea that phonological inventories have to have a basis in available, differentiable phonetic sounds. There are important considerations, like the prediction that if you have [i] and [ɪ] in a language you cannot also have [e] (the sound in French *été*), though you can have [ɛ] as in English *bet*, and so on. So the basis is not just the inventory but its accompanying constraints. These constraints may not just be production constraints: the role of perceptual discrimination in forming what is possible in language in general, and in any particular language is also very important. It is hard to imagine a general phonetic theory that is not about both production and perception and how they relate to each other.

The argument about how sounds must be able to be made reliably different and perceptually discriminable holds not just for different languages, of course, but also between accents within a single language. Accents are particularly interesting because of the way in which they are usually mutually intelligible – which is what we would expect given their common underlying origin. This origin is perhaps best modelled as an accent free pronunciation (phonology and phonetics) which does not exist in any speaker, but which forms the highest node in the hierarchy relating accents. The general form of this tree is

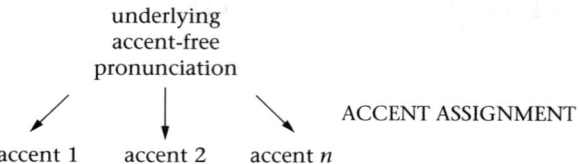

The diagram is overly simple because it does not include an account of the phonological and phonetic derivations; the idea is simply to show how accents relate to each other *via* a common underlying pronunciation. The hierarchical arrangement goes toward accounting for mutual intelligibility and provides a means of relating accents without introducing spurious notions such as 'continua' of accents.

Two dimensions to speech production theory

There are two dimensions to our understanding of speech production, and these can be expressed in the form of questions:

1. The mechanism focussed dimension asks, among other things:
   a. What are the *general properties* of the speech production mechanism?
   b. How are the acoustic, aerodynamic, neuro-physiological (motor) and cognitive aspects of the mechanism to be modelled in as much as they underlie the acoustic signals *perceived* to be speech?
   c. What does the mechanism, and the way it works, *offer* for the purposes of linguistically-based communication?
   d. What are the *constraints* at all levels on what the mechanism can offer?
2. The linguistics focussed dimension asks, among other things:
   a. What *use* does the human linguistic communication system make of the available mechanisms for producing an appropriate acoustic signal?
   b. To what extent is the *linguistics* constrained by the design or use of that mechanism?

These questions can be refined in a number of ways and are fundamental to understanding how the mechanism of speech interacts with the demands of the linguistics of speech. Clearly speech production, as a linguistic phenomenon, cannot make impossible demands on the mechanism, but the interaction between the two, and the constraints are by no means obvious. For example, 1a. is about the way the mechanism is constrained in what it can offer the linguistics, and 2b. is about the way the mechanism, whatever it can offer, constrains the linguistic potential.

The purpose of phonetic descriptions

Many researchers have seen a major purpose of phonetics research in describing the sounds of the world's languages, sub-divided of course into the sounds in particular languages. From this it is possible to spot some basic patterning, often observing for example overlap in segment inventories between languages. Statistically based observations about the distribution of sounds among languages, to identify language families and so on, are then possible. A more demanding pursuit with the same goal, from our more synthesis-oriented approach rather than analytic point of view, would be the development of ideas about what *could* be a sound in a language, and what could not. Perhaps a notion of *preference* and *constraint* on the occurrence of sounds would be as productive as observations about distribution – since the next obvious stage in the investigation of the sounds of languages is to try to explain *why* the sounds are what they are and *why* they distribute in the particular ways they do, assuming they do not do so randomly.

So, beginning with the description,

- what exactly is it that we want to describe?
- what exactly will be our method of representation?
- and how exactly will the representation be derived?

Continuing with the representation:

- what will the representation itself 'mean'?
- will it have a meaning which extends beyond the observations it is based on?

We shall see that how we represent the objects of our observations and how they relate to each other acquires its own meaning as the theory is developed. That meaning, of course, hinges on the purpose of our theory – it is about what we want our theory to inform of us of. So, to take one or two simple examples, we might characterise sounds in terms of some feature matrix and this would enable us to spot classes of sounds defined by common features and perhaps common behaviour expressed in general as, for instance: 'All members of this particular set of sounds share these five features and behave in this way when they occur in this or that point in the phonological hierarchy'. The choice of representation has cast light on the meaning of the behaviour of particular segments. Another example might be the wrapper representational concept to which we return repeatedly. Wrapping utterances in a succession of hierarchically organised 'concepts' (for example 'expression' or 'prosody') draws out a specific meaning assigned to the hierarchy: the hierarchy itself means that specific types of phenomena can occur in speech and be related in illuminating ways.

If our concern is with the language or accent *per se* we need a description which does not reflect any idiosyncrasies of any one speaker. The problem is how we define what is to be included – perhaps what is used generally by the language community, and what is to be excluded – perhaps what is used only by a subset of the language community and which has no linguistic significance. We shall need to ask how large a group of speakers has to be before what this group does actually becomes of general phonetic interest for the language or dialect. The problem could be put the other way round: we could decide what is of phonetic interest – say, a particular variant – without mention initially of the size of the group which uses it. Another problem here is that the usage may not be entirely consistent in the sense, not that it is not itself patterned, but in the sense that it is optional *within* a pattern.

Thus, for example, some speakers of English regularly fail in certain phonological environments to release word- or syllable- final plosives. When they do *not* do this the result may be random or its patterning may be conditioned by a-linguistic factors. It might be argued that unreleased plosives have no significant role in English, though several millions of speakers may well use them. It is not a question of the fineness of the transcription either. The question is usually resolved on an individual *ad hoc* basis, whereas using some notion of fineness would involve setting a threshold which applied across the board.

This is a real problem. Clearly the speech organs vary between people and inevitably this must result in variations to the soundwave. The aim is to determine what is significant linguistically, and this needs careful definition. For example, *extrinsic* allophones (Chapter 3) may be deemed to be significant, but *intrinsic* allophones deemed to be insignificant, though occasionally we may want to draw attention to what an individual speaker is doing even if there is no linguistic significance; this will happen in the case of pathological pronunciation, for example.

Description and classification

Most descriptivists would agree that at a phonological level we are concerned with classification, contrast and opposition: purely linguistic dimensions of speech production. But it is not just phonological oppositions which need handling in the phonology; sometimes phonology needs to draw out processes which add some nuance to a sound – producing a planned extrinsic allophone for phonetic rendering, but which may have little contrastive content.

Contemporary phonology goes beyond early ideas about classification; and for us it is at least about characterising and explaining the processes involved in generating utterance plans. Earlier, phoneticians examining the 'functional phonology' of the sounds and articulations they were describing tended to equate classification with identifying phonemes, seen originally as abstract labels on groupings of sound variants and later as highly abstract objects underlying the entire phonological structure or system of a language. It is easy to see why when feature systems were introduced into phonology their 'values' at this classificatory or contrast-centred level might reflect 'discrete terms', if not necessarily being fully binary.

Several phoneticians of the 1960s were clear that they wanted what they called 'continuous' feature values in *phonetic* descriptions. Of course, continuous is a special case of discrete; it describes an infinite number of points infinitely close together. But this is perhaps not what they meant. Somehow these phoneticians wanted, quite properly, to emphasise that phonetics as a rendering process is intrinsically continuous in nature and produces a truly analog and 'shaded' acoustic signal, but to emphasise also that phonology is not continuous and has no intention of accounting for these shadings while they are linguistically insignificant – in their terms, of course. The awkwardness of the exchanges between phonologists and phoneticians on the subject then, as even now in some quarters, barely hides a paradigm shift in the discipline from *descriptive and analytical* to *explanatory and synthetic*, from simply describing *what* people say to full-scale modelling of *how and why* they say it.

We quote from Ladefoged (1993), who tries to reconcile the positions by saying what a synthesising rather than descriptive phonology would be like:

> A complete description of the sound pattern of a language would be one that took an abstract representation in which features are used to classify sounds, applied all the phonological rules, and then showed

how the output of the phonology could be used to produce speech. (p. 271)

This is the paradigm shift. Phonology would be about characterising that part of a speech production model which accounts for cognitively sourced processes which derive ultimately the abstract plan on which phonetic rendering is based. Phonetic rendering is the process which takes the utterance plan and turns it into articulation and sound. At last we have a truly *hierarchical* approach to modelling speech – as speech production with a cognitive phase which is logically prior to a distinct physical phase, each a sub-hierarchy contributing to speech production.

Ladefoged is clearly pointing toward a model which

- has phonology as logically, if not temporally, prior to phonetics,
- is comprehensively generative in nature, involving a phonological explanation for phonetic observations,
- allows in principle for phonetic explanation of many prior phonological processes.

Classical Phonetics included none of these. The phonetic explanation of some phonological process was just possible, but only really intended after the fact because some phonologists saw the need to discuss approaches such as natural phonology (Stampe 1979) in which phonological processes were rated according to how well they accorded with phonetic and other expectations. In as much as a model in some sense is the exemplification of some aspect of a theory, any speech production model formally constructed hierarchically and with a view to meeting the condition of explanatory adequacy marks a commitment to a theory of speech production which might *include* the surface descriptions of Classical Phonetics, but which truly transcends this early approach.

Speech production models

Early speech production models were far from explicit. Öhman's numerical model of coarticulation (Öhman 1966, 1967) points the way along with a number of other papers on details of coarticulation and data analysis of the period. The beginning of speech technology around this time also forces the introduction of true computational modelling – an innovation in phonetics which thus joins computational linguistics in wanting to produce more explicit accounts of the discipline. The best and most open speech synthesis model of the time was, in our opinion, that produced by Holmes (Holmes *et al.* 1964) because it explicitly builds in as much as possible of the phonetics of the time making along the way its own contribution to phonetic theory: in the area of coarticulation modelling, for example (Chapter 2). Unfortunately the phonetics model available was limited in scope to the Classical Phonetics approach. One further notable contribution to the paradigm shift was the work by Kim (1966) whose synthesis model foreshadowed later approaches to computational modelling in phonetics.

Levels of abstraction

Cognitive processing is an integral part of speech production; but which aspects of speech are cognitive and which are physical? Speech segments are sometimes said to have a certain *status*. In the Classical Phonetics tradition the term might be used to refer to the notion of phonemes *vs.* allophones. Allophones are variants of phonemes and were regarded as systematically different ways of pronouncing sounds belonging to the same phoneme. Phonemes are abstract concepts, not actual sounds.

However, segments can have four levels of status, not just two. Besides the phoneme level there are two distinct levels of allophone. A sound variant can have

1. *no significance* – it is a randomly occurring variant;
2. *phonetic significance* – it is systematic, does not necessarily contribute to the identification of morphemes, is derived usually physically within the phonetics;
3. *surface phonological significance* – it is systematic, but does not necessarily contribute to the identification of morphemes, and is derived cognitively within the phonology;
4. *underlying phonological significance* – it contributes to the identification of morphemes.

In an explanatory speech production model the objects at level 2 are intrinsic allophonic, whereas at level 3 they are extrinsic allophonic. Phonemes (or underlying segments which are 'merely' classificatory) exist at level 4. Levels 3 and 4, being phonological are abstract and cognitive. Each level has a different degree of abstraction, with level 1 being the least abstract and level 4 being the most abstract. We need this concept of levels and status to explain systematic use of status change in languages and accents (Chapter 2). Briefly, different languages will identify sounds at different levels; so the status of sounds (intrinsic allophonic, extrinsic allophonic or extreme classificatory) can vary between languages.

Duration – timing

The concept 'duration' presents a difficulty for some phoneticians (for example Laver 1994, p. 431) when they try to equate the timing of a physical event with a linguistic abstraction of that event. Typically attempts to discover the start and end points of phonological units fail because there is no one-to-one correlation between such abstract units and any physical units. The rendering process which equates utterance plans with acoustic signals is itself non-linear and parametric, with the physical parameters often asynchronous. Thus attempting to locate the beginning of an abstract segment among a number of parameters starting at different points in time is absurd. Fowler (1980) made much of this point in accounting for co-production (Chapter 3).

Articulatory Control

The static anatomical model which forms part of Classical Phonetics describes where the articulators might be positioned to produce a segment. Nothing is said about how the articulatory configurations of the vocal tract are achieved, and nothing about the mechanism or functioning of any control system for articulator movement.

- We can see by examining the phonological feature labels in Distinctive Feature Theory, for example, how often one discipline or part of a discipline can lag another. Thus, even in *The Sound Pattern of English* Chomsky and Halle (1968) base their feature set partly on this early anatomical model, although both theoretical and experimental phonetics had already progressed to a more dynamic control model. In fact, in phonology up to comparatively recent times we find little to reflect the progress in phonetics. And the reverse is also true: too much of contemporary phonetics fails to take into account the considerable developments in phonology since *Sound Pattern*.

In terms of the post-Classical approach to speech production theory *movement* becomes the centre of focus: there is a shift from modelling the static properties of articulation to a more dynamic approach involving *time*. The articulators move – indeed x-ray videos and other modern imaging techniques seem to present a picture of almost *continuous* movement, especially of articulators like the tongue and jaw which are involved in almost every 'segment'. We must begin though by being very careful: we may observe visually (perhaps with the help of those *x*-rays or other experimental techniques) movement of, say, the tongue, but in fact the tongue is the name given to an anatomical organ the movement and shape of which are not *directly* under control. Beneath the surface of the tongue and other articulators lies a complex musculature, and it is this which is controlled to produce movement and shape.

Even the contraction or tensing of a single muscle is more complex than it might appear visually. A muscle consists of a sheath or outer covering beneath which are hundreds of individual muscle fibres. It is these which are ultimately under innervatory control from the brain's motor cortex. Muscle fibres are *recruited* to participate in the overall muscle contraction.

Models of speech production

Speech production can be modelled from different angles. Thus a model based on, say, the distinctive features of the Prague School and later the generative phonologists would approach areas of speech production from a strictly *linguistic* direction. The Haskins Labs based proposals put forward by Liberman *et al.* (1967) developing a model which envisages rules for transforming cascades of strings from phonemic representations all the way down to the acoustic signal is also predominantly linguistically oriented. But there are also models based in *acoustics*, *biology* or *psychology* which tend to address different areas of speech production rather than the entire subject area. Thus Fant's (1960) Acoustic Model of Speech Production addresses the development of the acoustic signal in speech, with considerable detail of the source/filter model, but with very little attention to linguistics. Biological models have addressed the effects of biological status on speech prosody and segmental rendering, as have psychological models, with the latter in particular dealing with speech perception – often built on a biological or acoustic appraisal of speech hearing.

The Liberman *et al.* model foreshadows the modern parametric approach. The starting point of speech production in this model is strings of phonemes which by processes 'above' speech constitute a highly abstract representation of the sound shape of some meaning to be conveyed by the speech. These are quickly transformed by a cascade of abstract phonological processes into a representation which these days we might refer to as the *utterance plan*. The conversion from this, effectively extrinsic allophonic, representation is not one-to-one and tries to account for the observed continuousness of the acoustic output by hypothesising that it is the parametric nature of the physical speech production process which accounts for apparent overlapping of segments. They are proposing something very similar in type to the later proposals of Fowler (1980) regarding the co-production of speech segments. The 'neuromotor commands' for individual segments are issued in such a way that they result in a kind of staggering of the muscular response, and it is this overlap of neuromotor commands which provides the explanation for the apparent overlap of segments at the acoustic level. Thus there are two non-linear processes at work:

- parallel issuing of neuromotor commands associated with 'whole' abstract sequential segments – the main innovation emphasised by Liberman, and
- parallel delivery of commands associated with the component parameters of the abstract sequenced segments – the main innovation picked up and developed by Fowler.

Serial ordering – the Lashley/MacNeilage legacy

Discussions of the serial ordering of speech first emerged with Lashley (1951), later picked up and developed by MacNeilage (1970) and others, continuing to the present time. Clearly speakers issue *motor commands;* the motor command is an abstract concept meaning significant or coherent sets of neural signals issued by the brain and ending up with the appropriate contraction of the speech musculature. But

1. it is not necessarily the case that these commands are issued in the order apparent in a left-to-right phonological characterisation of the utterance plan (using modern terminology);
2. it is not clear how the sequence, if it departs from the phonological sequence, is *controlled* or whether it becomes partially parallel rather than wholly serial;
3. it is not clear exactly how speakers might adjust motor commands to take account of the fact that the start point of articulator movement varies so considerably with phonological linear context.

The basic problems are

- how to model the fact that a serial representation somehow ends up with a parallel effect, or an effect best represented as parallel, and

- that it cannot logically be possible to completely specify a motor command in advance if the system does not know where an articulator is to move from – it may already have been where we now need it, or it may be a long way away in articulatory terms.

More graphically:

- How can we account for how the apparent invariance of the input to motor control turns into correct articulator movement whether the speaker is upright *or* standing on their head?
- How can there be anything akin to invariant motor control specifications in some 'motor control centre' under these conditions?

Speakers can even articulate perfectly when performing cartwheels – a feat which has to involve constant 'awareness' of the continuously varying angles of gravitational pull; for example, in one moment the tongue is falling 'down' and needs lifting, but in the next moment it is falling 'sideways' and in the next it is falling 'up' and needs pushing down, and so on.

The solution proposed by MacNeilage (1970) was to hypothesise that motor control is in terms of *spatial configurations* rather than in terms of the motor commands needed to achieve those configurations. The reason for the proposal is simple: the spatial configuration is more robust in specification than the sets of signals needed to achieve it.

The case for an *acoustic representation* could equally well be argued along the same lines. Today we might prefer (Chapter 7) a 'perceived acoustic representation' rather than a representation of the actual acoustic signal: this hypothesis takes into account that the speaker's goal is more likely to be the listener's perception of the signal rather than the signal itself.

MacNeilage's spatial targets need to be *internalised;* that is, they need to have been set up in advance. They are delivered serially as prescribed by the linguistics dominating them – in modern terms, the utterance plan. Short-term intramuscular feedback (the gamma reflex arc) probably provides the necessary adjustments to deal with the current state of the vocal tract mechanism. Note that longer-term feedback enabling a context sensitive adjustment of motor commands from segment to segment is not hypothesised as playing a role in MacNeilage's model – essentially an open loop model.

Lashley's approach to serial ordering

Lashley (1951) hypothesised that

- there are several independent sub-systems in speech production and these interact dynamically to produce the appropriate articulation;
- these sub-systems correspond to
  - the speaker's intention (which he called the 'determining tendency', the 'store of images and words'),
  - the motor organisation, and
  - a device responsible for temporal ordering.

The difficult point for phoneticians is Lashley's suggestion that temporal ordering itself is not inherent in the idea, the word, or the motor organisation – but that it is controlled and imposed. The temporal ordering device is a syntax, a device responsible for pulling objects together in a specific order. In his description it is responsible for word ordering, and hence, in a hierarchical arrangement, the ordering of motor actions. The model Lashley puts forward is an open loop model, though the systems within it are constantly interacting.

Ordering in Öhman's early model of coarticulation

Öhman's model (1966, 1967) hypothesises that 'phoneme' objects (our extrinsic allophones) have intrinsic properties as part of their *static* specification, properties which do not include information with respect to ordering. He hypothesises a *dynamic* treatment of phonemes to blend them in some way to achieve continuous speech. For Öhman temporal ordering is the result of movement from vowel to vowel, with consonants dropped onto this basic vowel continuum. Öhman's model does two things:

- it accounts for the coarticulatory effects he observed
- characterises a dual control mechanism, separate for vowels and consonants.

Öhman was focussed on explaining coarticulation, and perhaps for this reason he does not give a full account of how he expects the underlying ordering of vowels to be achieved, and is unclear about how consonants are dropped onto the correct place in the vowel continuum. As for most phoneticians the organisation of the segment sequence is simply given by the rules of the underlying phonology – a view which raises more questions than it answers.

Rhythm and temporal ordering

Researchers agree that rhythm is related to temporal ordering, but hypotheses vary as to the nature of the relationship. There are basically two possibilities:

- rhythm is controlled by a dominant agent, perhaps using some biological 'clock' to establish the relative timing of segments in rendering the utterance plan (Chapter 6); or
- rhythm is a surface observed phenomenon which is the product of the sequencing of phonetic objects, each with its own intrinsic timing (Klatt 1979).

Computational models of speech production tend to show that Klatt's approach results in an intolerable cumulative error in long phrases or sentences (Tatham and Morton 2005), and although differing in detail most researchers prefer the hypothesis that rhythm is independently generated (either biologically or cognitively, or by some cognitive interpretation of a biological clock). However, both approaches have difficulty in explaining the processes which result in the temporal 'telescoping' effect on unstressed syllables when they are surrounded by relatively regularly timed stressed syllables. Stressed syllables tend to occur at regular intervals, though the effect is usually thought to be more a *perceived* phenomenon with a less robust physical correlate.

Lashley's control mechanism

Lashley argues for a higher level control mechanism imposed on spatial motor movements. This is not dissimilar to our Cognitive Phonetics Agent which acts mainly as a supervisor overseeing the phonetic rendering process. Lashley suggests in effect a hierarchical structure for the model in which

- speech is not adequately characterised by a simple stimulus-response chain model;
- the overall organisation is hierarchical in structure;
- there is an overarching mechanism which controls the serial ordering of speech.

A timing mechanism external to the control system needs to be invoked also; the provision is for a biologically rooted clock to provide an independent reference for rhythm. Note, though, that the clock is not itself the source of the rhythm: rhythm is *patterned* timing, not timing itself. Note also that Lashley in effect denies the idea that a biological clock itself might be the source of a trigger moving from one speech segment to the next in an open loop fashion.

For Lashley all serially ordered movements (biological) or behaviours (cognitive) are organised within a hierarchical control system: in the case of language this is a *production syntax*, as opposed to the descriptive syntax of linguistics. Speech is organised temporally in much the same way as sentences are organised by a syntax.

TM (Chapter 6) takes this further. The exemplar sentences produced by a Chomskyan grammar are simultaneous, in the sense that all components (words) are produced together in a *descriptive* hierarchy, not in the serial order of a *production* hierarchy. When sentences are processed for speech they need to acquire an internal serial order. Following the assignment of production word order, the speech serial ordering is provided by the hierarchical structure of the speech production model, beginning with phonology, but organised within the wrapper architecture for subsequent rendering.

Action Theory

Speech production theories which support the layered model were criticised by the new Action Theory (Fowler 1980) on several grounds:

- speaking does not consist of the handing on of information for re-encoding layer after layer through the entire speech production process;
- the amount of information that would have to be added during such a translation or re-writing process is too great and too complex to be plausible;
- the neuro-physiological mechanism for action and how it functions in speaking has been misunderstood and wrongly modelled.

These claims form not just a weak departure from earlier established theory, but constitute the basis of a radically new way of looking at speech production. (For a critical review of Fowler's proposals see Lindblom and MacNeilage 1986.)

Action Theory suggests that information processing at the cognitive levels of phonology and early in the phonetics is not in terms of the detailed representations (for example bundles of distinctive features) we had been used to in linguistics. Much more it is a comparatively simple handling of broadly based labels (like spatial or acoustic targets) describing *gross* effects of articulation. One might imagine instructions like *Do vocal cord vibration!* or *Do vowel-ness!*. A characteristic of such instructions is that they lack detailed information about *how* to do the actions specified. Action Theorists would claim that this detailed information is itself contained in the way in which the articulatory system itself is structured in terms of its internal messaging system — so does not need to be specified as part of the higher level instruction. The mechanism itself 'knows' the detail of the processes it is involved in, in much the same way as the objects in the object-oriented programming paradigm incorporate the detail of the processes they are involved in – see Tatham and Morton (1988) which introduced object-oriented paradigm into the TM computational model of speech production explicitly for this reason, following precisely and acknowledging the arguments put forward earlier by Fowler and elaborated by other proponents of the approach (Saltzman and Munhall 1989).

The articulatory mechanism (that is, the whole neuro-physiology and anatomy of the system) is said to be arranged in structures. These are invoked in the theory as 'coordinative structures'. A coordinative structure is a grouping, say (though not necessarily always), of muscles which embodies well defined 'working relationships' between them. In some sense the muscles in a coordinative structure cooperate to fill out and perform the appropriate details of a gross instruction.

How this cooperation or coordination within the structure operates is described in the model by equations governing the working relationships between the component parts of the structure. Using the more usual terminology of computer modelling, we would say that a coordinative structure is *internally* programmed to behave in a particular way (hence our adoption of the object oriented paradigm for this part of the model). The component parts are not directly or independently controlled. Each operates in conjunction with its colleagues in a well defined way which can be described using an equation.

The speech control system *knows* that the appropriate detailed contractions, etc., will take place according to the local arrangements as defined by the equations governing the relationships between the structure's components. So it need only issue very gross instructions designed to do no more trigger the coordinative structure's own internal program.

Structures (along with their programmed *intra*-cooperative abilities) are recruited and marshalled by the system to execute the simple linguistic requirements, or perhaps, better, the requirements which we characterise in speech production terms, since there might be other details which are irrelevant to our model. In addition, structures are *nested:* that is, one structure may itself, together with other structures, form some super-coordinative structure.

Tuning

The individual components of a coordinative structure, including low level structures which form a super-structure, although standing in a well defined relationship to other components of the structure, are capable of having that relationship altered by a 'tuning process'. That is, the internal workings of a coordinative structure can be adjusted: their internal programs can be interfered with. However, because of the way in which any one component of the structure relates to all the others such tuning will result in some correlating adjustments made automatically among the remaining components of the system. That is, a coordinative structure, certainly in the TM model, is in principle self-organising. If one area of the structure is re-tuned the other areas will self-organise; it is a property of each local program contributing toward the behaviour of the structure that external interference is internally compensated. This does not mean that external interference, even benign tuning, is negated, it means that it is potentially optimally accommodated – leaving scope for the tuning signal itself to be less than optimal. Fowler has little to say about this property of structures and the tuning mechanism, but in the TM model tuning is the mechanism for *supervising* the structure's performance – it is the way to optimise coordinative structure behaviour. This aspect of the TM model is dealt with in Chapter 6, but note that optimisation does not mean obtaining a behaviour that most closely matches any underlying target.

Time in the Action Theory model

The notion of some degree of cooperation between muscle groups or between mechanically linked portions of the vocal apparatus is certainly not new, but before Action Theory had been little more than a relatively vague idea in speech production theory. Action Theory does however add an important new idea: one of the crucial properties of a coordinative structure is that it exists in time. Surprisingly the idea of introducing time into describing speech is fairly novel. Chapter 3 describes how time has become central to coarticulation theory since its beginnings in the 1960s, but before then time had been sidelined to a tiny role, and appeared only in a very abstract way. Only in post-Classical descriptions of speech does time take up a role on the stage of speech *production*, and eclipse the earlier predominant interpretation – that of simple object sequencing. Previously, reference to time was either concerned with what we might call 'notional time' or to perceived *relative time* – 'This segment is longer than that segment'.

In Action Theory much of the timing detail of an articulatory gesture which had hitherto in cascading rewrite theories been assumed to be calculated (and therefore the result of cognitive activity) is treated as an actual property of the structure itself. Tuning is possible, as with other (spatial) parameters, but the basic timing of the elements within the structure is still a given property of the structure itself and the internal workings of its coordinative activity. The notion that time is added at such a comparatively low level in the system is new. It is important to realise that timing in Action Theory is not the timing of the boundaries of sequenced segments, it is more the timing of the articulatory gesture's component parameters. The articulatory gesture is a composite of parallel parameters which are not synchronised with respect to the individual start and stop times. The way in which these parameter times 'slide over' one another is what *explains* co-production. The basic notion is explicitly adopted into the TM model.

- Notice that 'time' is ambiguous. It can mean *clock time* – an abstract concept enabling us to measure the *physical timing* of events (when they occur with respect to one another) and their individual timing (that is, their *durations*). *'The time duration of the vocal cord vibration associated with this vowel following a [p] in English, is 125ms and it is timed to start 25ms after the release of the stop.'*

Usefulness of the Action Theory model

Proponents of Action Theory have been somewhat rash in their claims as to the effect it has on traditional (generative) phonology. Would it, for example, virtually *eliminate* it? It is understandable that detailed linguistic considerations have not yet been answered by Action Theory since its proponents are for the most part neuro-physiologists and psychologists rather than linguists, or if they are linguists they are phoneticians concerned with the new explanatory approach to speech production. It would seem that some processes accounted for in generative phonology are better modelled as properties of the phonetic rendering system. So, for example, processes such as the nasalisation of inter-nasal vowels in words like *man* in English, or the apparent lengthening of vowels before [+voice] consonants in syllables, are better explained as part of how speech is phonetically rendered rather than phonologically described (Morton and Tatham 1980). Phonology is however different from speech production theory in the sense that it usually is confined to an aoristic account of processes which might characterise exemplar utterance plans – an essentially *static* account. Fowler and the original proponents of Action Theory would be much less worried by traditional phonology if it had been seen as an account of explainable processes accounting for actual utterance plans – an essentially *dynamic* account.

Arguably Action Theory is essentially a physicalist theory of speech production in that it is attempting to take into account more of the detail of the actual mechanisms involved and show that when this is done it has serious consequences for the way the input to the system, and therefore the higher levels as a whole, might be formulated. There are attempts to partially reinterpret the physical model abstractly in an attempt to accommodate some of the observations in the area of Cognitive Phonetics – the area of phonetics which is strictly not physical, but also not phonological.

Task Dynamics

Task Dynamics is a re-naming, refinement and slight re-orientation of Action Theory focussing on articulator movement and defocussing any prior phonological stage (see Saltzman and Munhall 1989). It focuses on the task, emphasising dynamics which are specific to the task, rather than to the articulators involved.

The task in TM is a constant on one side of the specifying equation:

$$T = v_1 \cdot v_2 \cdot v_3 \cdot \ldots \cdot v_n$$

where v_1 to v_n are variables within a specific grouping of such variables (a coordinative structure in Action Theory terms) working together to keep T (the task) constant. Equally in Task Dynamics such a goal would comprise a *pattern* of articulatory action directly related to a critical *area* of the vocal tract – a place where constriction is possible – to achieve a linguistically significant *articulatory gesture*.

As with Action Theory we are dealing technically with what is known as a damped mass-spring model. In such a model in speech production the mass is said to be 'critically damped' in the sense that the spring component 'drives' the mass toward a pre-requested target – a position of equilibrium of the system. This asymptotic movement (the damping contribution) comprises the articulatory output of the *gesture* – a one-dimensional trajectory toward the specified target.

Articulatory Phonology

Articulatory Phonology (Browman and Goldstein 1986) adopts the gesture focus of Task Dynamics. However, unlike TM, the articulatory gesture is thought of in Articulatory Phonology as a *phonological* object. In a hierarchical architecture, Articulatory Phonology meshes with lower level Task Dynamics, feeding it on occasion with gestural structure information which is *pre-organised* into linguistically significant tasks. This is what we might call a 'sequenced event' approach, though the detail of gestures reveals, as with Action Theory, a temporally complex parallelling of gestural components which, as before, explain co-production phenomena.

Browman and Goldstein acknowledge that time in phonology is purely notional and that phonetic rendering (the job of Task Dynamics in this approach) requires the introduction of clock time. The problem for them, and *all* other researchers in the field, is how to relate notional and clock times. It must be realised, however, that this is fact one small aspect of the much more general problem of relating abstract phenomena with physical phenomena and the intractable mind/body relationship problem.

Although the main objective of Articulatory Phonology – to produce a fused approach to phonology and phonetics – fails, it nevertheless brings forward a number of innovations which are important and which have influenced subsequent modelling in speech production. Among the achievements are

- the introduction of a formal framework for characterising correlated and synchronised, though not fused, production models in phonology and phonetics;
- the use of a formal parametric approach based *in general* on true articulatory features rather than the abstract phonological features of mixed origin used in generative phonology or the inconsistent place/manner features of Classical Phonetics;
- the introduction of a formal set of *specific* phonetic parameters (the so-called vocal tract variables) based on a consistent property of the vocal tract throughout its length: the speaker's ability to set up constriction and hence impedance to the airflow;

- the formal rejection of the prevalent 'anatomical parts model' for articulation as exemplified in Classical Phonetics.

The use of a time-locked parametric model for phonetic rendering of the phonological plan elucidates pointedly the co-production explanation of observed coarticulation introduced by Fowler in her Action Theory. Whereas Fowler spoke of the overlapping features of segmental articulation, Browman and Goldstein are able to show formally exactly how the features telescope temporally as they render the utterance plan – simultaneously characterised as the underlying phonology.

As several researchers have done, Browman and Goldstein (1989) observe that there are differences in co-production between different languages. They explain this as deriving from the way in which gestures may be set up differently in different languages. There are two significant aspects to the explanation here:

- the parameters themselves which underlie the gestural dynamics may be different;
- the phasing relationship between parameters will differ between languages.

They hypothesise that the gestural setting for specific languages is learned, and that the mechanism for the acquisition is the tuning process which sets gestures to their language specific values. The explanation here is a little vague, but it could be said to tie in with the notion of *cognitive intervention* in biological processes borrowed from biopsychology and introduced into speech production theory by Tatham (1971), Tatham (1986b) and Tatham and Morton 2004, 2005. What is not apparent in the Browman and Goldstein formulation is the notion that any actual act of dynamic rendering will need to be monitored and *supervised* from the co-production point of view if the coarticulatory variations observed under different conditions of expressive content are to be explained. TM goes further in claiming that *all* speech production is so monitored and supervised to enable simplification of the utterance plan input (Chapter 6).

Speech production theory – changing direction

Action Theory (Fowler, from 1970s) and Cognitive Phonetics (Morton and Tatham, from 1980s) have each sought to redefine the scope of phonology and phonetics.

1. On the one hand Action Theory had taken many of the phenomena previously associated with phonology and cognition and placed them at the periphery: they became intrinsic to the motor control system and lost their origins in cognitive phonological processing. In particular these now low-level processes became part of the internal functioning of coordinative structures.
2. On the other hand Cognitive Phonetics introduced *cognitive* processing into the domain of phonetics – previously reserved for physical processes. The point here was that there are many phonetic phenomena which are intrinsic to the physical mechanism (co-production and coarticulatory processes) which are nevertheless amenable to limited cognitive intervention – cognitively driven constraint could be used to modify physical processes to provide systematic alternates. Examples cited here were
    - variation in the way different dialects of English succumb to such phenomena at the phonetic level – for example inter-nasal nasalisation of phonologically oral vowels in a word like *man* [mæn] *vs.* [mæ̃n], or
    - provision of promoted *contrastive* phonological segments – for example the systematic manipulation of aerodynamic constraints on vocal cord vibration following plosives to provide different 'lengths' of aspiration for contrastive purposes in the English pair *tad* and *dad* [tʰæd] *vs.* [dæd].

Unifying the approach

There are a number of fronts on which the problem of unification of the phonological and phonetic models so clearly drawn out by Browman and Goldstein needs to be tackled. It is not a simple matter to unify two such different theories:

- phonology is entirely abstract (though it does attempt to derive some explanation from the phonetic area particularly in contemporary formulations) and deals with cognitive processes associated with what we know of the sound patterning of languages and how we plan the phonetic rendering of an utterance, and
- phonetics is almost entirely physical (though, of course, it derives its 'instructions' concerning what physical actions to perform as part of the rendering process from the phonological area).

Ruling out explicit segmentation

Browman and Goldstein reorient the model away from chunking into a parametrically based account in which the continuous behaviour of the vocal tract parameters is emphasised irrespective of how this behaviour does or does not synchronise between parameters. The notion of continuous behaviour implies, of course, that progression through time now becomes central to the model – a foreground consideration, and the notion of segment chunking is relegated to being just a background consideration. Several phoneticians in the 1960s had pointed out that as soon as the modelling goes beyond the simple description of acoustic signals and vocal tract configurations it becomes less relevant to think of speech production in terms of a sequence of segments (Tatham 1971). These phoneticians pointed out that it is more productive to consider how the various parameters of speech work together a-synchronously to produce the acoustic signal. Browman and Goldstein are responsible for formally developing this idea.

In general linguistics, though, the idea was developed much earlier. In the 1940s it formed the basis of Prosodic Analysis – a phonological model proposed by Firth (1948). This phonological model also had much in it which foreshadowed modern non-linear phonology (Goldsmith 1990).

The Gestural Score

The graphical notation of Articulatory Phonology makes much of the idea of parallel parameters unfolding in time. The term used by Browman and Goldstein to describe the notation is *gestural score* by analogy with a musical score which sets up parallel staves running from left to right across the page to indicate how the various instruments in a band or orchestra play together. The call their staves *tracks*, and these are used to represent the tract variable parameters.

The other side of the coin is seen in the Classical Phonetics attempt to characterise too much at the phonetic level using concepts like the phoneme which properly belong in phonology. While modelling what they *perceived* Classical Phoneticians claimed to be modelling aspects of actual physical speech.

5
Speech Production: Prosody

Introduction

The terms *prosodics* and *prosody* refer to a dimension of speech which goes beyond individual sounds and how they are might be strung together. As the term *suprasegmental* implies we are concerned with phenomena which either linearly span or hierarchically dominate segments. There are three main suprasegmental features which need to be examined to understand prosody in speech production and perception: *intonation*, *stress* and *rhythm*. These are the traditional terms from Classical Phonetics (Chapter 1) and, in line with most terms in that theory, effectively focus on our *perception* of correlating physical phenomena. Prosody has a linguistic dimension: it can be used to differentiate for example between declarative and question sentences in *John's gone home.* and *John's gone home?* by delivering the sentence embedded in a different intonation contour. It also has a function beyond this linguistic one – the conveying of expressive content (Tatham and Morton 2004). The prosodic features are used to signal speakers' attitudes and emotions. In our terminology a speaker's utterance is wrapped in its prosody, which in turn is wrapped in its expression, thus (using XML [Sharma and Kunins 2002] notation):

```
<expression>
  <prosody>
    <segmental utterance/>
  </prosody>
</expression>
```

The terminology is a little ambiguous here because *prosody* is used both for linguistic and expressive content; the reason for this is that the cognitive features of prosody (intonation, stress and rhythm) and their physical correlates (fundamental frequency, amplitude and timing) are used in particular ways to express both.

Spanning – an intonation example

We might ask how we might say the English sentence *Matt fell off his bike*. Perceptually the intonation assigned to such a sentence generally falls in pitch from the word with the main focus, *Matt*, to the finish, provided the sentence is uttered as a statement of fact. The intonation is said to be falling if the speaker is confident of the assertion being made. But this same five word sequence can, without changing their order, be made to express the same speaker's total lack of knowledge as to whether Matt has fallen off his bike or not: *Matt fell off his bike?* In speech the sentence would be given a perceived progressively rising intonation, indicating to the listener that a question was being asked and that the speaker was short on information about what has happened to Matt.

This is a clear example of the power of prosody over the simple basic meaning of the words themselves. The listener instantly assigns meaning beyond what the words themselves express, and is able to tell something about the speaker. In the sentence with the falling intonation information flow about Matt's fate is from speaker to listener, but in the sentence with rising intonation the listener learns that *they* are to supply the information and that the only information flowing from the speaker is at best that they are in some doubt about Matt's fate.

This is not the only way of asking a question in English, and in fact it is not the preferred way. The more usual way is to transform the syntax of the sentence to produce the sentence: *Did Matt fall off his bike?* Note, however, that *Matt fell off his bike?* and *Did Matt fall off his bike?* do not have exactly the same meaning. In some other languages altering just the intonation is actually the usual way of doing things. So comparing French with English using the *John's gone home* sentence we could have:

French	English
Jean est rentré. [statement]	*John's gone home.* [statement]
Jean est rentré? [preferred query form]	*John's gone home?*
Est-ce que Jean est rentré? or *Jean, est-il rentré?*	*Has John gone home?* [preferred query form]

In the statements in both languages we find that the perceived intonation is falling from the word *Jean/John*, whereas in the questions the perceived intonation is rising from *Jean/John*, although in English the form which uses inversion can have falling intonation. Not all languages contrast statements and questions in this exactly this way – but most have ways of expressing query and uncertainty, and indeed other feelings and emotions, using variations in prosodic patterning.

Prosodic effects

Prosodic effects, then, span more than one individual speech segment. In the abstract terminology of linguistics and perceptual studies we are dealing with stress, rhythm and intonation; in the physical terminology of acoustics with correlating patterns of amplitude, timing and fundamental frequency variation. Part of the task of speech theory is to expand on this correlation and explain it. In linguistics the basic unit which is manipulated for these effects is the syllable, and these prosodic effects are usually modelled in terms of the syllabic structure of utterances.

Rhythm

Linguists have traditionally identified two different kinds of languages with respect to sentence rhythm. Both have what the Classical Phoneticians called *isochrony* – that is, both time sentence utterances by noting the equal spacing of stressed syllables within a phrase or sentence. Those languages (like French) which do not have word stress variation (i.e. have all syllables equally stressed within the word) have every syllable therefore spaced equidistantly in time; but those languages (like English) which do have word stress variation have their stressed syllables delivered on an equally spaced basis, with unstressed syllables being fitted within the dominant regular arrival of primary stressed syllables.

This is a clear and classic example of the nonlinearity in the correlation between an abstract characterisation of speech based on perception and the acoustic signal which triggered the perception. The correlation is partly nonlinear because the perceptual process is nonlinear (Chapter 8). We discuss elsewhere (Chapters 3 and 6) the dangers inherent in models which, coming from either an abstract or a physical viewpoint, ignore this nonlinearity or, worse, ignore each other. That isochrony identifies a strong cognitive awareness of a particular rhythmic patterning in speech and that it is hard to find in the acoustic signal should be neither a surprise nor an excuse to avoid trying to relate the two. Speakers and listeners of all languages readily report this awareness (Tatham and Morton 2002).

Intonation

Intonation is perhaps the most complex of the prosodic phenomena to be assigned in speech production – and consequently it is the one most likely to fail in terms of predictive modelling. There is no model yet which does not generate errors, though some are better than others (and see below).

The correlation between abstract and physical prosody

In the descriptive model of Classical Phonetics we can speak of the assignment of prosodic features. At the physical level we are more likely to speak of measuring the features. The simplest correlation equates length (patterned as rhythm) with duration, pitch (patterned as intonation) with fundamental frequency and prominence (patterned as stress) with amplitude or intensity. Some phoneticians have brought physiological features into the correlation as well: thus stress involves patterns of varying degrees of muscular contraction. Aerodynamics figures also in some models where stress is correlated with patterns of air flow and pressure variation. Most models of prosody focus on the correlation between cognitively based assignment of prosodic features and their associated acoustic properties. The correlation is almost never completely linear.

For us there are two types of variation: there is the variation inherent in repetitions within one speaker and between speakers for any one segment object, but there is also the variation of intrinsic duration between different segments. This is not entirely irrelevant. If we fail to capture in our description that [ɛ] is shorter than [u], for example, we fail to capture the fact that speakers of English are disturbed when [ɛ] is made long and [u] is made short. They may not immediately be able to say *why* they are disturbed, but the fact that they are means that something that they know has been violated. It is the same with stress – there is intrinsic variation in intensity of different sounds, and speakers are aware of this; it must therefore figure in our description of the phonetics of the language. It has been pointed out (Gimson 1989) that listeners need assign only two or three degrees of stress to what is, in fact, a speaker's 'infinite number of degrees of variation'.

Linguistic distinctiveness

Returning to segment length though, and just to reinforce the point that we do need to account for the details of variability, let us consider the example of how vowels appear to have greater duration when they occur before syllable closing consonants which are phonologically [+voice]. This is almost certainly a universal phonetic phenomenon. However, still keeping within the traditional approach, in some accents of English a final plosive may well be unreleased, effectively rendering the plosive acoustically silent. Yet despite this, listeners can readily distinguish between *bat* and *bad* – [bæt̚], [bæd̚] – presumably because they can detect the vowel length difference and, importantly, use this linguistically. We could say that the universal *phonetic* rendering effect of apparent increase vowel duration has acquired *phonological* status because it is being used in a distinctive way in this accent. To tighten up the terminology a little we might say that the incidental difference in the [physical] *durations* of the [physical] *vocal cord vibration period* in these two words enables the perception of a [cognitive] *length* difference for the [cognitive] *vowels* resulting in the assignment of either a [cognitive] *voiceless* or a *voiced plosive* to the final period of [physical] *silence*. We can go further and say that the featural difference between the vowels has resulted in 'feature transfer' – the assignment of different features to adjacent segments previously not showing the difference. That is, the silent period is now perceived as having the status of /t/ or /d/.

So if we use the criterion of distinctiveness to decide whether or not to ignore some variation, descriptions of one accent might ignore features which are significant in another, just as descriptions of languages differ in terms of what segmental and prosodic effects are included or not. A theory of accent (Chapter 4) would have difficulty here because of apparent inconsistency in trying to explain the conflict between phonetic and phonological effects if both were derived from the same accent free underlying representation. There are abstract distinctive phonological features and there are physical phonetic features. What a theory of speech production needs to account for is when and how variation in the physical properties of speech are usable and used for phonological purposes. This applies to both the segmental and prosodic aspects of speech.

Syllables

Classical Phonetics has difficulties with the concept of syllable – the unit we need to model prosody adequately. Phoneticians have often defined syllables functionally in terms of a particular language – this would be a contemporary basic phonological definition matching well the notion of psychological reality. But also there have been attempts at phonetic definitions which fail to link into the functional definitions. Researchers recognised that there is psychological reality to the concept of speech segment and to the concept of linear groupings of these. For example a word like *barter* is recognised by speakers and listeners as having four 'speech sounds' grouped in two 'syllables', thus (in many accents of British English) /bɑ·tə/. However defining the concept was problematical despite the introduction of different definitions from two different domains: syllables are

1. functional groupings of segments (abstract, phonological), or
2. segmental groupings whose boundaries are defined by regular fluctuations in airflow or acoustic signal amplitude (physical, phonetic).

If phonetics renders phonological plans and if syllables figure in those plans, there should be some phonetic correlates. Notice that there is a possibility (recognised by most phoneticians and others) that there are phonological syllables *because* of the way speech production is organised. Clearly there are general phonetic constraints on phonology and it may well be that phonetic syllable existence and organisation is one of them.

Syllable structure: constituent segments

In descriptive phonology segments group into syllables according to a clear hierarchical system which can be illustrated by a tree structure with syllable as the node dominating, to the left, an optional onset and to the right a rhyme. The rhyme node dominates, to the left, an obligatory vowel nucleus and, to the right, an optional coda.

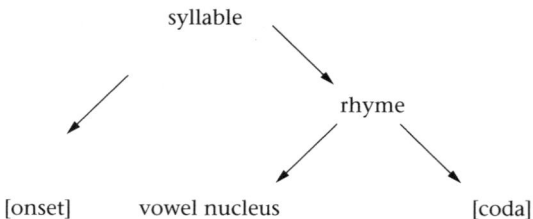

A linear characterisation of the surface of this structure (in English) gives us: C_0^3 V C_0^4 – a syllable is a sequence of three objects: from zero to three consonants followed by a single vowel followed by zero to four consonants. The vowel nucleus remains obligatory, but the surrounding consonants vary in number.

Additionally laterals (/l/ and /r/) and nasals (/n/, /m/, and /ŋ/) are said to be able to form the nucleus of a syllable – usually when the syllable is unstressed and preceded by a plosive. In the rendering process the plosive releases 'into' the lateral or nasal. Examples of words where this can occur are: *sudden – Sutton, medal – metal;* notice that in these it is possible to distinguish between the voiced and voiceless versions of the plosives. The lateral or nasal can be preceded by other consonants; so: *level, brazen, several* (/sɛv·r̩l/). Note that in some accents of English *several* might well be /sɛv·rʊ/ in the utterance plan, and words like *wall* (/wɔ·ʊ/) might well be described as bisyllabic. There is a long standing discussion as to whether we have a syllabic /r/ in words like *member, better* (in North American and some other accents of English), and we ourselves see no reason not to call the /r/ here syllabic in some speakers to be consistent. Similarly, from a historical perspective, a word like *chevals* (*horses*) in Old French, originally /tʃə·vals/, but then /tʃə·va·ʊs/, later to become /ʃə·vo/ in most contemporary versions of Metropolitan French and /ʃə·voʊ/ in some Canadian variants – *chevaux*) has the same problem distinguishing between vowel and consonant categories. Note that we are using slant rather than square brackets here to indicate a symbolic representation at the utterance plan level rather than the post-rendering level. That is, these are extrinsic rather than intrinsic allophones.

It may be best to say that continuants can form the nuclei of syllables, whether they are within the category vowel or consonant in the usual classification. The problem arises for those who want to say either that all syllabic nuclei are vowels (in which case the transcription and the thinking behind it has to insert some kind of central neutral vowel (say, /ə/) prior to the consonant – and clearly some speakers do this audibly, though perhaps most do not), or want to define vowels as those elements which can act as syllabic nuclei.

There may be no harm at all in saying that there are elements which can be either vowels or consonants depending on their syntagmatic arrangement within syllables. Notice, for instance, one of the examples above: *several*. Here the /r/ is the onset to the syllable and the nucleus is the /l̩/, but we also find the word *leveller* which can be pronounced: /lev-lr̩/ where the /l/ is the syllable onset and the /r̩/ is the syllabic nucleus. Probably the argument is futile, and all that matters is consistency in the descriptive system, unless there is any other *external* reason to prefer one solution to the other.

Syllables – definitions

So, as we have just seen, it is not difficult to define a phonological syllable. On the surface it is a sequence of phoneme-sized objects exhibiting a distinctive underlying hierarchical structure. We call them phoneme-sized to avoid calling them phonemes or extrinsic allophones, since they can be either of these depending on which level we are looking at. The diagram above showed the hierarchical relationship preferred by linguists between the various linear elements. Only one element is required: the vocalic syllable nucleus. The underlying structure of syllables is, as a framework, quite common among the world's languages, though the number of onset or coda consonants may vary between languages. Some refinement of the definition is needed, as we just saw, to cater for what the Classical Phoneticians called *syllabic consonants* such as /l̩/, /r̩/ and the nasals. In fact although these consonants are not quite sonorant enough to aspire to vowel status they can, on occasion, be *promoted* to serve as vowel nuclei. The use of the term 'promotion' implies higher status for vowels: this is based on the fact that the vowel nucleus is not optional, whereas the surrounding consonants are. That some consonants might have this dual status is an important concept in our model, where the notion of promotion figures prominently. It is generally agreed that in idealised speech (that is speech with normal speed and no stylistic or expressive content) there is a progressive increase in sonority though the sequence of onset consonants toward the nucleic vocalic peak, with a decrease in sonority as we move through the coda consonants toward the end of the syllable. In practice, expression and deletions or reductions sometimes appear to violate this rule – which has been primarily formulated with exemplar (Chapter 6) phonology in mind.

There are phonological syllables and there are renderings of these. We could call the renderings (or the phonetic objects subjected to rendering processes) phonetic syllables. Although speakers and listeners are able to report the syllabic count for an utterance there is sometimes confusion as to whether they are talking about phonological or phonetic syllables. Thus a word like *separately* might be reported as having three or four syllables by speakers and listeners who regularly pronounce the word [ˈsɛ-prət-li] – that is, the word might have three phonetic syllables and four phonological syllables (depending at which level in the phonology it is looked at). There are a number of apparent anomalies in speaker/listener reporting which are due to a preference for reporting the syllable count either before (underlying phonological) or after (derived phonological or phonetic) any syllable deletion or 'collapsing' processes. It might be interesting to try to determine whether there is a difference in reporting depending on whether the deletion is phonological or phonetic.

Syllable juncture

Researchers (Lehiste 1970, among others) agree that syllables are the basic units for suprasegmental *analysis* (in a descriptive model) or *synthesis* (in a speech production model) making it important to have a clear means of identifying them and determining their boundaries. At the phonological level there is no difficulty in principle in identifying boundaries: a boundary between syllables occurs where the coda of syllable 1 stops and the onset of syllable 2 starts. The problem is deciding which segments in the string of consonants belong to syllable one and which to syllable two. Consonants which, all things being equal, could be part of the offset of one syllable, or part of the onset of the next syllable are usually called *ambisyllabic*, and the resolution of any particular assignment of a consonant to this or that syllable may end up for linguists or for lay speakers a matter of preference. But why not? We would be foolish to expect everything that human beings do to be able to be characterised by regular rules! Ambisyllabicity rarely causes confusion for lay speakers, and rarely is there any ambiguity caused by not being clear as to which syllable a particular consonant belongs. Listeners may well be scanning utterance chunks, perhaps using a moving window, rather than concentrating on a syllable-by-syllable perceptual strategy: in any case there are other, non-phonological cues to help solve such problems in real life.

Prosody – focus on segments detracts from good prosody models

Some researchers working in the area of suprasegmentals or prosodics draw attention to how this focus on segments detracts from the development of good models of prosody. This is especially true if prosody is seen as a system imposed on the segmental structure of utterances – an approach characterised by statements such as: '*The utterance can be said with a falling intonation to indicate that the speaker is making a statement or with a rising intonation to indicate that the speaker is asking a question.*' The approach pivots around the segmental utterance and what prosody is to be fitted to it.

Traditional models of prosody

The traditional way of regarding the relationship between syllable segments and prosody involves the idea of fitting suprasegmentals to strings of syllables. The assumption is that there is some kind of logical priority for segments. We see in Chapter 6 that we prefer to think of the prior *independent* existence of prosody, and include in the model the notion that *syllable strings get fitted to an existing prosodic structure*. Hence the hierarchical approach with prosody dominating segments, and the use of the wrapper model – with prosody wrapping segments. We will stay with the traditional view for the moment in order to discuss the various models which fall within that view.

Ladefoged's expression of the viewpoint is one of the clearest (Ladefoged 1993): prosodic features 'are characterized by the fact that they must be described in relation to other items in the same utterance' (p. 15). This is to underline the fact that they are *supra*-segmental. However it is perfectly possible to described intonation and other prosodic patterning without referring to specific segments. In doing this we would be characterising abstract prosodic generalisations. Though when it comes to talking about a single intonation pattern or a particular example of rhythm, it would be necessary to refer to *which* syllable takes sentence stress, or where the intonational downturn at the end of the sentence/statement might occur, or how particular unstressed syllables fitted into the rhythmic structure of a particular sentence.

But we should not be tempted to say something which assumes that prosodic contours are fitted to the segmental structure of a sentence or a even a class of sentences. It is better, we believe, to speak of prosodic contours first in the abstract, and then *to fit sentence instantiations to them*.

Thus we see two needs:

1. the independent characterisation of prosodic features or their 'contours' relating to sentences, phrases or some other run of syntactic domain – a static or exemplar account, and
2. the description of a formal relationship between individual properties of the contours with particular segments in an actual phrase or sentence.

Tone

Some researchers classify tone as a suprasegmental feature. This is not necessarily the best classification since as far as we know, despite the fact that tone when rendered involves a fundamental frequency contour, it is wholly described within the confines of a single syllable segment. Tone is however a parameter of syllables which comes under pressure when wrapped within particular prosodic contours; that is, prosody tends to alter tone. But because, say, a falling tone on a syllable is constrained by the rising intonation contour into which it must fit, this does not make tone a suprasegmental feature any more than it makes the length of syllable or element within a syllable a suprasegmental feature.

We can define tone as a prosodic feature if the focus is on the sub-syllabic unit, but define it as a segmental feature if the focus is on the syllable unit. Similarly with stress and duration (abstractly: length). In any case it is the patterning of the features which constitutes the prosodic feature itself: intonation is the patterning of abstract pitch, stress is the patterning of abstract prominence, rhythm is the patterning of abstract length. All three might be more precisely defined as the assignment of the relevant patterning – a definition which clearly and deliberately avoids any suggestion of a linear relationship between these abstract features and their physical correlates.

Features for prosody *vs.* features for segments

In general most researchers would agree that the features for characterising prosody are different from those needed to characterise segments. However this may not be the case in some circumstances. So for example it is necessary to speak of vocal cord vibration and fundamental frequency when speaking of *individual* segments:

- Are they planned to be voiced or not?
- Does fundamental frequency alter with segmental context?
- How does micro-intonation (not a prosodic feature) work?

And also:

- Do some segments have intrinsically more intensity than others?
- Do some segments have greater intrinsic duration than others?

In fact, having stressed the need to model prosodic and segmental features separately, the two are not as separate as might be supposed. For example, the intonation turn down and the slowing down of rate – both perceived toward the end of a sentence/statement – are prosodic features which have an effect on several parameters of the individual segments spanned. And it is therefore true that these changes can be discussed in connection with what is happening to *adjacent segments* – and this is perhaps predictable, given the wrapping prosody. A discussion which focuses on adjacent segments is not the same as a discussion focussing on a group of spanned segments. On the one hand what is happening in each segment with respect to its neighbours is being described, and on the other the nature of the spanning contour is being described with respect to its segmental domain.

Perhaps it might be best to say that to establish baseline norms in an initial characterisation of speech, it is appropriate to treat separately prosodic features and the parameters of segmental articulation or the resulting acoustic signal. But as soon as we introduce the concept of prosody wrapping the string of segments we have to characterise the interaction between the two. To that extent the features of characterisation of the two phenomena are not independent since describing the interaction requires a common or overlapping set of features. Only really in the abstract can the two be separately characterised – and in this case the characterisations are on separate tiers. When the phenomena become united on a single tier, then the interaction is apparent.

We perhaps need a diagnostic for what constitutes a prosodic event. Table 5.1 shows the classification of the features involved in prosody – by segmental and by prosodic domains. Notice that features operating in the prosodic domain involve patterning which spans the domain. This patterning is often referred to as the *prosodic contour*. Cognitive intervention can occur in either domain: that is, there is intervention in *both* segmental and prosodic feature production. Similarly the specific cognitive intervention associated with limiting or enhancing coarticulation

Table 5.1 Classification of various features by segmental or prosodic domain

Feature or Phenomenon	Segmental Domain	Prosodic Domain
syllable (word) stress	X	
sentence stress (prominence patterning)		X
intonation (pitch patterning)		X
tone	X	
physical duration	X	
rhythm (temporal patterning)		X
physical coarticulation / co-production	X	
general cognitive intervention	X	X
cognitively constrained coarticulation / co-production	X(?)	X(?)

Table 5.2 Basic queries concerning feature domains, with appropriate responses

Diagnostic query	Yes	No
Is the feature confined to the domain of phoneme-sized elements?	segmental	next query
Is the feature confined to individual syllable domains?	segmental	next query
Does the feature's domain span multiple consecutive syllables?	prosodic	

or co-production might be either segmental or prosodic – this, though, is an area which needs further investigation.

The diagnostic will run something along the lines shown in Table 5.2. Here questions lead to yes/no answers suggesting whether the feature is segmental or prosodic.

We note that

- it is impossible to have utterance rendering – that is, a physical instantiation of an utterance plan – which is not rendered within a *prosodic wrapper*;
- prosody can derive from purely linguistic considerations, but is also the vehicle of expression;
- the instantiation cannot exist without being rendered within an *expression wrapper*.

Hence prosody is always present in speech and always has two sources – linguistic and expressive. Moreover the prosody exists logically independently of and prior to the utterance it wraps.

Syllables and stress

Stress, often without distinguishing between phonological and phonetic stress, has been modelled as a property of

- vowels (in some older approaches),
- vowels as syllabic nuclei, or
- entire syllables.

Our model opts for stress as a feature of the phonological syllable. It is important to distinguish two types of stress: word stress (a segmental feature) and sentence stress (a prosodic feature). The stress associated with sentences identifies the relative stress pattern among word stressed syllables with a sentence (or phase or some other syntactic subdivision of a sentence). The simplest characterisation of sentence stress (see Chomsky and Halle 1968 for the first really coherent description) involves identifying one candidate stressed syllable as carrying some kind of focus, or focal point, within the sentence. Since we are seeing that prosodic features interact, we discover that *which* stressed syllable is chosen conditions how the intonation pattern pans out and also has implications for the rhythmic pattern of the sentence. A more detailed characterisation would also describe the interactions occurring within sub-sentence domains, such as phrases.

Several researchers have investigated how phonological stress on words within an utterance plan correlates with features of the acoustic output from the subsequent rendering processes. Others have investigated articulatory correlates of stress, such as 'chest pulses', air flow and air pressure patterning, and muscle 'tension' within articulators. The most comprehensive and most often quoted work here is that of Fry (1955, 1958) who associated higher than expected fundamental frequency with a stressed syllable (correlating also with sentence stress), and greater than expected duration for the stressed vowel within the syllable and greater intensity for that vowel. Fry also noticed that on average unstressed vowels tended to be articulated more toward the centre of the oral cavity (using the Classical Phonetics two dimensional map of articulatory vowel space), prompting a variation of spectral content compared with fully stressed vowels. Classical Phonetics makes the observation that vowels tend to centralise when unstressed.

Fry's observations about vowel centralisation accords well with phonological processes in those languages or accents which call for vowel reduction in certain phonological contexts. Fry does not attempt formally to distinguished between those stressing variations which result from phonological planning processes and those which result from phonetic rendering processes. One thing we should not assume is that the rendering of phonological stress differs between languages: rather it is safer to assume that it is phonological stress itself varies between languages. The point here is that syllables may be unstressed because they are planned to be unstressed (more likely), or they may be unstressed because they are rendered unstressed despite their planning (less likely). Thus the centralisation of the unstressed vowel in the initial syllable of *content* (the adjective) in most accents of English – [kən'tɛnt] – is a phonological processes which does not apply in some accents of Northern England – [kɒn'tɛnt]. It probably has nothing to do with how some underlying extrinsic allophone /ɒ/ might be phonetically rendered. Briefly: the quality change associated sometimes with unstressed versions of vowel nuclei is planned, it is not a by-product of the rendering process.

Some researchers have defined word stress as a *perceptual* property based on the acoustic properties of a syllable. The acoustic variables which might contribute are:

- increased duration – perceived as increased length, and/or
- increased intensity – perceived as increased loudness, and/or
- 'unusual' fundamental frequency movement – perceived as pitch movement.

As a kind of shorthand, writers like Ladefoged refer to stressed syllables as being 'pronounced with a greater amount of energy' than unstressed syllables. However, we repeat that if this is how stress is defined – whether in perceptual or production or acoustic terms – it is the case that this stress is *not* a prosodic feature. It certainly is not prosodic simply because it spans the segments internal to the syllable. There are good reasons for not including syllable stress within prosodic features. One of these is the wrapper hierarchy. Prosody wraps all of utterances, and word stress is not a property of utterances, but a local property confined to individual syllables (unless it is expressive or contrastive stress or emphasis – Chapter 6).

Theorists who focus on a *perceptual* definition of stress need also to include *speaker* use of stress in their definitions. Speakers would need to plan increased length, loudness or pitch movement, and these would need to be rendered as some combination of increased duration, intensity or fundamental frequency movement. The reason for this is that the perceptual model needs to be part of the speaker/listener chain – what is perceived is generally what is planned by the speaker irrespective of the process of rendering and the actual acoustic signal created. A simple speech production model can refer to *intended* stressing, but a perceptual model needs to explain how stress is assigned from the acoustic signal which triggered it.

In the TM model a speaker would need to wrap these in some more abstract element such as <prominence> – in the sense that the speaker's goal would be listener detection of intended increased prominence. Phonologically it may not matter how prominence is actually rendered, so long as it is perceived. This is an important point of detail which we return to many times: the main goal for the speaker is adequate perception by the listener. In speech production and perception what is important is that the two should match: the speaker's plan should match the listener's perceived representation assigned to the heard signal. We see in the sections on Cognitive Phonetics (Chapters 3 and 6) that the rendering process is cognitively overseen to make sure this happens.

Prominence and stress

We are taking the view that a stressed syllable is one which is intended to be stressed by the speaker. It is marked as stressed in the utterance plan – that is, it is actually intended to be *perceived* as stressed. This of course rests on the assumption that the goal of the speaker is to enable transfer of the utterance plan to the listener, where 'transfer' means cause the listener to assign to the incoming signal a representation which is equivalent to the speaker's utterance plan.

Phonologically we usually think of syllables as being basically either stressed or unstressed. In addition some researchers find it productive to invoke different levels of stress. Because the stressing is phonological it has linguistic significance – it is not randomly applied. When some researchers speak of the stressing of a 'sound' they are presumably referring to the phonological stressing of a syllable.

The confusion over definitions and the various levels needed in speech production and perception models leads to a feeling that stress is not all that well understood. Researchers regularly raise such questions as:

- How does apparent increase in sub-glottal air pressure relate to the rendering of the stressed *phonological* syllable?
- Is heightened sub-glottal air pressure part of the rendering of the *entire* syllable (or its phonetic correlate) or just the *syllabic nucleus* (or its phonetic correlate)?
- Are planned sounds which potentially call for vocal cord vibration (phonologically [+voice] sounds) *all* involved – vowel syllable nuclei and their surrounding consonants?
- Are sounds within the syllable but which do *not* involve vocal cord vibration also rendered with increased sub-glottal air pressure?
- What is the timing relationship between the beginning of increased muscular contraction (associated with the heightened 'push' on the lungs) and the start and stop of the *phonetic* syllable?
- What about the relative timing of any increase in 'energy' associated with the muscular contractions for articulators *other* than those used in increasing the sub-glottal air pressure for the stressed syllable?

Researchers have observed coarticulatory effects in speech (Chapter 2). A coarticulatory effect is an observed distortion of the surface waveform – one cause of this is co-production or the overlapping of articulatory (muscular) parameters during the rendering process. Depending on whether a coarticulatory (surface) or a co-production (underlying) viewpoint is emphasised we can also ask:

- Does stressing have an effect on the results of co-production *via* a rebalancing of the relative dominance of phoneme or syllable-sized segments? That is, do the overlapping or co-produced parameters of segments telescope to bring about a change in the hierarchical structure of syllables?
- Coarticulation theorists would similarly ask whether coarticulatory effects are distorted by changes of stress in the phonetic syllable – coarticulation might be increased or decreased by variation in stressing.

There are clearly many questions to ask here which go beyond the simple idea of increased energy associated with a 'stressed sound'. Some of these are associated with the underlying production phonology of words and their component syllables and segments, some are associated with how phonological planning relates to the articulatory or acoustic signals, and some are associated with the perception of stress from these stimuli.

Laryngeal activity

Because of the increase in sub-glottal air pressure, some researchers have referred to a general increase in laryngeal activity in the production of stressed sounds or syllables. It is often not entire clear what such an increase in laryngeal activity might be. Perhaps

- an increase in rate of vibration of the vocal cords?
- an increase in amplitude of vibration of the vocal cords, which, together with increased sub-glottal pressure produces an increase in the amplitude of the resultant audio?
- an increase in the duration of vocal cord vibration?

Thus increased laryngeal activity could cause increased fundamental frequency and intensity of the acoustic signal; and it might also result in increased duration since increased 'effort' does not just mean increased *magnitude* of effort but increased effort over unit time – increased duration.

These are the acoustic signals and their underlying articulatory variables which contribute toward the perceptual assignment of stress.

The perceptual assignment of stress

Listeners perceive different degrees of stress, and are able to report this. The reporting is not necessarily direct, but given by indicating a perceived change of meaning – as with English words like *content* which alter their meanings depending on which syllable carries the phonological stress. The alternation in this word is between /kən·ˈtɛnt/ (adjective) and /ˈkɒn·tɛnt/ (noun); the slash brackets are used to indicate abstract extrinsic allophonic planning strings – that is, the reduced vowel in the unstressed syllable in the adjective is planned in rather than arising as a consequence of rendering (see above).

The question for workers in perception is just what are the relevant acoustic features which trigger stress assignment. Researchers like Fry and others have listed the acoustic properties of segments and/or syllables which correlate with listeners' *reporting* of stress – but what they have not done is provide us with an algorithm which shows explicitly how these acoustic features are differentially involved in the assignment process. In the TM perceptual model (Chapter 7) a symbolic representation is assigned by listeners, but clearly some stimulus triggers the assignment process. What it certainly is not is the prior existence of the representation *within* the signal. With researchers reporting multiple 'cues' for stress assignment the explanation of the process is clearly complex and yet to be explained in any useful way. We have referred elsewhere (Tatham and Morton 2005) to the development of computational models (engineered as 'speech synthesis') and we would eventually expect the algorithms in these models to be clear as to just how these multiple cues interact and, moreover, explain how the relative balance of the cues within that interaction itself seems to vary. Several variables are involved in the process, but their relationship is not constant: we need an understanding of what governs or explains this relationship: it is not enough to state its existence.

There is another aspect to defining stress in perceptual terms which needs to be considered. Some researchers have referred to the notion that stress is *signalled* by the nature of the physical signal – this is equivalent to our saying that the acoustic signal triggers the stress assignment process. But this should not perhaps be extended to a quantitative correlation. By this we mean that the idea of 'increased energy' does not immediately give rise to the correlating notion of the assignment of 'increased stress'. Indeed it is not difficult to find an example of lower energy – relative to the adjacent syllables – giving rise to the perception of an increased stress on the syllable. Of course 'increased energy' may mean increased with respect to what it would have been if the syllable had not been stressed; and this calls also on the notion of norms or targets stored within the listener. The problem is that we often perceive increased stress where in fact there is no such increase in energy (or at least not carried over into the soundwave). Examples might be:

- *Alabama* [æ̱lə'bæmə] – with high amplitude (underlined) on the initial 'wrong' syllable, or
- a non-reduced vowel in Northern British English – *content* pronounced as [kɒ̱n'tɛnt], where the [ɑ] is higher in amplitude (underlined) than the [ɛ].

In addition it is important to take into account that the assignment of stress, and perhaps any other representation connected with speech, is going to change if the listener or their internal perceptual 'environment' has changed. Consider the following diagram:

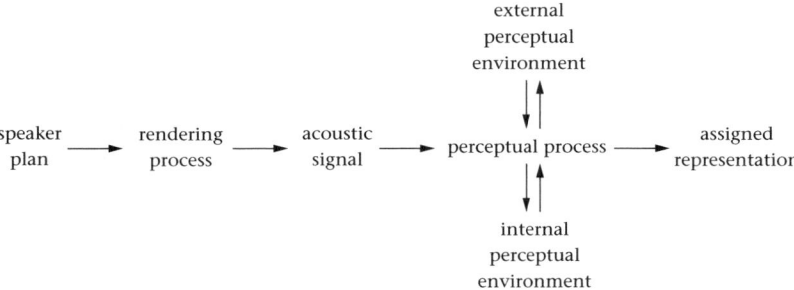

The diagram shows three input paths to the perceptual process: the acoustic signal as generated from the speaker's plan (but transformed *via* the rendering process), the influence of the listener's external perceptual environment, and the influence of the listener's internal perceptual environment. These influences do not detract from the speaker's goal of producing as near a match as possible between the speaker plan and the perceiver's assigned representation.

The assignment of a particular representation to an incoming acoustic signal should not be regarded as fixed: it is a variable process depending on several environmental factors. For example, the perceptual process may be 'globally' biased in general to interpret a particular acoustic signal in a particular way, or it may have been locally biased perhaps by some previous acoustic signal or some ongoing feedback or some internal change such as attitude or emotion. Perception is influenced by physical intervention from external sources and by internal biological and cognitive intervention. It is clearly a complex process calling for a complex model which cannot predict the outcome of the process without taking account of the various inputs arriving in addition to the plain acoustic signal.

Speaker planned stress may involve bringing into play all three acoustic parameters, often in different combinations. Similarly for the listener, stress may be decoded when one, two or all three parameters are adjusted in the way described (greater duration, higher amplitude, change of fundamental frequency). The exact combination and ratio of the parameters has not yet been satisfactorily modelled since there is so far insufficient data to enable an understanding of their relative roles. One reason for this is that the balance between these parameters varies, and the effects of the external and internal environments may well vary too dependent on, say, what the listener has just decoded.

Length

Length is not generally considered to be phonemic in English. And the *wood/wooed* distinction in most accents involves a change of phoneme not just a change in length. A parallel is the *bit/beat* distinction which is also a change of phoneme and a change in length. The point here is that the length difference is associated with the intrinsic set of properties of the different vowels: they differ on more features than just phonological length.

Some phonologists have introduced a vowel lengthening rule in their descriptive models for English and some other languages:

- Vowels lengthen when they are followed in their syllables by consonantal segments which are [+voice].

The rule is probably falsely assigned to phonology, and many phoneticians invoke this as a descriptive phonetic rule. In TM we could of course describe an apparent increase in the duration of the vowel, but quickly observe that an equally probable explanation is that what is thought to be vocal cord vibration associated with the vowel is probably more appropriately assigned to the consonant. Consider the waveform renderings of *bad* /bæd/ and *bat*/bæt/ in Figure 8. Appropriate phonetic transcriptions for these might be [bæd˺] and [bæt˺] indicating the unreleased [d] and [t] common in many accents.

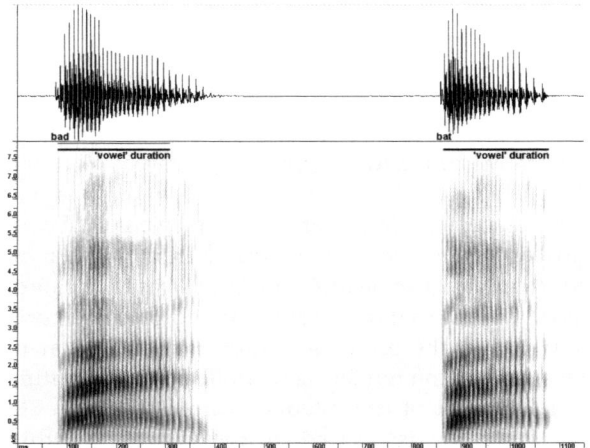

Figure 5.1 Waveforms and spectrograms of *bad* and *bat*, with the final plosives unreleased. Note that the greater duration of vocal cord vibration in *bad* can be assigned to the final 'devoiced' consonant rather than to the 'vowel'. If this is the case the rule which lengthens vowels before voiced consonants is too simplistic, since the vowel section of the vocal cord vibration is approximately the same in both *bad* and *bat*.

The phonological argument goes like this:

1. because of a rule in English phonology – voiced consonants devoice in syllable final position (the actual rule is slightly more elaborate than this simple statement) – there is no actual phonological distinction made at the plan level (the output of the phonology) between the final alveolar plosives; but
2. because listeners can still readily distinguish these words (even when there is no plosive release) it must be the logically *prior* rule – vowels lengthen before voiced consonants – which cues them to perceive the distinction; and so
3. the lengthening must be phonological.

The phonetic argument, however, goes like this:

1. because of a universal coarticulatory rule – vocal cord vibration tends, during phonetic rendering, to fail partially in planned [+voice] plosives as the intra-oral air pressure rises to a critical level – only the initial part of the stop phase of the plosive will show vocal cord vibration;

2. listeners have no difficulty in detecting the vocal cord vibration failure, at least in part because it happens to them, and assign the planned category to the remaining fragment or residual of the [+voice] stop; and so
3. there is no increase in vowel duration, and the partial loss of vocal cord vibration in the stop is phonetic in origin.

The phonetic argument rests on empirical data – the observed vocal cord vibration *after* the plosive closure – and invokes the aerodynamic facts surrounding so-called 'spontaneous voicing'. Thus, whereas the phonological solution needs to suppose that there are no phonological features rendered into the soundwave, the phonetic solution explains that in fact there is enough residual of the rendering of a phonological feature to trigger perceptual assignment of the intended category. In the TM model the perceptual procedure is assisted by the inclusion within perception of a *predictive speaker model* which enables the listener to understand the partial failure of vocal cord vibration as a *loss to the consonant*, not a gain to the vowel.

A possible counter-argument invokes the situation in languages like French where a final [d], along with other planned [+voice] consonants will *not* lose its vocal cord vibration, thus implying that vocal cord vibration failure is not universal. However, the argument becomes spurious when we invoke the *additional* cognitive intervention in the rendering process clearly apparent in such environments – not just in French, but in other languages including English in many environments.

Segments have intrinsic phonological length, which for English is perceptually binary – segments are either long or short – and intrinsic phonetic duration which is different for every segment. There are problems with establishing the intrinsic properties of phonetic segments; these are akin to the basic problem of trying to establish some kind of 'target' set of properties. Experimentally it is virtually impossible to determine target properties directly and even a kind of 'reverse engineering' or 'inverse filtering' would be enormously complex and completely outside our abilities at the moment. Such a technique would involve removing from a carefully observed output signal (articulatory or acoustic) the effects of:

- expressive content;
- over-arching prosody;
- local or segmental linguistic context determined by the production phonology;

- effects of cognitively derived intervention or supervision;
- motor control effects – including feedback, coordinative structure re-balancing if necessary, contextual co-production effects, external mechanical constraints hampering motor control;
- mechanical effects – predominantly coarticulatory effects induced by inertia.

Since there is not enough known about any of these effects to construct a computational model which could extract the original target from its surface manifestation there is no chance for the moment of reverse engineering. And in any case it is only a *reasonable guess* that the notion of underlying target is viable.

A general question might arise for phonetics research concerning how we might increase our understanding of all these effects. Here all we can do is invoke the standard methodology of the black box paradigm shown in the diagram. The problem is that to successfully model the processes in the black box we need to know at least the nature of the output (which we can in principle determine by careful experiments) and the nature of the input. We know very, very little about the input. Unfortunately this unbalanced approach almost removes the black box paradigm from our investigations; the most we can come up with is plausible and reasonable hypotheses as to what might constitute an input to the system, and hope that consistency of solution enables us to increase our confidence in the hypotheses to the point where we can be fairly sure that we know enough about the input.

| unknown, but amenable to hypothesis | dependent on knowledge of the input; a few known | surface effects knowable in principle; some known | surface effects largely known or knowable in principle |

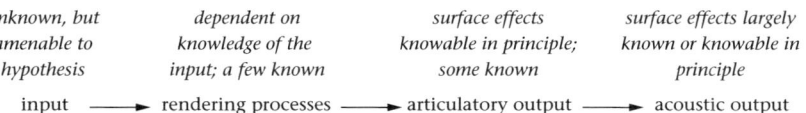

input ⟶ rendering processes ⟶ articulatory output ⟶ acoustic output

The intrinsic lengths and durations of segments, and other intrinsic properties, vary of course from language to language. Thus the surface $[i]_{French}$ in French *pipe* $[pip]_{French}$ is shorter than the surface $[i]_{English}$ in English *peep* $[pip]_{English}$. French vowels are said to be all intrinsically phonologically short, but there is clearly a durational hierarchy among them. There has also been a temptation among phonologists to allow French the vowel lengthening rule, though the explanation here is certainly the same as it is for English (see above). Some languages do, of course, have contrasting long and short versions of the 'same' vowel and sometimes of consonants (for example so-called geminate consonants).

There is a tendency for long vowels to become diphthongised. There is evidence, for example, that even in Metropolitan French vowels which are 'lengthened', say in words like *faire*, become diphthongised, and a pronunciation of this word as [fɛər]$_{French}$ is not unusual – and sometimes the process even extends to deleting the /r/. Diphthongisation occurs regularly in some French speakers in Canada.

The metrical organisation of speech

Phonological pause length might also provide linguistic information, and it certainly provides expressive content by interrupting a listener's prediction of prosodic flow or 'rhythm'. The insertion of pauses around non-function words and in other places is an expressive highlighting device. The metrical organisation of utterances – that is, *structured* temporal organisation in our terminology – involves perceived quality, length, loudness and pitch; these are rendered as spectral content, duration, intensity and fundamental frequency, but not on a one-to-one basis. All the features of prosody at the cognitive and physical levels seem to be involved in the metrical organisation. This could either be because

1. what happens in the temporal dimension influences what happens to these parameters – that is, the involvement is a coarticulatory consequence of the rendering mechanism; or
2. the rendering of temporal structure involves invoking these parameters as part of the process of turning the utterance plan into sound.

For 1 some researchers have postulated an independent clock to which speech events are locked in some way: we call this the *metronome hypothesis*. Such a clock would issue marker events at equal intervals, and the utterance would be timed according to groupings of such marks into larger units. This would mean that, whatever appears on the surface, there is an isochronic system underlying timing, and surface timing intervals can be measured in terms of this system's isochronic units.

For 2 we need some underlying timing plan which is not necessarily locked onto an independent clock – though it may *reference* a clock. Such a plan could include isochrony, but this is not a *sine qua non*.

In terms of our basic wrapper theory (Chapter 6) it would be necessary to establish where in the hierarchy the timing wrapper inserts. Call this the *planned timing hypothesis*.

In some sense the hypotheses are very little different. In 1 the emphasis is on the clock itself which might be seen as dominating the rhythm of speech, whereas in 2 a timing plan makes use of a clock, perhaps, by *fetching* timing rather than *fitting to* it. Notice that *timing* is structured time involving events which are not themselves part of that time. As an example we could mention another highlighting feature involving rendering, say, an important word or phrase at a different rate from the surrounding context: the timing manipulation invoked as a highlighting strategy makes sense only with reference to the timing fetched for the overall utterance context.

For some researchers (for example, Klatt 1979) there is neither an underlying clock not an underlying rhythm plan. Any apparent surface rhythm whether actual or perceived is the product of simply sequencing utterance elements. Regularities in timing observed at the surface (including the replication – like, for example, the fact that [e] regularly has less duration than, say, [ei]) are due to the cascade of intrinsic durations of segments modified by certain constraints. Among such constraints might be phrase or sentence final timing effects (progressively increasing duration of syllables), or within-syllable effects like the often cited (but see above) lengthening of vocalic nuclei if followed immediately by a phonological [+voice] segment.

But in the real world no segment exists divorced from a prosodic contour and adjacent segments in a string forming the utterance. The overall rate of delivery of the utterance affects the underlying intrinsic durations of segments. And segments are affected differentially. If, for example, a particular utterance is spoken rapidly not all segments are shortened in duration by the same proportion: vowels are generally shortened more than consonants. Double the rate of utterance and you do not halve the length of every segment in the utterance. Figure 5.2 shows the same utterance rendered at different rates of delivery.

Stressed syllables form the basis of rhythmic structure

Most writers relate rhythmic structure to the patterning of stressed and unstressed syllables in the language. The reference point for rhythmic units is the stressed syllable – with this beginning the unit,

146 *Speech Production Theory*

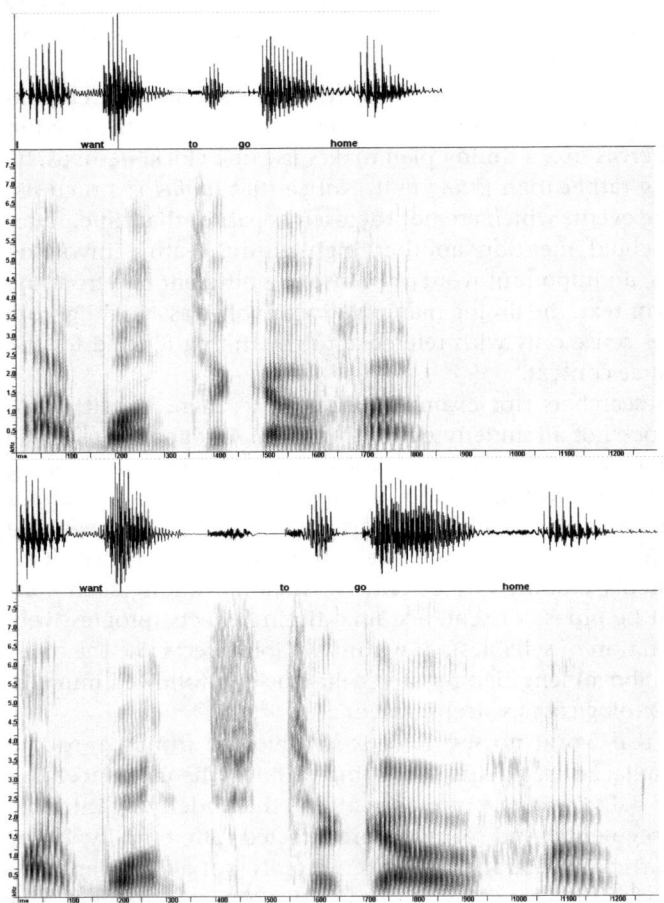

Figure 5.2 Waveforms and spectrograms of *I want to go home*, rendered fast and slow. Notice the unusual release of the final [t] of *want* in the slow version, and the way in which individual 'segments' are rendered differentially in the two versions.

with all unstressed syllables fitting in before the next stressed syllable begins the next rhythmic unit. We make a distinction in our theory between *foot* which is the planned unit of rhythm, and *rhythmic unit* which we reserve for the rendering (the articulation and the acoustic signal).

Using this definition of rhythmic elements we can say that isochrony is the basic speaker-intended or listener-perceived equal length from the start of one stressed syllable to the start of the next one. Researchers working on the acoustic signal usually measure the *duration* from the start of the phonetic stressed syllable to the start of the next. The phonetic stressed syllable 'corresponds' to the phonological stressed syllable.

In languages where it is claimed there is no linguistically determined length variation (either phonemic or phonetic) as in Metropolitan French, all syllables are equally stressed. We can apply the same definition: a foot takes in just one syllable, and the rhythmic unit also takes in the rendering of just one syllable. Thus such languages are just special cases of stress timing, but conceptually equivalent to the Classical Phonetics trend to classify these languages as different – *viz.* being *syllable timed:* syllable timing is stress timing where the foot or rhythmic unit consists invariably of just one segment. It is clear, though, that this concept is a little unrealistic, and in practice even speakers of metropolitan French show a rhythmic structure to their speech based on differential stressing, and certainly Canadian speakers very often do stress the initial syllable of polysyllabic words. If speakers of Metropolitan French stress differentially they tend to stress the *final* syllable of polysyllabic words. In all languages, though, these ideas are really about some notion of *ideal* expressionless speech, that is, speech which has no expression wrapper. In practice all speech is expression wrapped, and it may be the expression which is responsible for those stressing patterns – both in terms of duration and amplitude – which apparently depart from the usual isochronic characterisation in phonology/phonetics.

Isochrony – the elusive basis for rhythm

A large number of researchers have exhaustively measured the internal durational structure of speech waveforms, and come to the conclusion that they can find no isochrony – that is, no tendency for the rhythmic units which correlate with utterance plan feet to have equal durations. We should say at this point that we ourselves see little mystery surrounding the notion of isochrony – it is alive, robust and well in utterance plans and perceptual representations. Since it is a cognitively based phenomenon we would not expect it – like anything else in speech in the utterance plan – to have a unique linear correlate in the articulatory or acoustic worlds. We have drawn attention to the kinds of constraint on translating neat isochronic plans into a metronomically paced rhythm in the acoustic signal.

Ladefoged (1993) points out that the traditional description of rhythm based on stress patterns needs revision, particularly because catch-all statements like *French is a syllable timed language* are not strictly true. However, we have to be very careful whether we are talking about utterance plans – where the traditional descriptions are more likely to be true – or the rendering of these plans – where the surface results appear at first glance to contradict the traditional descriptions. One reason for this is that the traditional representations do not take into account either the fact that utterance plans are rendered within expressive wrappers and *cannot* be divorced in real life from these wrappers, or that the rendering process in general is non-linear. So despite even the most recent findings referred to by Ladefoged it still makes sense to have a level of description (the speaker's utterance plan and the listener's assigned representation) which can serve as a baseline to enable us to talk about both the general properties of the rendering process and the particular properties of expressive rendering in respect of the resultant soundwave. Again, we emphasise that the final soundwave is a complex composite structure which is the result of a significantly non-linear rendering process. We would certainly not expect to find all speaker/listener *feelings* about speech directly correlated in some unique feature of the soundwave.

There is no reason to suppose that wide variability and the transfer of correlation between features at different levels should be any different for prosodic features than for segmental features.

Declination

Declination can be modelled as a universal constraint on an utterance's fundamental frequency, whereas the local effects are constrained by phonological requirements: the intonational or fundamental frequency plan is executed under the constraint of a progressive fall. From the linguistic point of view it might be argued that declination can be ignored, and this would constitute a claim about perception: listeners also ignore it. The *perceived* fall at the end of sentences, etc., is therefore *not* declination but a local fall *fitted to* the declination wrapper – the combined effect perhaps being more noticeable. The generalised hierarchical rendering structure in TM for rendering the prosodic contour plan relating declination, expressive prosody, intonation and other linguistic prosodic features can be sketched in XML format (see Tatham and Morton 2004) thus:

```
<declination>
  <expression>
    <prosodic_contour_plan>
      <intonation/>
      <rhythm/>
      <sentence_stress/>
    </prosodic_contour_plan>
  </expression>
</declination>
```

This fragment of the structure does not permit a clear account, at this stage, of *how* the prosodic features interact to produce a final planned prosodic contour. However it does permit us to emphasise how universal declination dominates the rendering hierarchy. The prosodic features are rendered within the contour plan, in turn rendered within expressive content – the whole rendered within the constraint of declination. As mentioned above there is no reason to suppose that all declination will turn out to be identical, within the range of variability of the phenomenon, partly at least because like other universal prosodic and segmental constraints there is some scope for overcoming or enhancing the constraints by cognitive intervention during the rendering supervisory processes (Chapter 6).

Views on declination

For Ladd (1984) however declination is not an intrinsic phonetic phenomenon, but the result of phonological requirement or planning. He goes further and asserts that it would not be correct to model declination as a phonetic effect on which 'phonological pitch' is superimposed. This view contradicts our view expressed above. Some researchers argue that phonetics has a minimal or even *no* role here, and that declination is an entirely phonologically driven phenomenon. Obviously with two tiers behind the effect – a phonological one and a phonetic one – it could potentially be either; it needs empirical – that is, experimental – evidence to support the one or the other. However we must be careful in assigning the effect to phonology simply because it variable: to do so would fall into the same trap as those phoneticians who feel obliged to call coarticulation an intended phenomenon simply because it varies (*cf.* the Cognitive Phonetics explanation of the variability). It may be the case that declination is very similar (Tatham *et al.* 1998).

Prosodic Analysis

Firth's (1948 and other publications) approach to Prosodic Analysis focuses strictly on paradigmatic relationships within linguistic structure, sharply contrasting these with syntagmatic relationships. A syntagmatic approach highlights the contrastive play, for example, between phonemic and extrinsic allophonic segments; whereas a paradigmatic approach might highlight the more dynamic sequential objects or events in language. Classical phonetics and a great deal of contemporary descriptive phonetics focuses on segment objects at the expense of dynamic structure, or considers the two to be different kinds of object, perhaps to be modelled quite separately. Firth was keen to emphasise the theoretical advantages of focussing on the way features dynamically span sequences of segment objects. The use of the term dynamic here does not necessarily imply the introduction of real time, simply a shift to an attempt to characterise the nature of feature spanning, rather than how whole segments might exist in a strictly syntagmatic relationship.

Using a very simple example just for illustrative purposes and invoking a fragment of a traditional distinctive feature-like approach we might represent the phrase *cats and dogs* thus:

	k	æ	t	s	n̩	d	ɒ	g	z
consonantal	+	−	+	+	+	+	−	+	
vocalic	−	+	−	−	−	−	+	−	−
syllabic	−	+	−	−	+	−	+	−	−
plosive	+	−	+	−	+	+	−	+	−
fricative	−	−	−	+	−	−	−	−	+
nasal	−	−	−	−	+	−	−	−	−
voice	−	+	−	−	+	+	+	+	+

In the diagram we see a fragment of a traditional distinctive feature matrix, but with highlighted 'continuous' features spanning segment and even syllable and word boundaries. Even Distinctive Feature Theory (Jakobson *et al.* 1952) permits the observation that there is much to be revealed about the structure of utterances by focussing on the parallel spans of features rather than their segment-by-segment contribution to the makeup of individual phonological objects.

Prosodic features obviously span runs of segments, but within the segmental structure there is a feature structure hidden by the traditional object–symbol approach characterised, for example, by representations of the International Phonetic Alphabet type. The static segmental approach might tell us that it is important to recognise that we could develop (given enough data going beyond this fragment) generalisations like:

- there are different types of consonants;
- consonants are not also vowels;
- vowels are syllabic nuclei – are [+syllabic] in this usage of feature labels;
- occasionally some consonantal segments are [+syllabic];
- vowels are voiced;
- nasals are voiced, but other consonants need not be.

These generalisations are not necessarily good ones and they might be different given more data: they are simply an illustration of remarks which can be made about data presented in this way. And similarly, if we shift our focus away from the columns of the matrix and onto its rows and concentrate on the notional dynamic *flow* of featural properties we might observe that:

- vocalic zones are punctuated by consonantal zones;
- consonantal zones can span multiple segmental elements, but vocalic zones do not;
- there is a 'contour' of movement between [+syllabic] and [−syllabic] zones;
- voicing easily spans syllable zones – it is not an alternating feature tied to [+syllabic] zones.

Firth of course has not been the only theorist to bring the dynamic featural approach to the forefront of the descriptive modelling. In more recent times Browman and Goldstein's Articulatory Phonology (1986) sets out a model which rests on articulatory features and which includes both static (to represent phonology) and dynamic (to represent phonetics) characterisations of an utterance. They attempt to blur the conceptual boundaries between the static and dynamic properties of speech. Although the attempt is not perhaps as successful as might have been intended they do point one way toward an important and fresh re-appraisal of our approach to modelling speech production.

At roughly the same time Tatham and Morton (Tatham 1986, Morton 1986a,1986b) introduced their Cognitive Phonetics. In this model we see an attempt to capture both static processes and dynamic processes in an integrated approach which is in many ways different from that of

Browman and Goldstein. Tatham and Morton do not imply that phonology is basically static and phonetics dynamic, rather they emphasise that it is important to recognise both areas and to afford each both static and dynamic properties. The way these static and dynamic 'planes' interact is central to TM theory, and the model explicitly places segmental objects, events and processes *within* a hierarchically organised prosodic structure. One advantage of the approach is that it readily lends itself to modelling expressive content transparently.

Prosody and parametric modelling

Firth's Prosodic Analysis leads us straight to the perhaps striking observation that even in a simple, idealised model with binary values for the parallel features or parameters synchronicity is rarer than predicted by the sequenced whole segment approach which Classical Phonetics focuses on. Firth is concerned with horizontal division rather than vertical division of speech (articulation or the acoustic signal); for him it is much more important to recognise that the horizontal parameters unfold not necessarily entirely synchronised with each other. Classical Phonetics had emphasised the largely *cognitive* nature of the synchronicity of features when characterising speech segments, as indeed does modern phonology. Such an approach in phonology regards the segment as a 'simultaneous' object, itself having no beginning or ending (in the physical sense), let alone any of its component parameters.

We must be careful to avoid confusing Firth's emphasis on a parametric characterisation of speech which was explicitly designed to highlight the non-synchronous nature of segments, with the Prague School (Trubetskoy 1939) or Generative (Chomsky and Halle 1968, in its classical 'linear' guise) phonologies' emphasis on features as components of simultaneous segments. Despite our simple diagram above, the two are not directly comparable. The characterisation of segments in terms of features was intended to enable generalisation of behaviour within the segment sets, to show how by reason of their feature composition segments could fall into predictable classes and types of behaviour. Firth's parametric characterisation was intended to highlight continuity of parameter behaviour beyond segment boundaries and to emphasise the asynchronousness of segment behaviour at the feature level. His formulation succeeds admirably in this direction and modern attempts to capture the same approach – for example, Articulatory Phonology (Browman and Goldstein 1986), but there are others – pale somewhat in the light of Firth's Prosodic Analysis. One clear and obvious difference between Firth and others emphasising the parametric approach is Firth's overarching prosody – in TM terms, his prosodic wrapper.

The Prague School paved the way for the Generativists to focus on features as a sub-phonemic unit, but the approach is confined to the abstractions of phonology and is of little use at the phonetic level of utterance rendering. Aside from the fact that there is no clear pathway between phonology and phonetic rendering, the heaviest constraint on using the approach is in fact the overall approach itself, which is static in nature. Immediately a dynamic perspective is introduced the orientation *must*, we believe, explicitly following Firth, turn on a different axis – the horizontal rather than the vertical.

For Firth and others the dynamic element in speech is much more important than for the more traditional of phonologists – including the Generativists (who come after Firth, of course). Firth extends the dynamic element to include all parameters of speech from voicing to nasality to lip configuration to tongue height, and so on.

Traditionally we think of the prosodic features of stress, rhythm and intonation as being dynamic in the sense that they span segments, are 'suprasegmental'. But this is a misuse of the term *dynamic*. Traditionally phonology treats all aspects, including prosodics, as timeless abstract objects, and this treatment – their modelling – is static. Firth was able to treat temporal dynamic objects in the abstract. But it is a mistake to equate *abstract* with *static* as a *sine qua non:* physical objects can be characterised both statically and dynamically, as can cognitive objects. It just so happens that traditionally physical objects in phonetics are treated dynamically (for example, the modelling of coarticulation) and abstract objects in phonology are treated statically (for example, the modelling of assimilation). And importantly in this respect, Firth and the prosody school buck this approach. As we have observed, in modern times the most notable approaches to attempt this are the Articulatory Phonology model, and the Cognitive Phonetics model – both of which attempt to unify phonetics and phonology as a speech production model, and incorporate both static and dynamic perspectives in their theories.

Prosodic effects on segmental articulation

If prosody overarches or wraps segmental processes we would expect there to be prosodic effects on segmental articulation: prosody is dominant and the segmental articulation fits within this. We shall see that it is fairly clear that there is a hierarchical organisation to these effects, correlating with the prosodic hierarchy. We must be careful not to speak here of linear sequences of words within phrases or other syntactic groups, but continue to emphasise the hierarchical nature of the model.

The hypothesis thrown up by a model of hierarchically organised prosody is that segmental rendering will be constrained in agreement with the hierarchy. We shall see that in turn prosodically constrained segmental rendering provides cues to the perceiver's assignment of a prosodic structure to the heard acoustic. Another way of saying this is that by the mechanism of prosodic constraint on segmental rendering, each 'segment' (of whatever 'size') assigned to the acoustic signal conveys not just information about the identity of the segment, but also its place in the utterance's prosody. Some researchers into the prosodic effects on segments tend to stop here, but for TM, featural spanning of segments and how this is constrained may well be the major 'segmental' contributor to prosodic assignment.

Two characteristics of prosodic influence on segments are often cited:

1. *Strengthening* – often referred to as a tendency to resist target under- or over-shoot, and an increase in the segment's duration. In TM this is a feature of focused improvement in rendering – a managed tendency toward increased *precision* of articulation. The improvement is not *directed* since it is not part of the utterance plan, but it is cognitively *managed* since it has a role to plan in the overall stability of the utterance and the robustness of its contribution to the assignment of a successful perceptual 'solution'.
2. *Domain-final lengthening* – often referred to as durational increase toward the end of higher prosodic domains like intonational phrases. The syllable is given as the lowest prosodic domain (that is, syllables are the *units* of prosody), with sentences and sentence groupings like paragraphs as the highest.

A third, weaker characteristic of prosodic influence which has been noted in some speakers (see Fougeron and Keating 1997) is:

3. *Precision* improvement in vowels toward the end of the higher prosodic domains, increasing the precision distance between phonetic syllable endpoints (corresponding to their onset and coda consonants) and their vocalic nuclei. What is important here is that some speakers enhance the local syllabic contour. In the TM model this means that they in effect enhance 'focus' of phonetic syllables by increasing the difference between the boundary segments and the nuclear segments. The observation by Fougeron and Keating is

particularly important because it means that there can be differential variation in precision *within* the syllable with a very specific result: the throwing into relief of individual syllables within a string of syllables – in this case progressively within particular prosodic domains.

In TM *precision distance* refers to the difference between the precision achievement of two compared segments or other objects (prosodic, for example). Precision in any one object refers to the *range* over which it can retain significant functional robustness, running from full target rendering to minimal target rendering. *Precision range* and *precision distance* are two of the rendering parameters carefully managed by the Cognitive Phonetics Agent or CPA.

In the context of the TM model the CPA is responsible for supervising the phonetic rending process, and it is easy to see that the CPA can (and would want to) influence the precision of articulation of segments taking into account factors such as potential ambiguity. But the increase in precision noted by researchers in various prosodic contexts is not obviously for this reason. Emphasis and expression also call for increased precision, but once again, this is not particularly so in these cases. The interesting question is to what extent the claim that prosody is basically *responsible* for any increase in precision is valid for these contexts. General strengthening or precision increase takes place in

- accented syllables,
- at the end of some prosodic domains, and
- in vowels (more specifically) toward the end of some prosodic domains.

It looks as though it may be best to remove accented syllables from the usual grouping. A syllable is accented for stylistic or other reasons, but the other two cases are of a different type – they are incidental to such reasons of style or expressive content.

In the case of effects correlating with positions in prosodic domains we might ask whether it would be appropriate to think of the increase as a kind of coarticulatory function. To put this another way: we can appreciate that accented syllables are accented for a deliberate purpose – that is, this is an *extrinsic* phenomenon – but it is harder to think of the other two as other than a (managed) involuntary effect – an extrinsically controlled *intrinsic* phenomenon. It could be argued that the increase in precision is there simply to mark the domain boundaries in some way – though pausing and the intonation pattern are also doing this.

The basis of intonation modelling

Researchers are divided as to where intonation fits in speech production theory: Is intonation appropriately modelled as a phonetic or phonological phenomenon?

- a phonetic model will emphasise the dynamic aspect of the signal – especially its continuousness; but
- a phonological model, because of its cognitively-oriented symbolic basis, favours discreteness in the representation.

One or two researchers summarise the phonological/phonetic distinction in terms of the quantitative emphasis of phonetics and the qualitative emphasis of phonology. Carmichael (2003) has a comprehensive statement and evaluation of the two approaches. We summarise our understanding of her position as follows:

- *Phonetic models* of intonation provide an explanation of the intonational features of the acoustic signal – especially the fundamental frequency. Random variability is excluded, but all *systematic* variability introduced through physical constraints are included. But, since a phonetic model is based on *physical* features it cannot be expected that an explanation of *linguistic* features would be included. At best, such models explain the acoustic signal, given an appropriate linguistic characterisation as its input – the prosodic wrapper of the phonological utterance plan, in TM terminology. In principle it should be possible to reconstruct the acoustic signal (but without non-systematic variability) from the model's output.
- *Phonological models* may *consult* the acoustic signal, but only to prompt an immediate data reduction process for deriving a discrete symbolic representation. Because of its phonological nature such a model is of direct relevance to listeners and perception. Listeners assign phonological representations to acoustic signals, and it is for this reason that phonological models are often about the processes involved in this assignment. For speech production the focus is on prosodic interpretation of semantic, syntactic and pragmatic features to specify the *prosodic wrapper* for the utterance plan; in perception the focus is on the processes involved in assigning an appropriate symbolic representation to a waveform such that semantic, syntactic and pragmatic features can be processed.

The emphasis with phonological models is therefore on what is *linguistically* important, the underlying representation corresponding also to what is *perceptually* relevant.

- Phonological models tend to de-emphasise the actual signal itself and work on symbolic representations.
- Phonetic models emphasise the acoustic signal, explaining the movement of fundamental frequency through the utterance – but not, in a truly phonetic model, in terms of the linguistics of the utterance.
- Phonetic models de-emphasise the linguistic features which may underlie the signal.

Both phonological and phonetic models of intonation can be linearly oriented or hierarchically oriented, with linear models emphasising the surface context of events, and hierarchical models emphasising the underlying structure and the contexts revealed within it. However, it seems to us that most phonological and phonetic events are truly explained *only* in terms of an underlying structure which is more complex than any purely linear analysis could tell us.

Intonation in TM

The linguistically oriented model of prosody developed by Tatham and Morton (Morton *et al.* 1999, Tatham *et al.* 2000) insists on full computational adequacy (Tatham and Morton 2004) for such an important and complex area of speech production theory. The approach incorporates a phonological intonation model which is non-linear in nature, and in doing so pays special attention to the dependencies between symbolic representations and their physical renderings. One reason for this is that the model implements the principles of Cognitive Phonetics with respect to cognitive control of intrinsic phonetic or rendering phenomena, whether they are segmental or prosodic in origin. Another way of saying this is that the model recognises that there are some phonetic processes (distinct from phonological processes) which have true linguistic significance.

The model makes the claim, and is designed to capture it as a fundamental principle, that many of the physical processes involved in speech production are cognitively represented. For this reason the approach can be said to move forward research ideas by tying in with both the general acoustics and aerodynamics of an utterance. The model goes further than simply attempting a direct link between the phonological representation and the fundamental frequency contour, as did Pierrehumbert, for example (Pierrehumbert 1981). The general philosophy derives from Cognitive Phonetics and is summarised in Tatham *et al.* (1998):

> Our underlying principle is that in the human being there are physical processes intrinsic to the overall speech mechanism, and that some

of these processes are open to cognitive representation – such that they are able to enter the domain of language processing. (p. 1)

The TM model claims that the relationship between production and perception involves knowledge of *both* components within *each* component, and consequently there is a clear path toward explicitly relating variation in the soundwave with the cognitive representations and processes involved in both production *and* perception. The model *requires* that a linguistically relevant acoustic event (including those variations which are linguistically relevant) be explicitly identified in both production *and* perception. A corollary of this is that any two linguistically distinct phenomena (prosodic or segmental) have to be reliably and consistently produced and perceived as equally distinct. The overall claim is that our strict adherence to the correspondence between cognitive and physical phenomena points toward a *phonological* model for prosody, but one which consistently and transparently explains phonetic outcomes. We claim this is a fundamental requirement for prosody models.

Units in TM intonation

In the TM intonation model – implemented in SPRUCE (Tatham and Lewis 1992, Tatham and Morton 2005), our computational model of speech production – we mark lexical stress, sentence and phrase boundaries, and focus. Intonation is dependent on the syntactic structure of sentences within the text: this accords with most models of intonation, even though we are concerned with fitting sentences to a prosodic wrapper, not the other way round. The following are marked:

- sentence and intonational phrase boundaries – marked H (high) and L (low).
- smaller domains, syntactic phrases, are defined within intonational phrases – marked T+ (turn-up) and T− (turn-down).
- lexical stress for each syllable – marked S (stressed) and U (unstressed)
- sentence focus – marked F (focus) on a single syllable

F is a device for introducing simple modifications to an otherwise neutral intonation. In our description here we bring this out to indicate the basis of the mechanism for varying intonation for expressive and other effects – though, clearly, this single example marker would not be sufficient (see Tatham and Morton 2004). Although F is tied to a particular syllable in the SPRUCE implementation, it constitutes in principle an element within the generalised prosodic wrapper. Early versions of the TM model wrongly equated S and U with the H and L tones to be found in ToBI (Silverman *et al.* 1992) – see below. ToBI uses H and L to characterise *pitch accent*, whereas TM use S and U as markers of *lexical stress*.

long-term processes	H	high intonational phrase boundary
	L	low intonational phrase boundary
mid-term processes	T+	turn-up of pitch
	T−	turn-down of pitch
lexical markers	S	stressed syllable
	U	unstressed syllable
modifier	F	overlays pitch accent and expressive content

TM recognises in the model three *types of process* derived from the Theory of Cognitive Phonetics:

1. Linguistically irrelevant *incidental processes*: these have mechanical or aerodynamic sources and do not contribute information to prosody. They are independent of language, and for that reason can contain no linguistic information. However, although often considered to introduce noise into the system they are *perceptually* relevant because, while not linguistically systematic, they are nevertheless expected by the listener. They contribute to cueing that the speech is human and have some place in a generalised model of perception. Examples are breathing and other aerodynamic or mechanical processes associated with the overall mechanism involved in speech production.
2. *Phonetic processes* intrinsic to the rendering system and which can be manipulated under cognitive control. This is the process widely known in biopsychology as 'cognitive intervention', in which somatic processes can be cognitively altered. In TM the intervention process is handled by a dedicated agent – the Cognitive Phonetics Agent, of CPA. Although intervention takes place at the phonetic level it is nevertheless phonologically relevant; and in the production of an utterance such processes are carefully monitored and supervised by the CPA. Cognitive intervention is a managed or supervised process played out across the entire utterance scenario, including both prosodic and segmental rendering (Chapter 6 has the details).
3. *Phonological processes* extrinsic to the rendering system; these are deliberately manipulated and produce phonologically relevant effects. Although cognitively sourced and not subject to the kind of

biological constraints expected of phonetic processes these processes are still monitored and supervised in the production of an utterance.

The TM computational intonation model derived from our approach to prosodic theory has a tiered hierarchical structure reflecting long-, mid- and short-term information:

tier	information source
long-term	sub-glottal air pressure progressive fall – a *linguistically irrelevant* process – assumed to give a progressive fall in fundamental frequency
mid-term	intrinsic rendering process responsible for controlling the changes of air pressure, increasing or decreasing fundamental frequency (turn-up and turn-down)
short-term	manipulation of vocal cord tension, giving rise to local changes in fundamental freqency

The computational implementation of the prosodic model in TM focuses on:

- a philosophy of integration of phonetic, linguistic and computational elements;
- the establishing of detailed and explicit relationships between physical and linguistic representations – this contrasts with most models which focus on linguistic representations;
- an entirely knowledge based approach focussing sharply on the explicit manipulation of tiered data structures;
- extensibility directed toward incorporating variability, pragmatic and expressive effects (*Tatham and Morton* 2004).

The ToBI (tones and break indices) model

ToBI (Silverman *et al*. 1992) is an intonation model offering a *highly abstract* markup of text or waveforms to indicate linguistically relevant features of prosody. The model is fairly explicit, and rests on a number of criteria – it is to be

- a characterisation of *phonological intonation*, rather than its physical correlates; and so for this reason
- a *symbolic representation* of what *underlies* the acoustic signal, explicitly *not* a symbolic representation of the signal itself;

- in the spirit of linguistics – that is, it should represent distinctive information of a symbolic nature rather than any automatically detectable physical parameters.

Note the emphasis on a highly abstract characterisation of intonation, and the explicit rejection of the physical signal as the object of description. This does *not* mean that analysis cannot take place with the signal in mind; what it does mean is that the analysis is *not* of the signal itself. This is a very important point because there have been researchers who have attempted to apply ToBI directly to the acoustic signal.

A consequence of the explicit strategy for ToBI is that its characterisation of the intonation of an utterance has *then* to be properly rendered as the specification for the associated acoustics. In summary, the ToBI model is

- abstract, and high level,
- the result of analysis,
- requires a low level rendering.

However, because of the *distinctiveness constraint* it is not guaranteed that sufficient detail can be marked to avoid re-interpreting the markup before normal phonetic rendering processes are applied. Another way of saying this is that there is the probability that not all necessary phonological information is recorded in the markup.

Details of the ToBI model

ToBI is a high level or phonological prosodic model stemming originally from many of the principles of autosegmental phonology (Goldsmith 1990). An intonation contour specifies a strictly *linear* concatenation of what are called 'pitch events'. Thus ToBI characterises intonational data structures from a *surface* perspective. Occasionally there is reference to levels, but *formally the model is linear*. In this section we comment on some of our understanding of ToBI properties as intended, and also as assumed by users – there is sometimes a mismatch.

1. *Global* intonational contours spanning stretches of speech are described in terms of the pattern built up by local events or *local* patterns of a string of events. The continuous global event – the utterance intonation contour – is the outcome of interpolating local events. The word *continuous* is our way of expressing the internal integrity of the string of symbols assembled during a ToBI analysis.

This internal integrity is captured by the *explicit surface patterning* within the string, without recourse to any hierarchically organised underlying data structure.
2. Local pitch events, such as pitch accent tones and boundary tones, are regarded as 'targets' along the global contour. Compare this to an alternative and quite common approach where a global intonation contour is taken as a movement of fundamental frequency interpolated between identified points along the way.
3. Local pitch events, characterised by ToBI high level symbolic representations are, it is claimed, able to be linked with actual physical events. The problem is that it is theoretically *impossible* to link certain aspects of a time-governed physical signal with a timeless static characterisation. Loosely delimited stretches of signal can at best be *associated* with ToBI's abstract symbolic characterisation. This is not a criticism of ToBI which is truly in the spirit of phonological prosody; it is, however, a general warning against trying to identify temporal events in abstract representations derived in the spirit of linguistics – ToBI cannot really be pushed this far.
4. Although considered an analysis tool (that is, the symbolic representations are derived from the actual physical events), ToBI markup is often considered by researchers to be adequate for representing projected utterance fundamental frequency contours for, say, speech synthesis (chapter 10, Tatham and Morton 2005). Applied this way the most that could be expected is a smoothed or idealised *exemplar* physical contour, but *not* an adequate example of a contour which might really have been produced by a human being. The theoretical assertion rests on the fact that ToBI involves a lossy reductionist approach which *denies* the possibility of accurate reconstruction. There is a strong parallel here with attempts to produce utterance plans wholly from a static phonology: at best all that can be produced is an idealised exemplar plan bearing only a symbolic relationship to what actually does happen in the physical world. This is a serious point, and one that is frequently missed.

ToBI is useful as a simple characterisation of *phonological* intonation. How this related to phonetic prosody is not the business of the model *per se*. Although ToBI markup of a soundwave is based on some rules, they are probably not explicit enough to make for the reliable and unambiguous symbolic characterisations that might be required in any attempt to assemble a formal linguistic model of speech perception intended to be applied in a simulation for automatic speech recognition

(Chapter 10) – the system designed for human transcribers of an existing soundwave. Because of the lossy nature of symbolic representations of this nature, recovery of fundamental frequency contours from a ToBI markup is at best dubious, though might constitute an unintended and therefore unfair use of the system. At worst ToBI does rely to a certain extent on the transcriber's *tacit*, or inexplicit, knowledge of the relationship between soundwave and cognitive representation, making this a *hybrid system:* part objective and part subjective. To this extent ToBI markup of a soundwave is very similar to an IPA transcription – insufficiently defined, on mixed levels and too lossy to be of any real use for reconstruction purposes. This would *not* be a criticism of either ToBI or of the IPA if it were the case that the loss-inducing algorithm were fully explicit: but, unfortunately, it is not. The diagram shows the main problem areas:

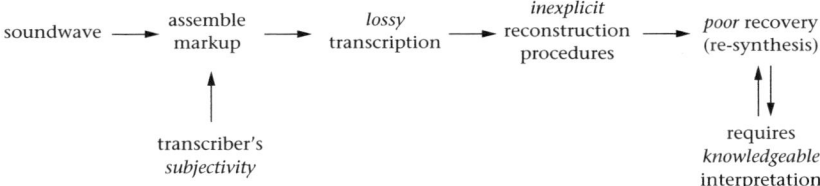

Part II
Speech Perception Theory

6
Dynamic Model Building and Expressive Content

Introduction

Models are abstract characterisations of some real world collection of events (which may well be a principled subset of the complete collection) which attempts, on the one hand to explain what has been observed (with recourse to external influencing factors), and on the other hand to predict future occurrences of similar events (Feynman 1995).

What levels of representation are necessary?

Researchers have raised the question whether we can move directly from a symbolic representation of linguistic objects to an acoustic representation, or whether we need an intermediary representation which is articulatorily based. In addition: Do we need a level of motor commands between the symbolic representation and an articulatory representation? Thus

symbolic representation ⟶ motor commands ⟶ articulations ⟶ acoustic signal

Cooper (1966) feels that the relationship between linguistic units or symbolic representations and motor commands is straightforward enough to be handled by a simple lookup table 'that would contain as few entries as there are phonemes' (p. 7). This is not correct because it does not make provision for phonological and surface underlying representations. The object set at the surface (the set of extrinsic allophones derived by phonological rule) is larger than the underlying object set (the set of minimally contrastive 'phonemes' – a misuse of the term). We feel that the relationships between symbolic representations and motor commands, and between motor commands and articulator movement are by no means as simple as implied by Cooper.

Modelling and the physical world

We are able to make observations about the output of speech production – the articulations and acoustic signals in the physical world – using the experimental techniques of the physical sciences, but we cannot characterise the input to the speech production process in the same way. If for example we hypothesise that the *symbolic* representation of the phonological utterance plan (the output of a production phonology) forms the input to speech production, we cannot perform experiments on it which are in any way comparable to the experiments we can perform on the output. There may be techniques developed in psychology which can be used (psychology because that is the wider domain within which phonology sits), but this abstract domain is not one which can be compared with any certainty to the output domain of the physical world. Linking the two domains in some kind of explanatory model therefore becomes problematical since the certainty of the two objects which this model links are out of balance. The paradigm only really works entirely satisfactorily if the two domains are graspable with equal certainty. Empirical data in phonology is not the same kind of thing as empirical data in acoustics: linking them is therefore, at the very least, difficult. A diagram illustrates the point:

input (unknown) ⟶ linking model (speech production) ⟶ output (knowable)

where the output is *knowable in principle* by empirical investigation, and the input is *unknown in physical terms*.

Some researchers have pointed out that we have at present only hypotheses as to the input units. But the situation is actually worse that this: we don't actually know that there *are* 'units' of speech to get to know. In any case this knowledge would constitute knowledge of an abstraction, which we can only reveal with techniques developed to access cognitive objects and processes. These techniques are not suspect here; what *is* suspect though is how, in the field of speech production studies, we can link these to the way we access physical processes. This problem is not unique, of course, to speech studies: it applies to all aspects of the study of human behaviour where we are able to access some physical output. What guides us in dancing, for example? Or in handwriting? Or in flying an aircraft? Or in the rapid hand movements required to play a fast-moving computer game?

Linguists have proposed units for their models, and these are units developed in linguistics for the analytical description of

1. observed output data (the written or spoken utterance, as in a phonetic transcription or a traditional pre-Chomskyian syntactic analysis), or
2. the hierarchical structure underlying the *potential* for output data (as in a Chomskyian phonological or syntactic analysis).

There is an interesting sense in which prosodic aspects are less problematical, perhaps because they seem to have a more direct relationship to objects or events in the physical world. But this says no more than that speech 'units' are whatever abstract units suit the purpose to hand. An important point to make is that, given the right experimental technique in psychology, it would be possible to assess the psychological reality of such units. For example, it is likely that there is a credible psychological reality for units such as syllable and phoneme, but a less credible psychological reality to units such as demisyllable or diphone, units sometimes adopted in speech technology.

Requirements of the model – feedback

Feedback has been observed to play a role in speech production, and so is one of the properties which need to be accounted for. There are three feedback loops which seem to play a role in speech production. This is usually demonstrated by experiments which inhibit the loop in some way to observe the production behaviour under conditions which deny feedback.

1. *Auditory feedback* – the loop takes in the acoustic signal made available *via* the air pathway between mainly mouth and ear or bone conduction *via* the mandible, and hearing – the peripheral physical processes of detection and analysis of the acoustic signal, as well as the transmission of the analysed signal to the auditory cortex along the auditory nerve. Suitable analysis also derives a time dimension from this signal. The cognitive interpretation of the signal, and subsequent cognitive evaluation of the results to provide a decision about adjustment of motor control *via* the normal pathways are also included. The loop can be regarded as being comparatively slow in round trip operation and may be appropriate for stabilising the

production of speech dynamics or prosodics. The diagram below illustrates the relatively slow acoustic feedback loop.

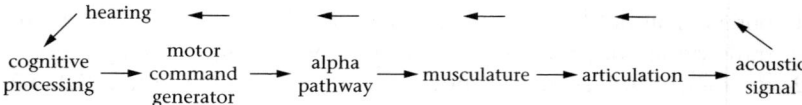

2. *Tactile feedback* – the loop takes in the detection of pressures within the vocal tract using arrays of pressure sensors on its inner walls and the tongue. These pressures may be slight (for example, the pressure of the air in the vocal tract), or involve the pressure of slight or heavy touch between two articulators. Timing can also be deduced from this signal at the cognitive level. The signal is relayed *via* sensory nerves to the brain and is at some stage appropriately cognitively processed to derive relevant information about the success of speech production, with a subsequent appropriate adjustment to motor control if called for. The loop can be regarded as being of medium speed and may be appropriate for stabilising the production of syllable-sized objects. The diagram illustrates the medium speed tactile feedback loop.

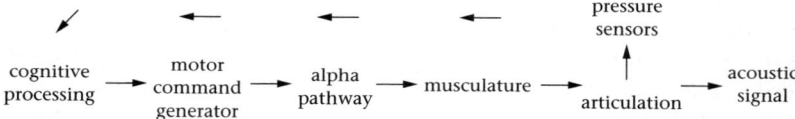

3. *Intramuscular feedback* – the loop begins with the detection of the rate of muscle stretch by muscle spindles (dedicated fibres within the muscles), basically signalling muscular deformation rates. The signal is conveyed to the spinal cord by the gamma neural pathway, there dividing into two separate channels. The more significant of these channels involves amplification of the signal at the spinal cord and its return *via* the alpha neural pathway back to the originating muscle, its regular muscle fibres and also into the particular coordinative structure network(s) in which the muscle plays a role. This loop is comparatively fast and capable of a contractile effect within the originating muscle which can counteract the detected stretch. The loop is designated 'reflex', involving no central cognitive intervention. The second channel the gamma signal takes when it divides at the spinal cord returns the signal to the brain for cognitive evaluation and, if necessary, cognitively originated motor action, or potentially re-setting of the thresholds within the gamma loop. The additional

transmission distances, cognitive processing and neuro-motor computations involved take the timing of this branch of the intramuscular feedback loop into the medium range, not dissimilar to that of the tactile feedback loop. The diagram illustrates the double pathway intramuscular feedback loops – fast and medium speed.

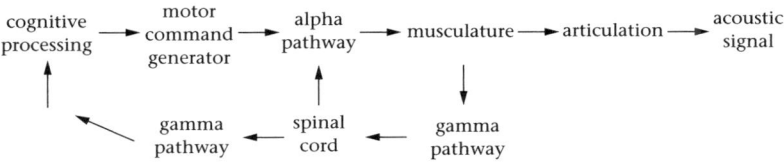

The speech production model

Whatever the actual objects or units of control (the muscle fibres, etc.) the *articulator* is the unit which seems to make most sense linguistically. At least one reason for this is the fact that speaker/listeners can discuss articulators: in contrast, they cannot discuss the musculature or neural signals. Although speakers are not entirely aware what they do with their tongues for example they at least know, without being taught, that the tongue is involved in speech. They cannot, however, discuss its precise positioning. There are some articulator details which are not discussable: the use of the vocal cords or velum, for example. Articulators make sense as the units also within the domain of psychology: their potential discussability means that they have some basis of 'reality' within the mind. Since linguistic processes are also cognitively based, it makes sense to relate the physical aspects of speech production to linguistic aspects *via* these common units. Articulators make sense as objects for our speech models at both the physical *and* cognitive levels.

Another physiological reason for making the articulators a pivotal mechanism in speech production theory is that they represent objects whose internal muscular 'structure' falls neatly into the coordinative structure basis of motor control (Chapter 4). Here we define a coordinative structure as a network of muscles which are capable of inter-communication and, based on this 'messaging', constitute a self-organising unit which enters into the overall motor control system as a directly controllable grouping. In the theory we have to regard the label attached to such a group as an abstract object. Thus if the tongue musculature is modelled as such a grouping (or group of sub-groups since some regard the tongue tip and root as independently controllable) then in some sense the tongue becomes an *abstract* object. Some researchers find this hard to incorporate into their theories because clearly the tongue can be seen and touched – it is hardly abstract for them. But functionally it can be regarded as abstract because its movement can only be directly influenced by accessing the muscular system 'within' it. In practice, once this idea is clear the duality of articulator status actually becomes very useful within the theory. In this section we have used the musculature of the tongue as our example, but of course there are several such structures involved in speech, and indeed there are significant *groupings* of such structures to obtain coordination – for example, the tongue-jaw linkage which can and does influence tongue positioning. The tongue height parameter of vowels is achieved by both tongue movement *and* jaw movement. Such groupings are referred to as *nested*.

What remains to consider in an articulator model is to what extent articulator objects are independently controllable. Phoneticians generally accept that they *are* independently controllable in general terms, but there may be many details of unavoidable interaction. For example, whether the jaw is already fully or partially open will influence the detail of how the lips are to be recruited for rounding, spreading and closure. The approach we take (with little or no experimental evidence) is that there is an independence of these lip movements as described and the jaw positioning as described, but that achieving the result is down to the stabilising and self-organising properties of the coordinative structures system. Thus the 'command' may be to the lip musculature for closure, and to the jaw musculature for half closure, how this actually pans out in terms of the detail of the contraction of the individual muscles is not the concern of the overall control, but of the *self-organising lower level system*. For now, we assume that it makes sense to call for lip closure with no high level concern for how this is to be achieved – it is a callable function *because* it has been found to be relatively independently usable.

Cognition develops models of speech processes

In TM theory we go a little further. The higher level cognitive processes involved in speech production are working on abstract *models* of relevant or significant parts of the low level systems. Several times in this book we refer to the human cognitive system as building and using models: for example, we feel that some speech behaviour can only be explained by assuming that the production rendering processes have access to an internal *model* of speech perception. The actual relationship between the model and the physical structure it represents is an important part of the motor control system and how we are to theorise about it. So that when a speaker wants to move the tongue upward this is modelled at a high level (monitored and corrected) before commands are issued to the lower self-organising system which will (perhaps slightly imperfectly) take care of a physical *reflection* of the abstractly *modelled* version.

Planes

Central to our speech production/perception model is the concept of 'planes'. There are two planes: the *static* and the *dynamic*. The concept enables us to separate out the knowledge base used in speech production/perception from the processes used to produce actual utterances.

Thus the static plane declares everything necessary to develop all possible utterance plans for all possible sentences in the language. In this case 'everything necessary' means the entire knowledge base on which the language depends. Although the information on the plane is held in *declarative* form, it could in principle be 'run' to output a phonetic rendering of all sentences in the language (an infinite set), or more realistically to produce particular idealised *exemplar* utterances. These are not actual utterances, but examples of what such utterances might look like, *all things being equal* – that is, as idealisations. There is no place here for variable factors such as expression and emotion, no place for violating rules and principles, no place for any of the variability associated with utterance rendering or idiosyncratic choices: the static plane is about *the language*, and only to the extent of generalising all possibilities does it reflect any actual utterances a speaker might produce. What the static plane does not house are sets of procedures for making specific selections from within all the conditions and options available.

The dynamic plane on the other hand is fundamentally *procedural* in nature. It houses the sets of procedures necessary for making selections from what is available on the static plane in order to produced *specific* utterances or instantiations of utterances. The dynamic plane is where the speaker/listener is modelled as a user of the language's knowledge base as declared on the static plane. One of the functions of the dynamic plane is to produce particular utterances within the general context of pragmatic and other constraints. Moving to the specific area of speech production, we could say that the requirement to speak a particular sentence depends on accessing the declared phonological and phonetic processes, but also on the nature of the 'wrappers' (Tatham and Morton 2004) being input to the dynamic plane.

The diagram shows the general linguistics model:

Static Plane [declarative]	Dynamic Plane [procedural]
a. general structure of the language – its grammar	a. shows how a specific structure is selected
b. all conditions and options for making choices within the grammar	b. selects conditions to enable specific choices
c. declares all possible occurring outputs, especially exemplar outputs	c. declares one specific output

In the diagram we show three levels arranged in pairs: under a. the static plane declares the grammar of the language (including the phonological and phonetic grammars – generalised declarations of what is possible). The dynamic plane enumerates procedures for selecting particular declarations and applying them to a specific case. Under b. the static plane declares conditions and options for making choices, but no indication of how these choices are to be made; this is the job of procedures on the dynamic plane. Finally c. on the final level is a declaration in principle all possible utterances – the putative output of 'running' the knowledge base, whereas on the dynamic plane a single specific utterance is output. In speech production this single output is produced by

- noting a-linguistic conditions derived from pragmatic (see below) and other considerations: these will be used to wrap the utterance output;
- taking in a single input sentence to be spoken, developing it into a specific utterance plan, and rendering it within the given wrappers.

Details of the speech production model

There are two static planes and two dynamic planes within the speech production model, one pair for phonological processes and one for phonetic rendering processes. Figure 6.1 shows the overall model.

Notice in the figure that the four planes are each contained within prosodic wrappers, or perhaps within a single overriding prosodic wrapper. This is because all segmental processes are carried out within prosody: prosody dominates phonological and phonetic structures and processing. In our terminology prosody wraps all speech production, and phonological processing and phonetic rendering are subordinate. Utterances are planned and rendered within the prosodic wrapper. Almost all traditional models have the relationship round the other

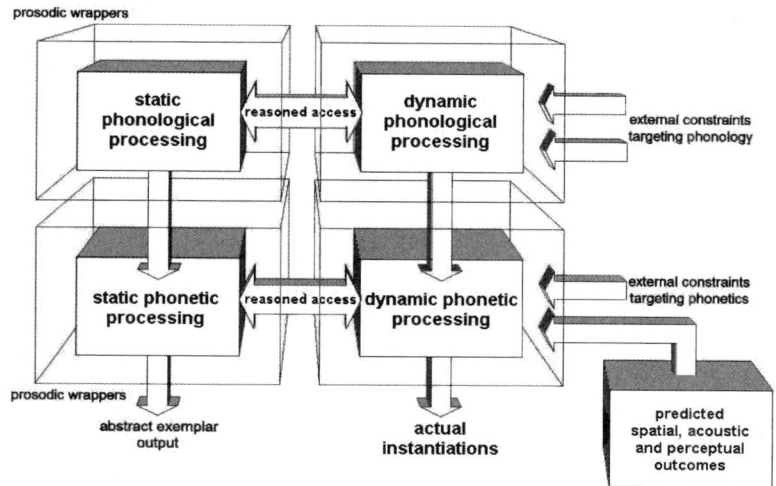

Figure 6.1 The *planes/wrapper model* in outline. Notice the abstract exemplar output from static processing and the actual instantiations output from dynamic processing. Notice how dynamic processing is constrained from external sources, and in particular how dynamic phonetic processing is constrained by the predictions of spatial, acoustic and perceptual outcomes of dynamic rendering (adapted from Tatham and Morton 2005).

way: phonological 'contours' are fitted to specific utterances (see Cruttenden 2001 for the Classical Phonetics view, and Silverman *et al.* 1992 for the ToBI view which is typical of contemporary approaches). The early and inspirational exception to the traditional approach and to which we have already referred (Chapter 5) can be found in Firth (1948 and other papers) where prosody is seen as dominant from an analysis perspective.

To the left of Figure 6.1 we find static phonology and phonetics, within their prosodic wrappers. These declare the entire phonological and phonetic knowledge bases, which can derive if necessary an abstract exemplar output useful for 'checking' the grammar and providing idealised examples of what the phonology and phonetics are capable of. In particular this is useful for enumerating examples of utterance plans (output from phonology), and how they might be rendered in an world devoid of pragmatic content. Classical Phonetics is in general found within this static, idealised world – it is about describing the possibilities for pronouncing a language. Generative Phonology and formal computational rendering models of the kind found in speech synthesis

(Chapter 10, and Tatham and Morton 2005) also locate within this static world. This is why 'running' Classical Phonetics fails to derive or explain much of the variation in real speech, and why speech synthesisers tend to output only exemplar utterances devoid of variation and expression.

To the right of Figure 6.1 we find the dynamic phonological and phonetic planes. Dynamic phonology assigns an utterance plan to a specific sentence produced earlier by the system; it does this within its prosodic wrapper. The procedures on the dynamic plane enable access to the corresponding static plane for the purposes of developing the utterance plan for this sentence. But notice that the processes have further inputs (to the far right) which convey external constraints – that is, constraints which are not strictly linguistic in origin. These constraints emanate, for example, from a pragmatic 'component' and other sources of expressive content. They constrain the dynamic procedures both prosodically and segmentally. For example, it might have been determined that a sentence is to be spoken with an attitude of authority or argumentatively: the phonological procedures develop the prosody and segmental content of the utterance *within these constraints* – technically, they are wrapped by them.

The output of dynamic phonology is a specific utterance plan wrapped in an appropriate prosodic wrapper which is now specific to any external constraints. In a sense this utterance plan is one of the infinite set which the knowledge base on the static plane characterises, but it has been arrived at by using only *specific* areas of the knowledge base and within the wrapper constraints.

The specific utterance plan passes to the dynamic phonetic procedures for rendering – producing the actual articulations and soundwaves for this utterance. Here again we find input channels bringing externally derived constraints specific to phonetic rendering. These might range from general environmental conditions, through to biologically derived constraints such as the general somatic tensing experienced by an angry speaker. These constraints bear on the phonetic segmental and prosodic rendering processes to produce speech with expressive content as well as linguistic content.

Supervision

A principal proposal in TM is the *Cognitive Phonetics Agent* (Tatham 1995, Tatham and Morton 2003), following the more general use of the term 'agent' in other fields (Garland and Alterman 2004, Luck *et al.* 2004). The CPA is a cognitive object which is designed to oversee and supervise phonetic rendering; for this purpose it is constantly polling rendering activity. Thus the CPA monitors, reasons about its findings and effects modifications of the speech output, depending on changes in context, *including the behaviour of listeners*. We believe strongly that phonetic rendering does not proceed 'blind' or in any sense automatically. Evidence from contextual variations in speech – ranging from constraints on intrinsic coarticulatory processes to subtle mood-induced variations in prosody – leads us to believe that logically posterior to the finalisation of an utterance plan its rendering is carefully managed to produce an optimum output. The output is optimised for promoting correct listener assignment of symbolic representations to the soundwave. The CPA, we claim, controls, organises, takes into account the limits of what can be done, instructs the system to modify constraints on the speech production mechanism – integrating with other information such as feedback from the listener's reaction to speech, or to the speaker's reaction to the listener's reaction in a conversation. All of this, of course, focuses on the phonetic dynamic plane. The CPA supervisory setup is analogous to a conductor's management of an orchestra's interpretation of an abstract printed musical score (in speech: the utterance plan): the conductor coordinates the musician's interpretation, guiding the way expression (in speech: pragmatic factors) is handled in terms of musical dynamics (in speech: prosody). The parallel is not, of course, exact, but the analogy is useful.

The CPA is responsible for organising the timing of inputs from various externally-derived information channels which call for specific phonological or phonetic effects associated with each utterance. It is clear in TM theory that failure to do so would destroy the coherence and integrity of a speaker's output, leading ultimately to perceptual disintegration. Immediate requirements can be met by repeatedly renewing requests to the dynamic phonology (and later the dynamic phonetics) to re-select from among the choices characterised on the corresponding *static* planes. Such renewed requests are, in our model, under the direction of the CPA.

In this role the CPA needs access to a timing device. Ivry *et al.* (2001) consider that one function of the *cerebellum* is that it operates as an internal clock. Its hypothesised role is the ability of the human to produce repetitive movements under voluntary control:

> Based on neurophysiological, behavior, and computational evidence, a number of theorists have emphasized a central role for the cerebellum in controlling the temporal aspects of movement. (p. 190)

They elaborate:

> ... the evidence strongly suggests a specialized role for the cerebellum in representing the temporal relationship between events in the milliseconds range. (p. 192)

Part of the CPA's task is to monitor the way phonological prosodic information is included in the plan, and also how phonetic prosodic rendering is carried out. In Tatham and Morton (2004) we proposed that expressive or emotive content should be encoded into the prosodics – the cognitive expressive content into phonological prosodics and the basic biological emotion apparent in the *state* of the physical system. The separation of cognitive and physical aspects here is deliberate, and is compatible, we believe, with current thinking in biopsychology.

Overall the task of the CPA is to monitor the physical system, and see that the utterance plan is carried out appropriately by phonetic rendering within the constraints of the various wrappers. But importantly the CPA is also monitoring how a generalised perceptual system might deal with the putative output, with a view to optimising the equation between production and perception. Another way of saying this is that the CPA has access to a running predictive model of speech perception which is trialling the *projected* output of the rendering processes. A re-entrant iterative system stabilises the acoustic output to a form predicted to be acceptable for perceptual purposes, given the utterance plan, expressive content requirements, ambient environment and other internal and external constraints.

The CPA will also track *actual* perception by observing the behaviour of listeners. There are bound to be imperfections in phonetic rendering, but many of these will be repaired by error correction procedures which are part of the perceptual process. The CPA will predict error correction, and observe when it fails, backtracking to improve rendering quality on a continuous basis if necessary.

This approach to modelling the speech production processes is relatively novel and attempts to characterise much of speaker/listener behaviour observed in the production and perception of speech as a *dynamic* event. It is fully explanatory in concept, and goes far beyond the static idealised descriptive models of earlier phonetics. It also reconciles the difficulties of explaining whether coarticulation is a voluntary or involuntary feature of speech: it is an intrinsic phenomenon whose manifestation is carefully managed to optimise the relationship between speaker and listener. More on the general theory can be found on www.morton-tatham.co.uk.

Predictive modelling – anticipatory cognitive processing

Cognitive Phonetics incorporates a device which can be defined as an *anticipatory system*. An anticipatory system is mathematically modelled in Rosen (1985) as

> ... a system containing a predictive model of itself and/or its environment, which allows it to change state at an instant in accord with the model's prediction pertaining to a later instant. (p. 72)

Such a system employs predictions in a 'feed-forward mode' to control events in the present. The CPA needs feedback from the listener, but also feed-forward to enable tuning of the physical system for the appropriate response. The CPA

- dynamically changes the physical settings of the current speech mechanism, and
- needs to predict short term events in order to fine tune the physical structures at the pre-motor stage.

Expressive content in speech production

Ideal speech communication occurs when the complete message is intended and known to the speaker. The speaker is able to convey the message, and the listener understands the intended message and provides feedback to the speaker that the message has been correctly received.

This assumes that the speaker

- knows what they think they are conveying;
- has a model of what the listener may feel on receiving the message

and that the listener

- can detect the entire message;
- has a model of the speaker's intended (and received) message.

But the *speaker* may be wrong on at least three counts, by being

1. unaware of conveying an attitude different from the one being attempted;

2. wrong about what the listener is feeling either about the attitude they are aware of in themselves, or of the attitude(s) they are *not* aware of conveying but one the listener *detects*;
3. unaware of an attitude the listener detects but which is not there, either revealed or concealed by the speaker.

The listener may be wrong as well by not

1. detecting the intended (revealed) attitude;
2. detecting the unintended (concealed) attitude;
3. being aware of detecting an attitude that is not there at all.

The medium of speech communication is the speech waveform which potentially contains *all* the information described in the language, as characterised by linguistics/phonetics. This waveform is a single entity bounded by the time of speaking; although it has been consistently described in the literature as consisting of two sections – the plain message with expressive/emotive content *added* to it (but see our wrapper hypothesis above: in TM the plain message is encoded *within* the expressive wrapper). The situation described formally here is too idealised: in practice rendering fails *frequently*, but is supervised to enable the speech waveform to be sufficient, if not optimised, for correct perceiver assignment of the speaker's intentions.

Listeners report that they can detect expressive/emotive content in the waveform. However, surprisingly researchers have *not* been able to point to a particular place in a waveform that can be labelled with any reliability as either plain message or expressive content. The results of these attempts have been to notice major changes in acoustic characteristics such as rate of change of fundamental frequency and rhythmic inconsistencies, and associate these changes with quite angry speech, or very sad speech – but the observations have been based on quite gross effects (Murray and Arnott 1993, Morton 1992). Tatham and Morton (2004) suggest an alternative approach in which expressive content participates *of necessity* in the wrapper architecture: that is, *all* speech has some expressive/emotive content. *All* the acoustic characteristics of the waveform are affected by the wrapper.

Expression is of two types:

a. *linguistically and cognitive motivated*, as in contrastive emphasis where the speaker wishes to correct a misunderstanding such as a misspelled word – *It's an 'f' not an 's' in the word 'feel'!*

b. *biologically motivated* where the entire biological system changes under the effect of an emotion reaction; the vocal tract is part of this overall somatic reaction, and the speech output is consequently affected.

Both types will be found in the waveform. We need to determine what properties of the waveform can be described and can be associated with these two sources of expression. The first characteristic of the waveform to take into account is its dynamic nature.

Supervision of expressive content

The supervision of expression follows the procedures outlined above for the general supervision of utterance plan rendering. The main domain over which the supervisor acts is the utterance (utterances can be short like individual words, or long like whole paragraphs). In expression, the units which change are the syllables *as* they function within larger units phrases and sequences of phrases, etc. Since expression wraps the utterance, the settings for successive elements (both prosodic and segmental) will be changed by the dynamically unfolding dialog requirements.

The CPA monitors the requirement for progressive change, signalling values and their management for ensuring continuously variable prosodic specifications: all organised, of course, on a parametric basis. The CPA, by changing the balance of the prosodic characteristics – say, from 'calm' to 'anger', along vectors such as 'happiness' and 'anger', can achieve the speaker's goals as supervised changes of 'intonation', 'stress' and 'rhythm' (abstract representations of combined prosodic parameters).

The dynamic nature of the waveform

The dynamic nature of the waveform reflects the dynamic nature of speech. Speaking is a time related event and occurs sequentially in time, an occurrence captured in the visual representation of the speech waveform. Expression is a dynamic *process*, changing in time as the dialogue develops. For example, we can begin an utterance calmly, then become either happy, or angry as in *'I thought we'd go to the beach, but the fog just rolled in and it's too cold and damp'*, in which the speaker may change the nature of the wrapper as the utterance unfolds. The expression wrapper is dynamic, just as is the segmental content of the utterance – though, of course, they are not necessarily temporally synchronised.

We suggest that is useful to characterise expression computationally (Tatham and Morton 2004, 2005). The general plan can be characterised as a sketch designed to associate abstract representations of expression as wrapping the plain message, with prosodics carrying the major expressive/emotive information, as in this representational hierarchy (characterised here in simple XML notation):

```
<expression>
    <prosodics>
        <utterance>
            <syllables/>
        </utterance>
    </prosodics>
</expression>
```

(For an explanation of how we use XML notation to declare expressive data structures in TM see Tatham and Morton 2004).

But the basic questions remain:

1. How can we model what in the waveform triggers the percept of expression (Tatham and Morton 2003)?
2. What constitutes a plausible model of the listener's assignment of expression to the heard signal, and can we assume that the 'decoded' outcome will be in most ways similar to the speaker's expression (intended or unintended)?

Variability in the waveform

The second characteristic of the waveform we must address is variability, an obvious and all-pervasive general characteristic of speech. No two waveforms are exactly alike, but we perceive *invariance* when the waveform triggers us to access our knowledge of the language. On the other hand, we suggest that *perceived* variations can be associated with elements of the utterance plan: either with syllable (or segment) elements or with expressive/emotive content arising from cognitive activity or as a product of the biological stance. For example, contrastive stress (as in the example above) will produce a waveform different from non-contrastive stress, but also variations because the speaker's vocal tract may also be in a particular biological stance at the moment. It is perhaps as well to remember that biological systems display variability to some extent as a result of their adaptive behaviour – they are dynamic systems. The task is to characterise the variability appropriately, not ascribe what the labeller might think is not invariant to 'random' variation.

- The point is that there are all the variations we have discussed in Chapter 2 – basically assimilatory, coarticulatory and random; but in addition there are cognitively and biologically induced variants (which may have their own local variation) which are down to the immediate nature of the expressive wrapper.

Some of these will arise as a result of constraint pressure. We suggest there is an abstract invariant object (the extrinsic allophone) specified in the plan, but which will undergo processing on the dynamic planes. It will be rendered as a surface object and may exhibit variation because it has been subject to constraints imposed by, say, phonetic coarticulatory phenomena or by the physical state of the speaker (for a fuller characterisation of the constraint hierarchy, see Tatham and Morton 2004, pp. 48–52). The result is that from one abstract (and therefore 'idealised') utterance plan, there can be many variations of that plan on the surface, and some of these variations are labelled (somewhat impressionistically) by a phonetician. Other constraints can be imposed by the phonology responding to a syntactic specification for say, contrastive emphasis, or during phonetic rendering because of pragmatic constraints specifying precision of articulation for clarity, or incorporation of feedback from the listener – under the general supervision of CPA.

We suggest that just as *all* utterances are expressive/emotive, *all* utterances contain variability derived from underlying invariant units specified by the plan; and that all physical variations are ultimately explainable by reference to the derivational history of the units and by reference to the state of the biological system at the time of the utterance. This is a complex model far removed from the invariance of Classical Phonetics descriptions or the overly simply models of coarticulation.

Prosody as information bearing

The prosody, a phonological description of features that overarch segments, syllables, words and phrases, is the 'vehicle' for expressive information. Generally in linguistic descriptions, prosodic features are described separately from the syllabic or segmental description. If expression is communicated by prosodic features, and all utterances have expressive/emotive content, then prosodic features are to be found in every utterance.

This is an approach different from that taken in most contemporary descriptions. These posit a 'neutral' prosody from which all expressive content is absent, although it is seen as a carrier of expression in *specific* utterances by those who research in the area of expressive/emotive content in speech. However, if neutral prosody is taken as an *idealised* form, what is the method these theorists put forward for mapping generalisations *from* observed spoken language *to* this idealised form? These procedures and the levels they represent are not made clear. Even proposed analysis (actually, transcription) systems like ToBI (Silverman *et al.* 1992) are quite inexplicit regarding the derivation of invariant labelling from continuously varying waveforms: that is, they are inexplicit concerning the processing knowledge of the perceiver.

Sources of expressive/emotive content

There is a great deal of literature on the cognitive sources of expressive/emotive content (Frijda 1993 and 2000, Lazarus 2001, among others), on the biological sources of emotion (LeDoux 1996, Rolls 1999, among others), on a system of mixed sources (Adolphs and Damasio 2000, Johnstone *et al.* 2001, among others), and on biologically sourced with *cognitive interpretation* (Scherer 1993, Panksepp 2000, among others). We suggest a model for taking into account the sourcing (Tatham and Morton 2004) in which a contribution to the characterisation of the utterance and the resulting speech waveform *must* include both biological and cognitive sources, no matter how tentative the hypotheses as they await empirical support.

The perception of expressive content

No one has yet produced a comprehensively plausible model of the perception of speech as segments, syllables, or prosodics that *includes* expressive content. That we *do* perceive speech is a commonplace, and that we can detect attitudes and emotion state by perceiving something we commonly call 'tone of voice' is also recognised. But describing what units are being perceived and what processes are occurring and how they integrate as part of expressively wrapped speech has not been done. In this section, we sketch an outline of a possible way to characterise basic and secondary emotive contributions to speech, and outline some questions that, if answered, might point the way to developing a model of perception of expression in spoken language.

An understanding of the production process has been discussed in models of 'production for perception', and the motor theory of speech perception, original and revised, in Chapter 7. The chapter also looks at other proposals for modelling perception. But in general these do not deal with expressive or emotive content.

- To move toward a more comprehensive approach which can include the perception of expressive content, we suggest beginning with improvements to the way we represent expression. Note that the representation of expression is *not* the discovery of how it is rendered in the waveform, but the abstract representation underlying that rendering, and is equivalent to the representation *assigned* to that rendering by the listener.

The vector representation

Expression can change in type and intensity throughout production of an utterance or during the course of a dialogue. We have recently proposed ways of modelling the 'expression space', as shown in Figure 6.2 (adapted from Tatham and Morton 2004). Emotions can be characterised parametrically as 'moving' within this space, increasing or decreasing intensity and combing with other emotions. The listener's task is to locate the perceived expression within this space in order to decode its 'meaning'.

Along with several researchers, we assume four basic emotions. The *speech* literature has been mainly concerned with 'basic emotions' such as anger, sadness, happiness, fear (Panksepp 1998). However, very little of actual human conversation or computer-based dialogue systems produce or require such clearly differentiated expression. Most

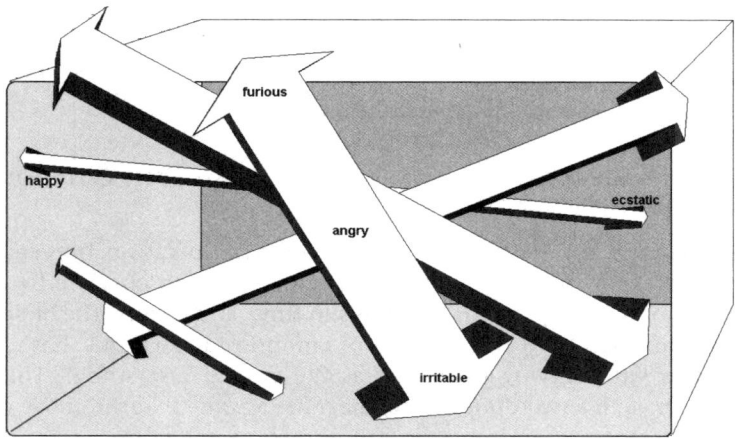

Figure 6.2 The emotion space, showing the furious-angry-irritable and happy-ecstatic vectors (adapted from Tatham and Morton 2004).

communication involves what has been referred to as 'secondary emotions' or 'blends' (Plutchik 1994, Oatley and Johnson-Laird 1998). In order to characterise these classes of emotion derived from the varying *intensity* of a basic emotion or *mixtures* of varying intensities of basic emotions, we suggest a vector based model. An early version of this proposal is outlined in Tatham and Morton (2004).

As a first approximation and a starting point, we can introduce an underlying idealised characterisation of the four basic emotions, each having a similar range and unlinked:

anger ↕   sadness ↕   happiness ↕   fear ↕   UNDERLYING TIER

In the diagram, that each basic emotion has a potential range is indicted by the vertical double arrow – each with the same range. In the next diagram, however, where we see how the objects on the underlying tier become instantiations at some more surface representation (a derived tier), anger and sadness become 'amplified' (though only moderately and differently – the different lengths of the arrows) and blended, whereas, happiness and fear are not instantiated.

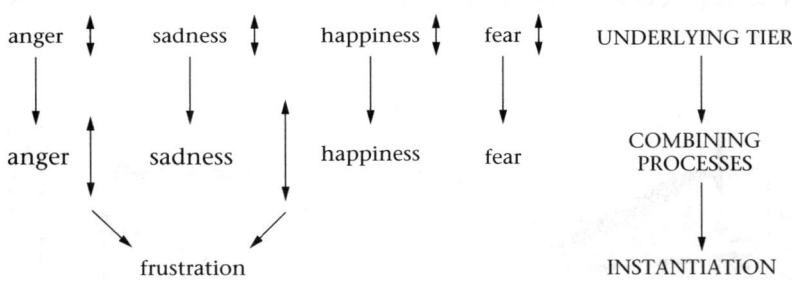

Happiness and fear may not be instantiated on this occasion, but remain in the system as potential emotions since we wish to characterise the dynamic nature of speech as it unfolds in time, and assume the biological systems associated with reports of emotion interact and that each can occur with varying intensities as the utterance(s) unfold. This is hard to show in a two-dimensional diagram: assume that the above diagram represents a snapshot during an unfolding utterance.

We hypothesise that anger blended with sadness result (by some formula unspecified here) results in frustration. This may not be true, but it is a plausible hypothesis for this example. Not only do two or more emotions contribute to secondary emotion, but also the intensity is the result of the amount of contribution of each. Thus it is the *relative* contributions of anger and sadness which contribute to the quality of the frustration – resulting in blends, which we might as listener-perceiver (or even speaker–perceiver in an act of self-awareness), for example, *label* as 'infuriating' or 'depressed with undercurrent of anger', and so on.

The theory identifies three sources of potential error in the model:

1. in the mapping from emotion vector space onto waveform parameters;
2. during mapping from waveform parameters onto the listener's perceptual emotion space;
3. in the variability among speakers.

The model is particularly vulnerable to 3, where the variability is so great that, for example, a narrow range of fundamental frequency in one speaker may indicate a large degree of sadness, but in another may be within this speaker's expected range. In this case, the listener's perceptual space (or the representation within it) would need to flexible enough to take into account the wide range of possibilities or other information needed to decode the speaker's emotion or attitude from the signal. This question, of mapping from speaker to waveform to listener in terms of production/perception space and trigger thresholds has not yet been satisfactorily addressed.

A parametric speech synthesis model would make an ideal test bed for the theory and its predictions, since it has the potential to formalise variability in the waveform in a constrained and manageable way, and since it, by definition, calls for a fully computational paradigm to handle representations and processes. Very little has been done along these lines to date, but we believe that there is here a clear pointer to future research.

The listener is active

Listeners do not simply react to speaker waveforms. They exist within their own psychological environment. What they perceive is not simply a function of the signal, but is also derived within the context of the listener's view of *self*. It is within this context, and the extent of the listener's knowledge and formalised experience, that the perceptual solution is assigned. Thus the listener's response can vary on occasion, dependent on contextual shift. And during a dialog/conversation, the listener's internal state can also change (see Tatham and Morton 2004, pp. 61–4 for a formal statement).

What does the listener model need?

The minimum scope for the listener model is the capacity and 'experience' to assign straight phonological patterns, including segmental or syllabic, and prosodic representations. The model most speech researchers work with is discussed in Chapter 7. Also required is a knowledge of the syntactic constructions, the most likely pragmatic sketches arising from experience and shared culture, and, we suggest, an awareness of expressive emotive content.

Some questions that need answering

Using the speech model outlined in Tatham and Morton (2003, 2004, 2005) which suggests an expression wrapper enclosing a prosodic wrapper, itself enclosing syllabic and segmentally based characterisations of speech, we ask:

a. Do we perceive (assign) the wrapper first or the syllable/segment first when listening to spoken language?
b. Does the perception of one of the above affect the perception of the other?
   - If the overall expression wrapper is not detected, will the utterance be more difficult to perceive?
   - If the prosodic wrapper is defective, how much might this affect perception of expressive content?
c. What are the units of prosody perception? The current descriptive model in phonetics describes prosodic features as changes in intonation, stress and rhythm patterning. The acoustic correlates (based on observations of what speakers *produce*) are said to be changes in fundamental frequency, intensity and rhythmic unit timing – though not in a linear relationship with the abstractions of the phonological tier. But how accurate are these mappings for *perception*? Are there other characterisations that might be more appropriate?
d. We have called for dynamically based modelling, but what exactly does this mean? An utterances is time-dependent; speech is produced in time, the acoustic features unroll in time. So the events under scrutiny are clearly dynamic, but are their descriptions? All too

often 'dynamic' is interpreted as a time-based series of static descriptions. We are reminded that the static frames of a movie are only 'dynamic' under very special, illusionary circumstances: their rapidly sequenced projection, and that even then 'movement' is down to 'persistence' constraints in vision. We have seen that static descriptions masquerading as dynamic characterisations fall short of adequacy in production models. Are there similar limitations in perception modelling? Is perception a 'rolling' activity which requires a dynamic model? Or can a model of a series of static descriptions account for the ability to perceive and understand expressive/ emotive spoken language?

e. How do we model the dynamic exchanges of feedback between speaker and listener – and between these and the predictive models of each other that *each* runs continuously during conversation?

There are several different ways of modelling a speaker's utterance plan, and how it is derived and subsequently rendered – for us under careful supervisory control, but always in the context of delivering a signal which is designed to be perceived. Listeners have strategies for dealing with this signal to assign to it a symbolic representation with the goal of matching the speaker's plan. Listeners' strategies, their use of feedback and the way they deliver feedback to the speaker have not yet been, in our view, adequately modelled. The essence of communication – *conveying* thoughts and ideas in an environment of feelings, attitudes and beliefs to another, and becoming *aware* that there has been communication – and how it occurs, is still open to new approaches to modelling. But one thing is becoming increasingly clear: the theory works best when the speaker/listener experience and what lies behind it are approached as a whole. Clearly there are many points of entry into the system, and several disciplines, some dealing with an abstract world, some with a physical world; it is this which prompts us to call for a coherent unifying metatheory to avoid conflict.

Pragmatics in phonetics

One source of variability in the speech waveform can be modelled as introduced by pragmatic considerations (Morton 1992, 1996). We discussed earlier two other possible sources: linguistic expression (a cognitive source), for example, contrastive emphasis, and a biological basis, for example the physical stance of the speaker.

Pragmatics is about how the context of the dialogue influences what is said, and how it is said (Levinson 1985, Grundy 2000, Kearns 2000). Pragmatic effects arise from the speakers' responses to dialogue context, to the context of what they wish to convey, awareness of the listeners' attitudes/emotions or what *appears* to be their attitudes, and the incorporation of predictions by both speakers and listeners of how dialogues or the current dialog develop. Pragmatics is also about the listener's ability to make inferences about what the speaker is saying in order to interpret both the intended and unintended meaning.

Contextual factors, described as pragmatic information, have been modelled by linguists using constructs such as *presupposition*. The term refers to what the speaker assumes the listener knows about the context that is not directly expressed. Take for example, the utterance *I'll leave at six tomorrow*. The listener may know that this is unusual, and that it means 6:00 a.m., and can tell this from particular information encoded in the waveform, which also triggers a range of attitudes and emotion about leaving on this occasion at this time.

Presupposition and entailment

The following example is based on Yule (1996, p. 25). Entailment is about additional information that can potentially be predicted from the utterance *in addition to the plain message*. For example, the speaker may say *They were away from the village for six weeks this summer*. A presupposition is probably that the speaker is talking about people known to both speaker and hearer, and that the speaker also believes that the information will interest the listener. Another presupposition is that the people could afford to spend such a long time away. The first may be correct, but not necessarily: the listener might not care, or in fact be upset for reasons the speaker has not presupposed, unless it is the speaker's wish to upset the listener. The second presupposition may be more incorrect in that the people involved may have been the guests of relatives or friends, or the holiday was combined with a business trip or conference, or there was a serious family problem.

What can be seen as entailment is that they had a break from routine, no matter what kind of break it was: it may have been costly but not necessarily; they have now returned. None of the presuppositions or entailments were actually discussed, but some information (latent or overt) about attitude and belief – and possibly emotion – can be described by linguists. The listener can follow up by inquiring about the speaker's beliefs that might presuppose the statement, and confirm the logical predictions of the entailments, and then add some of their own.

Inference

Inference is usually described as a listener 'process' leading to more information than might have been contained in the original utterance. Take the utterance: *There's that cat again*. The listener knows which cat, and what the speaker intends to communicate about the appearance of the cat. The listener will infer whether the speaker is pleased to see the cat, or irritated by its appearance. The inference process is seen to rely on shared experience which is triggered by the waveform – specifically by prosodic variation. The speaker knows how to access the phonetic dynamics and the listener can interpret these variations. Conversations and dialogues are complex interactions to describe, although they speakers and listeners generally manage to communicate what the want to without much difficulty. Remarkably they also communicate something of what they want to conceal.

In TM we model pragmatic effects as a specific source of variability in the speech waveform, not necessarily related to linguistic/cognitive or biologically determined effects. We have suggested that pragmatic effects lead to expressive content directly influencing prosody. Although it might be appropriate to model a separate input, we suggest that it may be appropriate to relate directly the cognitive and biological sources to pragmatic effects (Morton 1992, Tatham and Morton 2005, p. 309). For example, on a higher level, the choices of words and syntactic processes can reflect pragmatic effects (Levinson 1985, Grundy 2000, Verschueren 2003). Chosen words are encoded by phonology into the utterance plan. If 'emphasis' is required the cognitive linguistic feature of emphasis will be implemented on the phonological dynamic plane. The appropriate physical gesture will be assembled on the phonetic dynamic plane from the stored potential gestures.

If the speaker is happy or irritated, this might be revealed by their biological state at any point in time when speaking (Toates 2001, Tatham and Morton 2004, p. 280). In addition to word selection and phonological encoding to inform the listener not only about the basic message, changes in the biological state give information about the speaker's attitude and emotion, their attitude toward listener, and perhaps even modified to take into account the predicted listener response; this might be acceptance, agreement, pleasure, dismay, and so on. The speech waveform can trigger multiple responses in listeners, who then can change roles to become speakers; and the dialogue continues.

One of the major problems in the last two decades of speech research has been accounting for variability. Much of the variability has been ascribed to mechanical and aerodynamic effects as properties of the action of speaking (phonetic coarticulation) or to specific language-based choices (phonological assimilation, for example). However, we suggest that since listeners report sensitivity to expression and ease in detecting emotive content, a principled investigation of possible correlations between pragmatics and variability in the waveform might be productive, especially in utterances that do not vary except in terms of their prosodic rendering.

Language pathology and clinical neuroscience

Studies in this area are concerned with articulator control to achieve articulatory and acoustic goals; and with perceptual strategies and listener goal representations. There are many potential sources of error and failure throughout the system, but maintenance of the chain (as shown in the diagram) is paramount for the clinician.

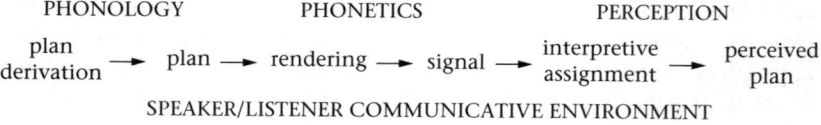

Expressive content and the overall communicative environment encompassing both production and perception do not as yet seem to figure with priority in research in this applied field: attention to wrappers in favour of out-of-context detail seems to be a contemporary focus.

Language teaching/learning

Currently this area seems to focus on the invariant units to be found in descriptive models of language. Variability is assumed to be constrained, although it is not clear as to by what, or how. There are parallels between this field of study and the clinical field, and much scope for cross-fertilisation, but such applied considerations must, if the theory is to be adequate, relate transparently to the parent disciplines involve. Currently pronunciation and perceptual training are neglected – perhaps on the grounds that other areas of language are more 'important' or more deserving of the teacher's time, perhaps on the grounds that once a learner can be more or less understood by a native speaker a law of diminishing returns kicks in, or, worse, perhaps on the scientifically unsubstantiated grounds that learning a better than adequate pronunciation is 'impossible'.

The simulation of speech – speech technology

There is much contemporary interest in simulating expressive/emotive speech, since this feature is thought to contribute significantly to naturalness (Tatham and Morton 2004, among others). But results so far have proved disappointing, simply because the necessary information and backup theory are not yet available to contribute significantly synthetic speech algorithms. Currently the unit selection approach (principled concatenation of variable length pre-recorded waveform samples taken from a large database of recorded human speech) is the favoured technique, having met with good acceptance by users. However the technique is unlikely to produce natural sounding expressive speech at the current rate of development, since managing expressive content is poorly implemented. Modifying utterance prosodics to simulate natural expressive speech is not yet adequate (Tatham and Morton 2005). In automatic speech recognition, variability in the input signal continues to prove the biggest problem, particularly, once again when that variability comes from expressive content. The strategies for simulating perception are still poor in this field, and models of the acoustic signal still prove inadequate.

7
Speech Perception and Prosody

Introduction

Speech perception theories, like *all* theories, are based on observations which are often the result of experimental or general empirical work, including introspection. It is the *interpretation* of these facts by classification, description and explanation that enables a coherent theory to be built. As with speech production, there are two aspects to the perception of speech:

- the *physical domain* – the acoustic signal and the way the listener accesses this signal using hearing; and
- the *psychological domain* – the interpretation of what the listener has heard.

The study of the relationship between these two domains falls within the study of psycho-acoustics. The perception of speech may not quite operate in the same way as the perception of non-speech sound, so that the specific treatment of the perception of speech falls within the area of psycho-linguistics. The process of hearing concludes with a neural representation of the sound heard. This is a projection onto the auditory cortex which we call the neural representation, the linguistic nature of which falls within the area of neuro-linguistics. It is not understood how this projection now gives way to the cognitive activity of perception. The result of this cognitive activity is an awareness by the listener of a symbolic representation of what was originally heard.

The *hearing process* results, within the cochlea, in a conversion of the analog acoustic signal into a *neuro-digital representation* in which the original amplitude is coded by the frequency of neural spikes travelling along the auditory nerve to the brain, and the original frequency spectrum is coded in terms of the component nerves comprising the auditory nerve bundle. The *perceptual process* assigns a *symbolic linguistic representation* to the neural representation of the original signal.

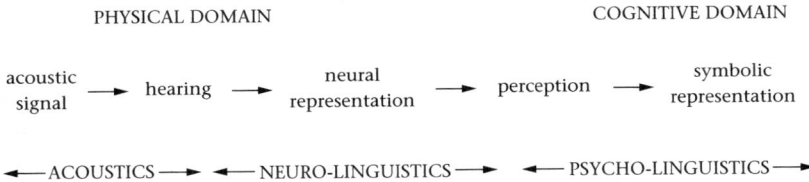

Consonants *vs.* vowels

Some researchers feel that the perceptual assignment of consonantal and vowel representations involves different processes. This view is based on the featural properties of the associated waveforms, including, for example the presence or absence of periodicity (usually deriving from vocal cord vibration) in the signal and the temporal distribution of the acoustic energy (for example, silent periods followed by the release bursts of a-periodic sounds associated with stops).

The assignment of consonantal representations may involve cues of relatively rapid transitions in the character of the spectrum, changes over short time periods of the signal's frequency distribution. A simple classifier (a computationally or mathematically based method of identifying objects) can 'recognise' periods of silence, bursts of signal with an a-periodic source, formant transitions in adjacent vowels, and so on. It is important to note that we are not saying that these features of the signal *are* the consonant, but that they form the cues by which the perceptual system is able to assign a consonantal representation.

Similarly, that a portion of signal is to be assigned a vowel representation may well often depend initially on the fact that the signal usually has a periodic waveform. The signal is normally continuous in nature, not exhibiting the discontinuities associated with stops, for example.

- Consonants do not have particular acoustic properties – they cannot because they are abstract linguistic objects. Stretches of acoustic signal may well have certain properties which can trigger the perceptual system to assign, firstly, generalised consonantal representations, and then perhaps particular consonantal representations. Such a model places the burden of recognition of this or that segment on the perceptual assignment process, not on the acoustic nature of the signal.

We shall see that there are two important reasons for characterising perception in this way:

1. The stretches of signal we associate with particular linguistic objects often vary enormously in their actual acoustic characteristics. The model needs to explain how perception can assign the same symbolic representation do differing signals.
2. The signal often does not contain the expected cues which would enable the simple *passive* classifier mentioned above to work properly. The signal is in some sense 'defective'. The model needs to explain how, provided this compromised signal is within certain limits, the perceptual system will nevertheless assign the correct symbolic representation.

In fact, on both counts the signal usually departs markedly from some abstract expected specification, triggering the perceptual system's active processes of representation assignment. It is for this kind of reason that we do not see perception as a process of deriving a representation from the soundwave – quite the opposite: the representation is not there to be derived. 'Correct' here means the representation the speaker intended the perceiver to assign.

It is a remarkable property of the human perceptual system that despite these sources of variability correct representational assignment and classification is possible. Human beings are said to be 'pattern seeking devices'. This means that they cannot help but seek patterns in incoming stimuli (not just speech, but visual and tactile signals, etc.), and are particularly good at assigning patterns to the stimuli. In contrast, one of the biggest problems in computer simulation of human behaviour is getting the machines to behave in this way. Normal computers are very good at arithmetic and logic but intrinsically poor at pattern seeking and matching.

The listener's perceptual goal

We begin with the assertion that the goal of the listener is to recover the speaker's utterance plan. It is important to note that we did *not* say 'recover the utterance plan from the soundwave': part of our hypothesis is that the soundwave does not embody the speaker's utterance plan. Perception is much more complex than a simple process of straightforward decoding of the soundwave back to the utterance plan which underlay it.

Perceivers, we believe, bring a great deal more to the perceptual process than an algorithm for decoding soundwaves. In fact we believe that their decoding algorithm, if viewed as operating only on the soundwave – that is, having just the one input – is probably quite poor and error-prone.

- In principle it would be possible to determine this empirically by asking listeners to decode speech signals without reference to any prior knowledge as to what a speech signal could be like; though such an experiment would be extremely difficult (perhaps impossible) to design and set up.

In the TM model speakers call into play a predictive model of perception as an integral part of their utterance rendering process. Rendering takes place in the light of predicted perceptual success, bearing in mind the extraneous factors (some linguistic, some not) impinging on the production/perception chain of events. Rendering is perhaps adjusted to a varying balance between ease of articulation and the listener's ability to repair defective signals.

The principle of sufficient perceptual separation

Often researchers refer to a principle of *sufficient perceptual separation*, but this is a little too simple. *What* is sufficient is a variable, and depends on a number of factors both linguistic and extra-linguistic. At any one moment the amount of 'separation' needed between differing elements in the signal can be thought of as predictable, though, from the listener's repair ability and the impinging 'noise' (unwanted signals or discontinuities in the signal). Remarkably the *speaker* is able to take all this into account and momentarily put themself in the place of the listener to produce a signal which is neither too robust nor insufficiently robust, but tailor-made in robustness to the listener's general environment *as it is now*.

Taken without considering how speakers and listeners interact to produce a satisfactory perceptual outcome, the principle of sufficient perceptual separation can be regarded as a tendency toward extravagance (for the sake of the listener) rather than economy (for the sake of the speaker). Perceptually, what matters is that sounds that affect the meaning of a word should be sufficiently distinct from one another. This can be achieved by maximizing the perceptual distance between the sounds that occur in a contrasting set, such as the vowels in stressed monosyllables. Thus the principle of perceptual separation does not usually result in one sound affecting an adjacent sound, as occurs with the principle of maximum ease of articulation. Instead, perceptual separation affects the set of sounds that potentially can occur at a given position in a word, such as the position that must be occupied by a vowel in a stressed syllable. However, the model is simplistic. The notion 'sufficient perceptual separation' implies separation to allow effortless (or 'passive') decoding, throwing the burden of ease of perception onto the speaker. But in fact we should be really thinking in terms of how sufficient the perceptual separation should be: certainly not absolute. Any utterance embodies problems for passive decoding – witness the extreme difficulties experienced by automatic speech recognition systems. What a speaker seems to do is produce a signal which is just enough to enable the listener, working hard, to assign an appropriate symbolic representation: and that is all. And the speaker knows just how much a listener can bring to the assignment process.

The conclusion for TM is that the speech production model has to incorporate a generalised predictive model of speech perception in order to function optimally. The data from speech production clearly shows that *precision* is a factor which is continuously variable, and that this precision or robustness correlates well and inversely with the level of noise imposed on the utterance or inherent in it (Tatham and Morton 1980). Noise here means anything which detracts from optimal perception and taxes too heavily the listener's repair strategies.

The perceptual task

The task of speech perception is to accept as input to the perceptual system the speech waveform coming from another speaker, and to assign to that waveform a phonological labelling, identifying the sequence of phonological elements used by the speaker to create the waveform. The goal is to label the acoustic signal with an appropriate phonological symbolic representation.

In Part I we were concerned with Speech Production, and we saw that prior to Action Theory the commonest way of modelling speech production was to assume that phonologically intended speech segments become blurred together as part of the production process. This blurring was called coarticulation. Theories of Speech Perception are concerned with how the listener in some sense reverses the coarticulatory process to recover the intended sequence of phonological elements. This does not necessarily mean a process of inversely filtering out coarticulatory effects, but of effecting a reversal by using the distorted waveform to assign a representation which is unaffected by the distortions themselves.

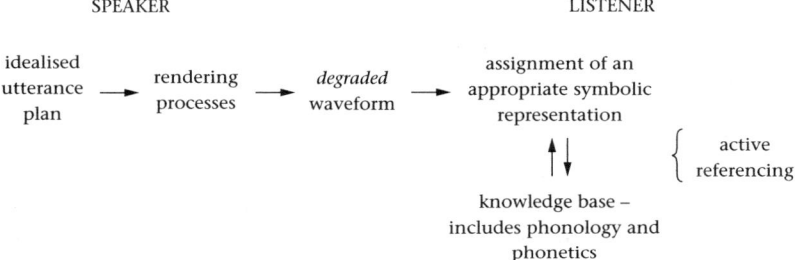

The diagram illustrates the basic model of speech perception. Speakers, working with an idealised abstract plan, submit this to a phonetic rendering process which produces a degraded waveform – one which is not a straightforward linear transformation of the utterance plan. Listeners assign to this an appropriate symbolic waveform using a process of actively referencing a knowledge base of the phonology of the language, the rendering processes involved and what can go wrong in this listener/speaker's experience. Such a model admits a 'sufficient perceptual separation', but notes that the separation can be far from absolute.

The general problem of speech perception

The main problem in arriving at a satisfactory theory of speech perception is accounting for the fact that speech soundwaves are not a one-to-one or linear encoding of a speaker's utterance plan.

Some researchers – especially those who model coarticulation as a deliberate active rendering process (Chapter 2 and 3) – suggest that in some way when the soundwave is produced the various features of the segments are spread around, merging segment with segment at the physical acoustic level. If this idea is accepted then in principle perception has simply to recover the features from the soundwave and re-assemble them to identify the original phonological segments. Such relatively passive theories of perception each try to devise an automatic filtering type of procedure to achieve this. Unfortunately four decades of research, and latterly the use of powerful computing facilities to provide models of perception based on signal processing (automatic speech recognition), have failed to come up with any really effective and plausible decoding procedure. In other words the hypothesis that the acoustic waveform is an encoding, however complex, of phonological segments and that those segments are consequently in principle recoverable by passive decoding, has so far defeated empirical verification. This does not mean to say that it will not eventually be possible to find segments in soundwaves, but for the moment alternative models are more viable. In our view it will never be possible to recover phonological segments from the soundwave because they are not there to be recovered.

So, the alternative hypothesis is that the soundwave is *not* a direct encoding of phonological segments. The segments are *not* in the acoustic signal and are *not* therefore recoverable from it – how could they be if they are not there to begin with? The segments are abstract and the signal is physical. Phonological segments are simply an abstract descriptive device devised by phonologists. A quite different perceptual strategy is therefore needed. In active theories of speech perception the incoming soundwave is used to enable the recovery of appropriate phonological segments not from the acoustic signal, but from within the listener's mind.

Speech is produced to be perceived by one or more listeners. There are a number of different speaker/perceiver temporal and spatial relationship scenarios. The major ones are:

1. speaker and listener are simultaneously present in the same location; for example a conversation is taking place between two or more people, or listeners are present but not interacting directly with the speaker – say, they are attending a lecture;
2. the listener is remote but simultaneous; for example a conversation is taking place over a phone connection, or the speaker is broadcasting to non-interacting listeners;
3. the listener is remote and not simultaneous; for example one or more listeners are hearing a recording – the speech is time shifted and interaction is not possible.

In these cases the listener may or may not in addition be able to see the speaker to gather visual cues which might assist speech perception.

Listening, like speaking, is basically a two-stage process:

- the predominantly passive process of hearing, followed by
- the predominantly active process of perceiving.

In *hearing* the listener must be able to detect and perform (in the inner ear) a signal processing task which pre-analyses, parameterises and digitises the signal before using the auditory nerve to convey it to the brain's auditory cortex. By and large this signal processing is passive, though some cognitively sourced intervention is possible, and results in a spectrally disassembled representation of the signal being projected onto the auditory cortex. The analysis performed by the cochlear/inner ear is functionally equivalent to the signal processing which underlies spectrographic representations used in acoustic phonetics research.

At its simplest, *perception* is the active assignment of a symbolic representation to what is heard. At this stage it is enough to underline that what does *not* happen is that the listener extracts some symbolic representation from the acoustic signal: physical phenomena cannot embody abstract representation – this cannot exist without the intervention of special and perhaps dedicated cognitive processing which brings to the act of perception information already held by the perceiver. There are many simple ways of illustrating this: for example, it is impossible to find word boundaries in the acoustic stream of a language not known to the listener. Word boundaries can only be assigned if the listener knows the language, its words, the phonological structure in general and how boundaries are characterised in the language. The listener also needs to know how acoustic signals convey any prosodic or segmental variants which might be down to style or expression.

Some researchers feel that it is unlikely that listeners proceed through a complete analysis or reconstruction of what they hear. Rather they jump to an early synthesis as soon as enough signal has been processed – a synthesis (or guess) at the 'meaning' of what they have heard, and often of what they are about to hear. An actual synthesis would not be necessary, but the synthesis model has the merit of being explicit. Complete synthesis would be called for if the listener were asked to report a final guess and not to act on a partial guess. Presumably the result is based on statistical probability – a weighted process of selecting from alternatives leaving the synthesis process. There are bound to be alternative solutions for the synthesis processes because the incoming data is by definition incomplete (or the synthesis process would not be necessary). Multiple solutions with probability indices attached may well be what comes out of the process.

Models of Speech Perception

There are two basic strategies which can be hypothesised for perception: passive and active. Passive strategies have little or no active listener cognitive intervention in the decoding process, whereas active strategies make cognitive intervention central to their operation. In active systems perception is seen as a process of *assignment* of a solution to decoding a message, rather than a process of *identification* of message content in the signal.

The generic passive paradigm

The signal is pre-segmented, and recognition is a process of matching and identifying the segments. The signal is directly accessed, and its content is appropriately labelled by a simple classifier. The assumption is that the signal is relatively simple and that the objects to be identified by the classifier are relatively consistent in their acoustic properties. Passive models also assume a high degree of robustness in the acoustic signal and in the speaker's rendering processes which create it. In other words, passive models require a deal of consistency in the relationship between the signal and the underlying utterance plan.

The classification process takes in the segments of the waveform and, by accessing known phonological segments, performs a simple matching process. The fact of known phonological representations – the phonological segments of the language – is what unifies the signal and the final phonological representation string corresponding to the speaker's utterance.

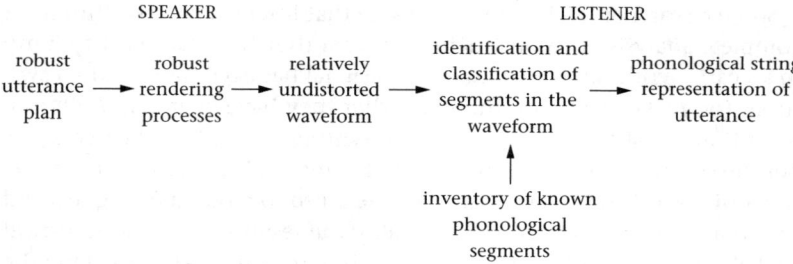

A few attempts at a passive model have gone so far as to claim that the phonological segments themselves are *in* the waveform; this would be an extreme version of the direct perception paradigm. A somewhat weaker version than the usual one, shown in the diagram, introduces alongside the known phonological segments a few basic phonological rules, like simple phonotactic rules. These would go a long way to making up for any shortfalls in the accuracy of the rendering process. Few researchers refer to other uses, but such an addition would also assist in decoding fast speech (with its deletions which can occur in late stages of the phonology or in the rendering processes) or some types of expressive speech.

The generic active paradigm

Passive models assume the acoustic signal to be simple and robust, revealing to the perceptual classifier its segmental origins. The active paradigm assumes conversely that the signal is complex. Proponents (and they are in the majority) of the active paradigm do not feel that the signal is simple enough to enable it to be decoded without much active intervention on the part of the listener. It is the nature of this intervention and what the listener needs to know within the perceptual system that forms the basis of active models.

In the active paradigm knowledge of the phonology of the language extends to a full model of phonological processing. The listener knows (since they are also a speaker) the entire phonological structure of the language, and this knowledge is brought to bear on the perceptual task. The relationship between the signal and the listener's final representation of the heard utterance is not seen as linear, but as a complex hierarchically organised system. It is this system which is responsible for producing an utterance plan: it is made available to perception as a hierarchical structure. In addition, of course, the listener must know of the non-linear processes in the speaker's phonetic rendering of the utterance plan. Many researchers fail to emphasise this – but a great deal of the 'failure' of the ideal representation results from the error-prone nature of phonetic rendering. Active models of perception make provision for 'making up' for phonetic weaknesses in rendering.

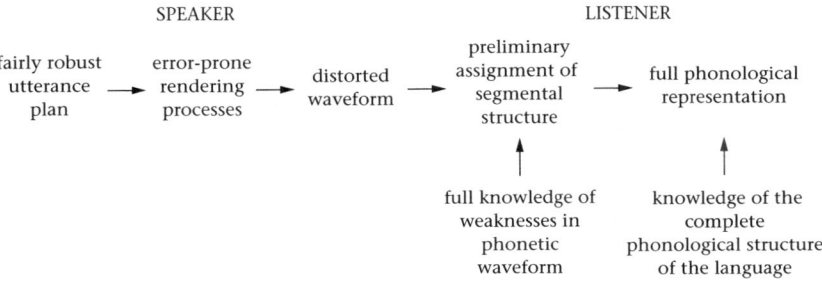

The diagram is a simplification of a typical active model of perception. The main points are included, however: the speaker's utterance plan is distorted in the phonetic rendering process to produce a distorted waveform. Perception involves the assignment of abstract representations which originate in the listener's mind, but which compensate for the distortions. Using knowledge of the phonological structure of the language, at the very least there is reconstruction of the speaker's utterance plan, and, in some models, a reconstruction of the entire phonological derivational history of the plan. The reconstruction is importantly a process of *assignment*.

Passive models – template-based models

Templates are idealised representations, usually of the acoustic signal; they are often to be found in automatic speech recognition systems (Chapter 12). The idea is to compare and match the incoming signal with templates stored in the listener's memory. The incoming signal is processed by a *comparator* against a scanning of the stored set of templates to find, in a simple model, an exact match, or in a more complex model, a *best* match. The important point about templates is that they are stored together with their labels. The success of the comparator in finding a match triggers the assignment of the found template's label to the acoustic signal. The main questions which arise include:

- Where did the templates come from? – how were they acquired?
- Does the template take the form of a 'recording' of a representative acoustic sample indexed with an acceptable range of variability?
- If there is a recording, what are its parameters? – it cannot be a raw acoustic signal since the brain has only access to a parameterised analysis of acoustic signals performed by the inner ear.
- Is the template, alternatively, an average of what has been heard before?
- How is the template store searched?
- How are templates sorted and indexed for searching?

There are many questions which need to be asked concerning templates, their form and how they are acquired and accessed. But in addition, a template-based model must say something about the relationship between an individual template and its neighbours, that is between templates and linguistic units since these effectively constitute their attached labels. Some researchers feel that we are not only able to assign labels to individual speech sounds but also to features of those sounds and linguistically significant *clusters* of sounds.

Any perceptual model needs to account for the observation that we can label linguistically significant objects and report their patterning. For example:

- parameters of segmental units, for example *voicing*;
- whole segments, for example *extrinsic allophones*, for establishing their patterned use;

- groupings of segments, for example the patterned use of *syllables*;
- prosodies, for example question *vs.* statement *intonation*, and
- expressively significant prosodies, for example angry or contrite *cues in the signal*.

Note the linguistic significance qualifier. Often in speech-oriented perceptual models properties of the acoustic signal which are *not* linguistically significant – that is, those that offer some basic contrast, or define some expressive property, as in the last example above – are not identified or even noticed.

A simple template model is hard to sustain in view of the fact that we frequently observe the perceptual system dealing with quite seriously degraded material. One possible way using templates would be for the system to come up with more than one hypothesis as to which template actually matches the input signal, and, working on experience, perhaps rank order them. The 'experience' could consist of some notion of frequency of occurrence *in a particular context*. That is, a *generalised* probability and a *particular* probability taking into account phonological as well as phonetic context.

So, for an example of hypothesising in a *phonological* context, consider how, given a run of three consonants at the start of a syllable it is entirely predictable that an 'unheard' initial consonant will be /s/ in English. This is due to the way consonants which open syllables are phonologically patterned. And for an example of hypothesising in a *phonetic* context: [t] can be recovered from an unreleased syllable final [t˹] given the relative duration of the preceding vowel and the particular changes to formant frequency during the final, say, 25 per cent of its duration.

Passive theories – filtering

Central to most passive theories of speech perception is the idea that the incoming signal is processed through *fixed passive filters*. Although there might on some occasions be active decoding of the waveform, but this is usually kept for extending the basic capabilities of a predominantly passive system. What these researchers are saying is that active cognitively determined processing occurs as an *extension* of passive filtering if the incoming signal is very indistinct or degraded in some way – normally in passive theories cognitive processing is not involved.

Some researchers have suggested that the normal way a listener perceives is to apply passive filtering to the signal based on the linguistic idea of distinctive features and their acoustic correlates. Detection and matching of the acoustic signal and the phonological representation can be carried out passively. Distinctive features are, however, elements within *abstract* phonological theory, but some acoustic phoneticians are keen to stress that very often they can be readily correlated with identifiable properties of the acoustic signal (Fant 1973). Fant's proposals are interesting because he makes the claim that basically production and perception are one and the same thing – they are simply alternative modalities providing for encoding soundwaves using the vocal tract at the output device and decoding soundwaves using the ear. In the brain (some would say *mind*) speech production and perception become one and the same thing.

Although distinctive features are used in classical phonological theory to characterise abstract phonological segments several researchers, including Fant, suggest that most of the time there are reliable acoustic correlates for the features. This idea attempts to bridge the gap between the abstract representation of speech and its physical representation. A speaker is said to map the phonological features *onto* the correlating acoustic features in the speech waveform, whereas the listener maps the acoustic features they hear back onto underlying abstract phonological features. Critical to this idea, of course, is the nature of the two mapping processes, and whether they are mirror images of each other. Speakers and listeners are sensitive to the correlations, which are readily accessed associations in the speaker/listener's mind.

Direct Perception (as opposed to 'mediated perception')

An extreme form of the passive approach is seen in the theory of Direct Perception (Gibson 1954). Applied to speech perception the Direct Perception theory suggest that the spectral and temporal analysis of the soundwave by the ear itself, and the characteristics of the spectral array representation of sound projected onto the auditory cortex constitute a sufficient analysis to enable awareness of the stimulus and its 'meaning'. Meaning here means an appropriate phonological representation. Cognitively mediated interpretation is considered unnecessary except in extreme cases of signal degradation. It is important to stress here the idea of awareness of a signal's phonological meaning – and the idea that this is *embodied in the acoustic signal.*

Understanding such a claim involves adopting a philosophical stance which is a little strange or unfamiliar to us in speech research. Along with

Fant, we might feel that it is true that soundwaves have certain readily identifiable, and perhaps relatively immutable, properties: the properties that can be regularly analysed out in a laboratory. For us however those properties do *not* include or characterise *phonological meaning*. A waveform or spectrogram, for example, is a *picture* of the sound associated with utterance but *not* of its meaning. In the view opposed to Direct Perception, meaning is something minds interpret from physical representations by a process of assignment and involves cognitive mediation.

Action Theorists, working in speech production, have explicitly identified themselves with the ideas of the Direct Perception theorists. Both minimise cognitive mediation in the processes of production and perception. Both give higher status to the passive properties of physical mechanisms than the 'translationists' (in speech production theory) or proponents of the active theories of perception. For the Action Theorist the *intrinsic* properties of a coordinative structure render it unnecessary to posit very much cognitive activity in phonology or phonetics. For the Direct Perceptionists the analysing properties of the ear and the format of the signal as projected onto the brain's auditory cortex (both essentially passive processes) make it unnecessary to invoke additional cognitive processing.

The Motor Theory of Speech Perception

The Motor Theory of Speech Perception is based on the claim that speech perception is an active process involving cognition and direct reference to the listener's speech production processes, or in the original terms, the articulatory patterns which might produce the heard signal.

The Motor Theory tackles the problem of unravelling coarticulation by proposing that the listener has knowledge of the way to produce isolated speech segments, and of the rules governing how they become coarticulated in normal running speech. Listeners have this knowledge because they do it themselves, though they are not, of course, consciously aware of what they are doing. The knowledge of the motor and coarticulation properties of speech – as possessed by the *listener* – are invoked as part of an *active process* of decoding the waveform into appropriate phonological labels. In the original 1967 (Liberman *et al.* 1967) formulation of the theory it was hypothesised that listeners actively reconstruct the actual 'muscle activation patterns' which they themselves have as representations of vocal tract gestures. The reconstruction invokes these muscle activation patterns in terms of sets of descriptors. Note however that the muscle activation patterns and the way they are stored constitute a static rather than dynamic representation. Coarticulatory processes are evaluated by reference to static linear context, rather than dynamic hierarchically organised structures.

The diagram shows how stored descriptors of muscle activation patterns for individual sounds generalised from the *listener's* own experience contribute together with coarticulatory descriptors to an active interpretation of the soundwave. The final output of this interpretation is a set of hypotheses concerning the string of the *speaker's* intended muscle activation patterns.

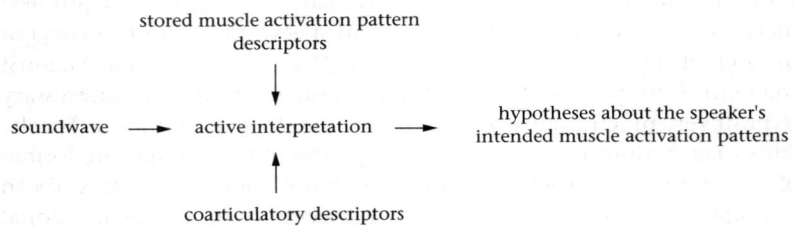

Because more detailed empirical investigation showed that such a reconstruction would *not*, in fact, reveal the kind of invariance needed to uniquely identify phonological objects, the Motor Theory was revised (Liberman and Mattingly 1985). The problem was that empirical investigations after the theory was put forward revealed that muscle activation patterns do not seem to be invariant.

The revised Motor Theory re-focuses away from the supposed invariant muscle activation patterns and hypothesises that the interpretation of the soundwave is in terms of the speaker's intended 'phonetic gestures'. These gestures (following the hypotheses of Action Theory) are *abstract* units which figure in the motor control of speech, and which are re-statements of underlying phonological plans (using our own terminology here). So, in the final version of the Motor Theory we find listeners actively reconstructing speaker plans for articulatory gestures according to a synthesis of their own procedures for speaking. It is not entirely clear whether the articulatory gestures are or need to be fully dynamic, as they are for example in Articulatory Phonology (Chapter 4) and TM.

The Motor Theory needs to re-interpret the listener's hypotheses about the speaker's intended segmental gestures so that a phonological representation can be assigned. The theory concludes with identified abstract gestures – but these are not phonological units. Without reworking the entire perceptual phonology in terms of those gestures, it will be necessary to include such an assignment stage in the model. Note that Browman and Goldstein were explicit about their attempt to rework perceptual phonology within their own gestural context.

Neither the early Motor Theory nor its revised version pay specific attention to prosody or to expressive content. These properties of speech are by their very nature dynamic, and it is almost certainly not the case that the Motor Theory, even if further extended, would be able to handle such complex issues. The theory originates in an era of static, motor target oriented modelling and would need re-focussing and redevelopment to cover aspects of speech beyond the simple segment-oriented description.

The Analysis by Synthesis Theory

The Analysis by Synthesis Theory is, to put it simply, the acoustic equivalent of the Motor Theory. It was devised by Stevens and Halle (1967) in an attempt to reconcile the apparent mismatch between the speech waveform the listener hears and the phonological labels which have to be applied to it. The difference between the two theories is that the Analysis by Synthesis Theory is concerned with bringing the listener's *acoustic* knowledge to the decoding process, whereas the Motor Theory is concerned with using the listener's *articulatory* knowledge.

Analysis by Synthesis Theory has the same problems as the Motor Theory when it comes to solving problems of the variability in speech. The theory is insufficiently rich to accommodate the interpretation of every source of variability, and in particular prosody and expressive content are neglected. In addition the model is, as with the Motor Theory, essentially segment oriented, though it does go beyond the Motor Theory in interfacing with the listener's phonology.

Hybrid models of speech perception

One or two researchers have proposed hybrid models, the basis of which is the hypothesis that listeners initially attempt a solution to the perceptual task by using some direct perception method. They use a more active approach only when the initial attempt fails.

There are problems, however with the hybrid compromise approach:

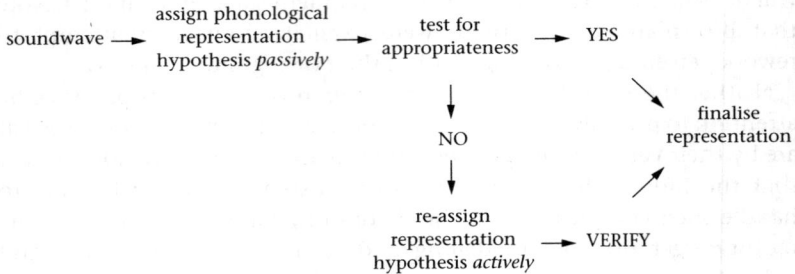

1. Firstly, how is the switching from the initial stage to the second stage thresholded? When does the speaker know that they have failed and need to move to the second stage?
2. Secondly, what time delay is needed for realising that the initial passive attempt has failed and that an active process needs to be applied to the same incoming data stream?

We know of no experiment which has successfully and reliably measured the timing of how speakers might switch approach on realising failure. What we might offer is the idea that active perception is the norm, but that the processes are arranged in some hierarchical way which make efficient use of the system in 'obvious' cases, moving to deeper but potentially more successful strategies as it becomes 'harder' to reach a satisfactory solution to the symbolic representation assignment task.

Categories

The TM theory shares properties with several general theories of speech perception. In particular there is the underlying idea that cognitively speech (and language) proceeds in terms of symbolic representations. Indeed all contemporary linguistics is built on this notion – sometimes quite explicitly, sometimes implicitly. The representation is based on categories which are there because of their functional roles within the language – or in our immediate case, within speech production and perception. In linguistics it is phonology which handles this functional role of the units of representation.

Clearly symbolic representations cannot be a property of the physical signal. They may have a psychological reality, if we are right, but not a physical reality. There may be general phenomena or, more precisely, *objects* in the physical signal which show a strong correlation with the abstract objects of a symbolic representation, but such a correlation does not extend to a definite co-existence and certainly not to identity. The abstract symbols of language are not objects to be found in the physical manifestation of language – such a possibility would be a serious violation of important scientific principles: symbols and the objects they symbolise cannot be the same thing. So, abstract symbolic representations are, by definition, a derivative of human cognition, and as such they are said to have *psychological reality*. That is they are both scientifically plausible and have a reality in the human being's mind.

One task of a theory of perception is to provide a robust linkage between the physical signal as its symbolic representation. A good start is to propose that the symbolic representation is assigned to the signal as the outcome of cognitive processing. Note that because the abstract representation cannot exist in the physical world it cannot be assigned as the *outcome* of a physical process; it can be only the outcome of a *cognitive* process.

The theory of Categorical Perception (Liberman *et al.* 1958, Repp 1984) is one attempt to model the assignment of discrete symbolic representations to the continuousness of the physical signal. We might also speak of a *mapping* between the two, but this does not mean an equivalence in any physical sense. Mapping, however, implies the possibility of setting out a passive algorithm which will enable one to be derived from the other. Assignment on the other hand implies a more active role for cognition: the algorithm is subject to variation depending on a number of environmental factors.

We must, however, be careful of the way in which we interpret the data from experiments such as those detailed in Liberman *et al.* (1958) and reviewed by Repp (1984). The classical experiments in categorical perception present graded stimuli to listeners asking them to identify what they hear. The fact that at some point on the vector there is a perceptual switch from one category to another does not imply that there *is* a boundary either in the stimulus or in the listener's mind. What these experiments claim to show is that perception is organised to input clines and output discrete symbolic objects. The assignment decision breakover points along a vector – where one symbolic label might switch to another in the listener's mind – vary of course with the language or accent. Another way of saying this is that listeners cannot label sections of the vector unless that know that they *can*, and that they have a suitable inventory of labels to deploy. The set of labels varies from language to language and accent to accent.

Direct Realism

Fowler's Direct Realism (Fowler 1986) theory, elaborating for speech on the generalised approach by Gibson (1954), suggests a linear relationship between a speech sound and, after a stage involving a representation of the articulation, the cognitive representation of that sound, thus avoiding any need for cognitive processes to make the link. The task of the listener here is to extract some detail of speaker's articulation from the signal being heard. Without cognitive mediation the listener is aware of a representation of the sound, and hence of an appropriate symbolic representation.

Direct Realism has serious difficulty in dealing with such phenomena as:

- defective acoustic signals due to failure of parts of the speaker's rendering processes;
- degraded signals due to ambient noise or masking effects;
- the listener's apparent ability to repair such 'damaged' signals provided they are intact to a particular threshold; even repairing the speech of hearing impaired speakers and other dysfluencies, as well as young children's speech;
- apparent collaboration between speaker and listener to achieve transfer of information – even under difficult conditions.

There is now little doubt that speakers are much more in control of their rendering of utterance plans than was previously thought. True, Fowler's Action Theory (for speech production) is almost certainly correct in assigning many rendering processes to self-organising neuro-motor structures arranged in a distributed processing array, but there is clear evidence of cognitive intervention in the performance of these biological structures. Fowler endows them, correctly, with properties wrongly thought earlier to be cognitive in nature, but misses the essential supervisory role of some *cognitive agent*. Precisely the same kind of criticism can be levelled at Direct Realism (for speech perception): of course there are *some* direct correlations between physical phenomena and their mental representation, but at the same time it seems fairly clear that the system's ability to run 'unassisted' – that is, without cognitive mediation – seems implausible.

Stevens' Quantal Theory

Stevens' Quantal Theory (Blumstein and Stevens 1979, Stevens 1989) suggests that the relationship between the acoustic signal and the physical configuration of the vocal tract is nonlinear. The theory singles out some regions of the vocal tract where relatively large changes of configuration result in comparatively small acoustic changes. Whether this quantal approach could be made to match up with perceived linguistic categories seems unlikely, given that the selection and assignment of categories is heavily language dependent. Moreover we do not feel that the converse can be the case either – that the physical quanta themselves can be explained by any direct reference to language. The existence of the quanta themselves is not disputed: it is whether they play a role in language which we question.

The quest for invariance

The Motor Theory of Speech Perception, Direct Realism and the Quantal Theory are all examples of attempts to build models which at some stage characterise invariant, and possibly unique, specifications for speech sounds. The empirical observation which such theories try to explain is that listeners are able to identify or assign symbolic solutions to heard acoustic signals, and that these symbolic representations come from a relatively small set of possibilities. The obvious first shot attempt is to propose a level of invariance in the signal, and then to develop models of how this might be linked to the invariance of the solution – that is: there is a unique symbol to be assigned because there is something equally unique in the signal. The relationship might be a direct one (Direct Realism), or mediated by a motor coding stage (Motor Theory of Speech Perception), or an acoustic analysis stage (the Quantal Theory and Analysis by Synthesis Theory).

The Associative Store Theory

The Associative Store Theory was developed in the 1970s and adopted as part of Cognitive Phonetics, and is an extreme form of an active theory of speech perception – see also Levinson 2005, p. 258, for more on the associative store. It is linguistic in as much as no physical mechanisms are described in the theory. The term 'associative store' is borrowed from the name of a type of computer memory common at the time. The memory arranged bytes in pairs in an array – with the second of each pair already stored. The essential property of this memory is its ability to input a new, but defective, byte into a blank memory 'slot' in the array, and output the corresponding stored *non*-defective byte as though this had been in the incoming signal. In Cognitive Phonetics the model focused on the observation that listeners are able to *repair* defective data – that is, they are able to report 'heard' data *as though it had not been defective*.

input byte	paired bytes		output byte
0	0	0	0
0	0	0	0
1	1	1	1
0	0	0	0
?	?→	1	1
1	1	1	1
0	0	0	0
1	1	0	0

If the model is viewed as a cascade of processes responsible for decoding meaning from the speech soundwave, the start of the overall process is some mental representation of the incoming soundwave. This representation may be degraded in the sense that it reflects errors which may have crept into the speech sounds by reason of poor production, poor transmission between the speaker and listener or poor hearing on the part of the listener.

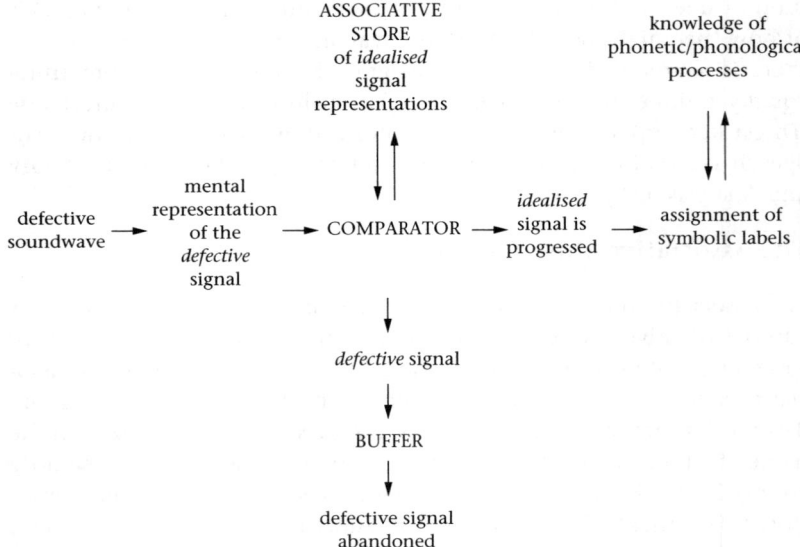

Central to the model is the comparator, a device for comparing a pair of signals. The comparator accepts a mental representation of the defective incoming signal and compares this with representations available in an associative store arrangement of idealised signals. These are predominantly language-specific since they have been acquired by exposure to this language. We do not discuss the acquisition procedure here. The result of a scan of the associative score is an *idealised* output which has been found as the 'best match' to the incoming signal. The idealised output constitutes a *repair* of the defective input signal; and it is this idealised signal which is passed for further processing in the form of an assignment of an appropriate symbolic representation. From this point on, if the listener is asked to report on what has been heard they will report the idealised signal not the defective one – it can be observed empirically that listeners *believe they have heard the repaired signal*.

What the listener reports as having been 'heard' is no more than a hypothesis which waits to be tested against the general context of the utterance(s) being heard. Occasionally this test will reveal that the repaired signal must be in error because it is logically inconsistent with the surrounding data. On occasions such as this the listener backtracks to a buffer where, at least for a brief period (corresponding to the intrinsic properties of short-term memory) the defective signal can be re-processed through the system.

The essential properties of this theory are:

- it is a cognitively oriented active theory;
- *two* input channels are available to the system – one carrying the defective 'signal' and the other carrying an idealised *repaired* version;
- potentially degraded input triggers a memory scan to retrieve a best-match stored item using associative store technology;
- a copy of the stored idealised item is passed for further phonetic/phonological processing;
- the original defective signal is discarded;
- perceptual awareness is of the item retrieved from store, *not* of the stimulus trigger item;
- the system is re-entrant, in the sense that failed solutions can be discarded and the perceptual process rerun to generate new hypotheses.

Thus the loss of stimuli is buffered for a short period of time, just in case they are needed again in the event of a processing error being detected or a hypothesised solution being rejected. The buffer is finite in length (i.e. there is a fixed number of pigeon slots) and therefore a limit on the number of stimuli that can be temporarily stored. Such a buffer is also known as short-term memory in the field of psychology.

So we add this detail to our characterisation of the Associative Store Model:

- the detection of an error during later processing triggers a rescan of the associative store by the comparator;
- the rescan is enabled by holding the original defective stimuli in a buffer before discarding;
- the buffer is finite in length, and operates on a first-in-first-out basis.

Similarity of production and perception

Some researchers feel that there is a processing scenario in speech perception which corresponds to a similar situation in speech production. There the utterance plan is prepared as the output to a tiered arrangement of cognitive processes. Once the plan is available it is 'handed on' for physical rendering to create the appropriate soundwave. Lindblom (1990) developed the production for perception idea that speakers aim to minimise their own efforts while at the same time providing the listener with a signal requiring the minimum necessary discrimination to resolve ambiguities. The model is plausible, but lacks a convincing discussion of the mechanisms and strategies which might be invoked, and does not involve the level of collaboration we suggest is necessary.

Speaker/listener collaboration (Cognitive Phonetics)

The TM Cognitive Phonetics approach develops the idea of speaker/listener collaboration further. The hypothesis is that speakers continuously run a model of speech perception which tests utterance plans before they are actually physically rendered. The idea is that the speaker works out what the rendered plan *would* sound like and how it *would* be perceived. The results of the test are fed back in an iterative loop to adjust the rendering process (if not the plan itself) to produce a signal optimised for the unambiguous perceptual assignment of a symbolic representation matching the original utterance plan. Rendering adjustment is performed in a supervisory arrangement under the control of the Cognitive Phonetics Agent (the CPA). The dominant motivation here is the speaker's goal of *successful listener decoding*.

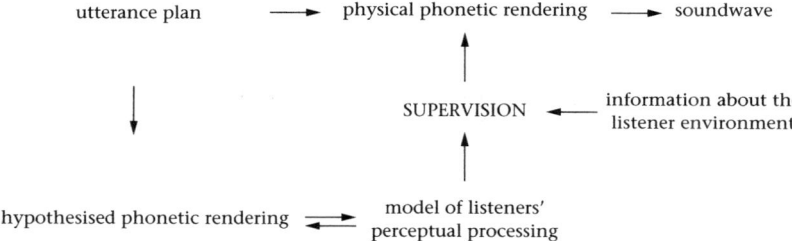

The model of listeners' perceptual processing is a *feed-forward anticipatory model* (Rosen 1985). In TM the idea of minimising speaker effort emphasised by Lindblom is played down and seems largely irrelevant. The reason for this is that we are not able to characterise effort either quantitatively or qualitatively. We cannot say whether this or that speech sound has more or less effort, let alone exactly how much that effort is.

In TM all speech is produced within an expressive wrapper (Tatham and Morton 2004), and as yet we are unable to characterise variable effort against the backdrop of expression. Does the increased precision of angry or careful explanatory speech require greater effort? Intuitively yes, but we do not *know* this yet in our science – the hypothesis awaits empirical support. But even if we did know that this or that speech sound needs greater or less effort, or this or that mode of expression requires more or less effort, how is this relevant to a model of speaker/listener interaction? For the sake of form we can conjure up reasons and explanations, but they would have little more status than conjecture. The 'principle of least effort' enjoys a wide following, but there is little if any solid evidence that human beings actually do manipulate their speech environment to minimise the expenditure of effort!

8
Speech Perception: Production for Perception

Introduction

Nooteboom (1975, 1983), Tatham (1970) and several other researchers introduced perception as one of the speaker's principal goals: speakers aim to be perceived; almost all speech production models have adopted this basic idea to account for perceiver-oriented variability in the acoustic signal. An example of a wholly speaker-oriented model can be found in MacNeilage (1970) where the goal or target is the articulation, with gamma loop control of contextual variants. TM has a different take on this: the goal is to provide a signal *optimised* for perception, where what is optimal may be a variable, since the listener's ability to perceive – that is, assign an appropriate labelling – is itself a variable depending on context and environment.

Nooteboom's (1983) speech production model includes a representation of auditory perceptual space. In this way, the speaker is able to draw on both spatial and perceptual representations of the articulation to compute appropriate motor commands to achieve targets. The motor commands are about movement from the current articulatory state.

- the speaker intends a particular spatial target;
- the articulatory mechanism is in a particular state – A;
- the speaker consults the representation in auditory space – B;
- the motor commands are computed for a revised target depending on A and B.

Speech Perception: Production for Perception 219

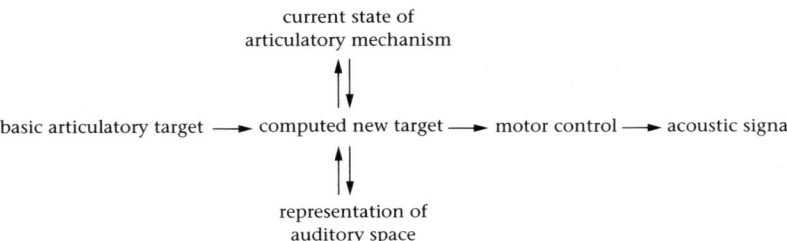

The model is essentially static in that it is couched in terms of targets and static representations. However, the inclusion of the speaker's ability to compute new targets partly by referencing the current state of the articulatory mechanism is a move toward a more dynamic approach.

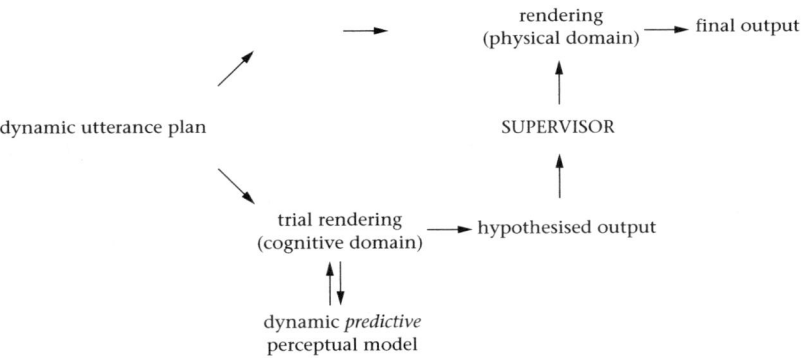

TM goes further (diagram above) and includes a *dynamic model* of speech, not simply representations of targets within some auditory perceptual space, but a model of the dynamic perceptual processes which assign symbolic labelling. The perceptual goal is the assignment of a correct or appropriate symbolic labelling to what the speaker has produced: the speaker, *via* a perceptual model, is able to compute the effectiveness of their strategy and make appropriate adjustments. Such an approach guarantees a highly successful perception despite linguistic and environmental variables, as well as perceptual contextually-dependent variables which may be introduced in the listener. The speaker is able to use the perceptual model to anticipate listener success and compensate in advanced for predicted failure.

Ease of articulation

Ladefoged (1993) feels that speakers 'often like to convey their meaning with the least possible articulatory effort' (p. 267), or perhaps the least necessary effort. Unless there is some special reason for the speaker to focus on articulatory precision (for example in the case of contrastive emphasis) they 'tend to produce utterances with a large number of assimilations', and there will even be whole segments deleted. One result will be that some differences between segments may be minimised. Ladefoged invokes a 'principle of ease of articulation', proposing that 'the main way of reducing articulatory effort is by making use of coarticulations between sounds' (p. 267).

Making use of coarticulation

For the speaker to 'use' coarticulation implies a voluntary push to actually produce coarticulation – implying that there are circumstances in which coarticulation does not occur. The literature has mixed feelings on these two areas: production for perception and ease of articulation. Both are perennial concepts, appearing prominently in the literature from time to time. Currently both are being focused on as 'principles' of phonetics in the popular Optimality Theory slant on phonology (Hayes and Steriade 2004, Prince and Smolensky 2004). The revisited idea is that phonology is constrained by phonetic facts and principles, and the model is conceived in line with most model building these days in the cognitive sciences and in linguistics in particular: that is, it is constraint based. But *of course* the cognitive objects and processes of phonology are phonetically constrained, and *of course* they conform to phonetic principles: how else could it be? – a point recognised and developed by phoneticians and phonologists since, and including, Sweet (1877). To our knowledge there has been no opposing view. The originality in Optimality Theory lies in its mathematical or computational rigour, rather than in its conceptualisation.

TM models phonetic rendering with coarticulation built into the dynamic gestural process and explained by factors outside linguistics. Ease of articulation and predicted perceptual success can switch in a degree of constraint on that coarticulation if we want to or need to. We believe that it is more useful for the model to be this way round because it asserts a baseline of coarticulation which is *externally* determined – it has nothing to do with linguistics. We can, though, if we so wish, constrain the baseline. Keating has the same idea (Chapter 3): there is a window or 'margin' expressing that there is always some submission to external coarticulatory forces by a segment, but that on any one occasion the segment will be produced within the window. The width of Keating's window has been determined empirically by examining exactly how segments behave with respect to how they succumb to coarticulatory forces. We have seen how other writers introduce the concept of a dynamic window – for example, Cho (2002) whose windows assume a dynamism dependent on utterance prosody.

Ladefoged wants to balance the *ease of articulation* principle (owned by the speaker) with the *sufficient perceptual separation* principle (owned by the listener). The point being that listeners, he feels, would 'prefer utterances that have sounds that remain constant and distinct on all occasions' (p. 268). This does not square with those researchers who believe that coarticulation assists perception. TM agrees with Ladefoged to a great extent: perceivers might also want to expend minimal effort in decoding what they hear. What we feel is necessary here is a model which equates the needs of speaker and listener to optimise the overall situation. The problem is that building such a model is by no means straightforward.

Targets – representations of which level?

It is possible to specify the target for each segment parametrically at any level in the hierarchy using articulatory, aerodynamic or acoustic parameters. Researchers often cite also the use of 'phonational parameters' which are used to render the 'conditions' under which utterances are to be spoken, meaning that expressive and general prosodic constraints apply.

What we may lack still is clear knowledge of how these three possibilities for representation (articulatory, aerodynamic or acoustic) relate in the *mental* processing of utterances. For the Cognitive Phonetics Agent to operate effectively there has to be knowledge of constraints at all three tiers in the model, since CPA controlled intervention is possible in terms of all three levels; at least we find it useful to have all three representations available in the model. We cannot say how a human being actually does these things. But we can hypothesise that there must be knowledge of all three levels of representation, and moreover there must be the means of *using* this knowledge to provide appropriate control and intervention at particular moments as the utterance rendering dynamically unfolds. But in addition there must be knowledge of perceptual processes and how these interact with the results of target combinations and constraints on *all three tiers*.

Adaptive Variability Theory

Lindblom's Adaptive Variability Theory (1983, 1990) has two basic ideas:
- speech is designed to communicate information effectively;
- speech is produced by a biological device which, like other biological devices, operates according to the principle of economy of effort.

Adaptive variability is all about the hypothesis that speakers are able to adjust how they produce ('render' in TM) speech according to the requirements of the communicative situation, which includes how perception works. This is quite similar to the earlier proposals of Tatham (1967 onwards). The role of perception is similar, though Tatham has rather more detail and attempts to explain the constraints on the system, discussing at some length the interaction between the cognitive and physical domains.

Coarticulation, proponents of Adaptive Variability Theory claim, potentially results in a reduction of perceived phonological contrast. The decrease is scalar depending where on the hyper-/hypo- speech continuum the event sits. This continuum characterises the range between resisted and intrinsic coarticulation. In Tatham's terminology this continuum runs from maximally enhanced through to maximally constrained, settling on the optimum value in the given utterance, once the phonological and other constraints have been evaluated. For Tatham's strict delineation of phonological and phonetic processes the decrease in contrast is essentially an alteration of 'trigger value' such that there is an *apparent* decrease in phonological contrast. What this actually means is that the difference between the planned utterance and the rendered utterance changes:

scale of coarticulatory control from *fully enhanced* through *neutral* to *fully constrained*
[enhanced]   1 ← — 0 — → 1   [constrained]

correlating scale of phonological contrast
[maximally decreased]   0 ← — 0 — → 1   [minimally decreased]

In Adaptive Variability Theory the rate of arrival of motor commands is what signals the intended duration of individual segments: the *durational plan* underlies the timing constraint. The durational plan is *not* part of the phonological utterance plan except perhaps in a notional sense because of the abstract nature of phonology. In the TM Cognitive Phonetic model marking of physical time is one of the initial phonetic processes which is carried out on the *dynamic phonetic plane* from interaction between the phonological utterance plan and the physical specifications held on the static phonetic plane – Chapter 6.

Articulator 'response' and its relevance to perception

Many researchers, in discussing their articulatory or motor control models, refer to 'articulator response', and we need to ask exactly what this means and how the term 'articulator' is defined. In the neurophysiology the immediate response to neural commands (that is, patterned 'meaningful' neural signals arriving along a motor neuron) is muscle fibre contraction within specific muscles, which in turn results in the overall contraction of those muscles.

Although muscle fibre contraction is an 'all-or-none', discrete or 'digital' response to neural signals, the contraction of whole muscles is analogue and scalar. At what point on a muscle's range of overall contraction the *response* contraction settles is a function of the percentage of muscle fibres recruited to the contraction and the rate of firing of the individual fibres.

Articulator structures in the sense implied by names such as 'tongue', 'lips', 'jaw', etc. are positioned and shaped by contraction of their intrinsic musculature. These articulator structures are responsible for overall vocal tract shape which in turn leads to the detail of the aerodynamic system's response: the output sound.

Articulator response – in the sense of vocal tract shape control to enable a particular sound output – therefore entails an entire hierarchical structure with a tight, but variable, internal system. That system is complex, involving nested groups of coordinative structures which are necessarily organised to be *goal oriented*. The final goal is the production of sound, though the goal of the utterance plan is to arrive at an *effective production/perception transaction* – that is, the communication of a linguistically encoded message.

In the TM model of speech production/perception it is the *plasticity* of the system originating in the sophisticated low level physical structure which enables coarticulation to be tackled head on. Lindblom's model however characterises the *surface effects* of this mechanism as observed experimentally in the final output, as do other models of coarticulation. Lindblom focuses strongly on this data, but the approach is essentially descriptive rather than explanatory – except to say that the observed variability in coarticulatory effects are down to interaction between production and perception. To have the required explanatory power Lindblom's approach, and its derivatives, would need to go beyond description of the surface mechanism and its effects, and show how the whole production system, from underlying phonology through to assigned perceptual representation – the act of 'recognition' – works as a coordinated whole.

The basic units for speech – segments again

There have been many proposals concerning the basic units for describing speech, though not all researchers make the proper distinction between units for *describing* speech (useful constructs of the phonetician) and the units people actually use to work with speech. Abercrombie (1967) seems to favour the syllable as the probable basic unit for speech – the result of a sequence of 'postures' of the vocal organs, though not in the simplistic way of a succession of discrete postures. We are more inclined toward the term 'gesture', with its greater emphasis on the dynamics of the utterance. A parametric characterisation of the syllable and successive syllables would emphasise continuousness more and allow for the parameters to start and stop asynchronously, thus providing a good foundation for explaining coarticulatory phenomena.

Many phoneticians of the Classical Phonetics era recognised the continuousness of speech, but sought to reconcile this with the discontinuousness of the segment-based descriptions by referring to segments as though they were points in time. The *obvious* alternative is that 'segments' are abstractions which underlie the continuousness of the physical phenomena associated with speech. Abercrombie (1967), for example, speaks of *consonants* as points in 'the constantly changing stream of speech' (p. 42) – an attempt to render the continuousness into an abstract static characterisation, but without making the leap also to a hierarchical perspective on the relationship between the segment and the physical signals. Abercrombie finds more difficulty with defining vowels (p. 55), but the same kind of idea is present, and we can think of vowels as perhaps short idealised portions of the physical signal. This is not an unreasonable compromise, given the general predisposition to adhere to linear modelling.

Segmentation for such theorists is literally the linear subdivision of the physical signal into segments. For the purposes of their descriptive model – that is, when it comes to providing labels – these segments, *as labelled*, are not necessarily as 'long' as the time between their boundaries: it is as though the physical time offered a framework for identifying an *idealised* object between the segment boundaries. Hence the unspoken assumption that somehow, by a process of abstraction, the ideal segment and its label are to found *within the dynamic physical signal*, though the label, being abstract of course, is not and cannot be itself dynamic. The segment is a static object with an appropriate label, derived by a process of boundary identification within the dynamic utterance – a consequence of adopting the linear paradigm. In more recent models we might prefer to think of a segment as a labelled static object *underlying* the dynamic utterance, or used to characterise the utterance without actually being a part of it. Thus neither segments nor labels are usefully to be found in the signal. Segments and their labels are sequentially assigned to an utterance in a simple model, and in the simple descriptive meaning of the phrase might be said in this sense to be 'derived' from the utterance. In a more explanatory approach we might say that segments and the labels are part of the underlying explanation of the physical signal, without of course being 'part of' the signal in any obvious sense.

Functional and physical definitions – potential conflict

A good example of the apparent conflict between functional and physically-oriented definitions: functionally /h/ is usually regarded by phonologists as a consonantal segment, in the sense that in languages like English it regularly forms the onset of a syllable and never the nucleus, which would make it a vowel. Physically though /h/ shares many properties associated with the phonetic rendering of underlying vowels rather than consonants, even down to exhibiting perhaps almost all of the characteristics of the following syllable nuclear vowel, though without the vocal cord vibration which normally correlates with vowels in most accents of English. A physically oriented description might speak of [h] as a 'voiceless vowel' or one devoid of vocal cord vibration in its rendering, and recognise that in terms of recognisable 'quality' (a catch-all term for the acoustic parameters which together trigger the perceptual assignment of labels for this or that vowel) there are going to be as many [h]s as there are renderings of vowels to follow them. The observation is moreover universal in the sense that such a model predicts that in all /h + V/ sequences in *all* languages the effect will be similar – [h] always assumes the quality, albeit without vocal cord vibration, associated with following vowel segment. Note, once again, that the alphabetic notation /h + V/, or, less abstractly for example [h + i ...] is incapable of implying any point in time where the [h] switches to the vowel. For a functional characterisation a point in time is irrelevant, for a characterisation of the acoustic a boundary-less abstractly labelled waveform (or some suitably imaged version of the waveform) is enough.

Segments – psychological reality

The idea that there are segments in the mind – that segments have a psychological reality – almost certainly arises from the way speech is represented in the speaker/listener mind when it is cognitively processed. That representation is invariably taken as being in terms of strings of objects which the speaker/listener correlates with the physical events which trigger them. The speaker/listener's *need* to make the correlation is so strong that listeners will report that they do indeed 'hear' the discrete segments – *which, of course, they do not*.

An object which is psychologically real is one which is recognisable and meaningful to a human being in the sense that it can form a unit which can be manipulated as part of a cognitively based system, such as speech. As an example we can cite the fact that /k/ and /t/ are objects which are psychologically real for speakers and listeners, whereas in physically rendering an utterance the fronting of [k] before a following [i], or the retracting of [t] before a following [ɑ] is *not* psychologically real – speakers and listeners are not normally aware of these details which creep into the rendering in a way which is not cognitively dominated.

As abstract objects segments are discrete; in no sense do they or can they blend into one another. The psychological reality of segments is clearly correlated with the way segments, and our ability to compare and contrast them, are basic to the way language works in terms of identity and opposition. Categorisation and the quest for identifying 'sameness' among objects detected by the senses is central to production and perception behaviour – certainly in speech and vision, and presumably in other modalities. Language is systematic in terms of the function of segments or units within its entire structure; it is this structure – the identifiable units and their relationships – which *is* language.

Discrete units in the cognitive world

It is commonly felt that language revolves around discrete and separately identifiable objects. All linguists have agreed with this view, and *non*-linguists seem to feel the same way and can report these feelings when questioned. So long as language is defined as a cognitive activity then this is probably true, but when we invoke the physical world then this association between language and discrete units does not necessarily continue to hold. One way of regarding cognition (which we can only characterise in an abstract way) is that it is really about modelling by the human being. What scientific method has come up with as a useful way of describing our universe is equally applicable, in our view, to how human beings proceed: it is as though they were scientists using a similar approach. Thus for a human being to comprehend the surrounding universe they have to model it, and it is this model which constitutes their organised cognitive perception of the world around them. If we extend the idea a little to cover a world which includes the brain mechanism itself we might say that cognition is a process of modelling brain activity – is an abstraction of brain activity (Lakoff and Johnson 1999). Neurolinguistics and psycholinguistics move forward slowly, but these are the areas where we would expect the linguistic aspects of brain and cognitive activity to be modelled.

Theoretical linguistics is perhaps too detached and too overly abstract to be helpful here. We are thinking of the way in which an abstract neurolinguistic model would itself have to characterise processes in terms of an abstraction involving just such discrete units, even though, like neuromotor processes in phonetics, the neural processes at the linguistic level may not involve discrete units. Put another way, just as the scientist models the universe as a simpler more manageable system, with little notion that the model might actually *be* the universe, so the abstract cognitive model necessary for human thought need not actually *be* the real world vehicle for such abstract processing. Because human cognition is in terms, linguistically, of discrete units it does not follow that non-abstract processing in the human beings is also in terms of discrete units. In fact, looking at what we do know of the brain and the motor system it might well be the case that we are in a position to state that it is not a system which relies on discrete units.

The units which linguists use as the basis of their models are structured – that is, form part of a system – in a hierarchical and linear fashion: that is, the structure may be characterised in terms of the relationships between levels in the hierarchy *and* in terms of the relationship between units within any one level. Some characteristics of language will lend themselves to one approach, others to the other approach, and some to both. Mental activity of any kind might in general be structured in this way, though brain activity does not necessarily have to adhere to the same approach.

Impossibility of isolating cognitive considerations from physical considerations

In phonetics it is impossible to isolate cognitive considerations from physical considerations. In fact much of the theorising in phonetics over the past half century has explicitly addressed the relationship between the cognitive processes of phonology and the physical processes of speech production. We feel there must be a relationship, but what that relationship is still defeats theorists; at the most we are able to characterise a rather loose correlative association between the two. Cognition and cognitive processes work to provide a human being with a model of what is going on physically when it comes to speech production and perception. The most we can hope for is that our models as scientists reflect this somehow. We come across this idea in the theory of Cognitive Phonetics where we try to model the way in which cognition intervenes in physical processes, and can easily be seen to be doing so.

Segment 'boundaries' and asynchrony

One argument complicating the definition of the segment is that segment boundaries are unclear, particularly if the segment is modelled parametrically. In an extreme case we might model a segment as a set of several tens of muscle parameters – one for each muscle used in producing speech sounds. From what electromyographic studies there have been, even with very small sets of muscles, it is clear that contraction begins and ends asynchronously. A number of reasons could be adduced to explain this:

1. the masses of the different muscles vary, and it would follow logically that to obtain some simultaneity at some point in a gesture the different muscles would have to begin contraction at different times;
2. some muscles will involve a greater degree of contraction than others, and this may take more time, so an early start is called for;
3. passive movement of a muscle by an adjacent muscle or muscle group may mean that it has less contracting to do;
4. in running speech a muscle associated with a particular segment may in fact be already contracted for the previous segment, thus calling for a later start.

In particular the last observation is important: a muscle may already be well on the way to the target contraction for a particular segment because that muscle was involved in the previous segment. What is important about this is how and where the calculation has taken place which leads to both *less contraction* and a *later start* to the contraction.

Two possible control models

1. If the processing for motor control is done at some high level, then the entire system must be known to the speaker, and in addition information about the current state-of-play must also be available to the speaker. This is the basis of any theory of speech production which rests on the notion of the independent controllability of gestural parameters – akin to the phonological notion of the independent controllability of features (Chen and Wang 1975).
2. If the processing is done at a low level, then there must be pathways available to conduct information around a low level muscle group which enables the group as a whole to behave toward a common goal. This is the basis of Action Theory, and the group would constitute a coordinative structure within that theory.

Segments may be more appropriately characterised in terms of parameters similar to those used by the Classical Phoneticians – a set based on the anatomy of the system. The same apparently asynchronous behaviour will be observed, particularly in terms of the timing of articulators already on the way to a particular gesture because of the way they have been involved in the previous gesture. Thus lip closure following a segment with a neutral lip position may well involve a gesture different in degree and timing from lip closure preceded by a segment with tightly rounded lips. A question at the high level would be how the system got to know that a different lip closing gesture is required. The very large number of contexts in which such gestures can occur in a way different from any single prescriptive target means that the status of static unique targets is called into question.

Uniqueness of segments as 'targets'

Segments as targets are usually taken as unique; that is, they have no variability. Whether targets are expressed parametrically or as whole objects, uniqueness makes sense at some highly abstract underlying level. At worst these unique segments constitute neat starting points from which to derive the more surface variants we can sense cognitively and measure physically. At best the uniqueness of segments constitutes a hypothesis as to the relevance of such segments in the cognitive system underlying physical speech.

Trubetskoy and the continuum of speech

Trubetskoy (1939) was in no doubt as to the actual nature of the acoustic signal of speech, and makes one of the earliest characterisations of the 'continuum' of speech and the fact that it 'can be divided into an arbitrary number of segments' (p. 13).

Trubetskoy points out that the phonetician in taking account of articulation and the acoustic signal will want sometimes to consider the underlying phonology – in treating, for example, 'distinctive oppositions of a sound' which need to be addressed in more detail than non-distinctive oppositions. It is unclear whether a phonetician could devise a comprehensive characterisation of speech without regard to its phonological structure. However, in our model, that regard comes from the fact that

- the input is the phonological plan;
- any cognitive manipulation of the rendering process will tie in (perhaps) with the underlying phonological structure of the utterance.

There is a difference between our approach here and Trubetskoy's. We are clearer that there is no phonetics (as a rendering system) without a prior phonology. He is using phonology to indicate what are the relevant areas of phonetics to investigate. That is, from Trubetskoy's point of view phonetics must *connect* with phonology, and, by extension, *constrain* phonology. However, within phonetics we *could* simply be making observations about the acoustics of speech sounds without reference to the utterance – we would need this, for example, in working out how to set up a speech synthesiser.

'Rule governed' processes?

Care must be exercised in using the phrase 'rule-governed process'. What is really meant is that whatever is *actually* going on it is suitably *modelled* as a rule-governed process. The reason for qualifying the phrase in this way is that a model centred on rules is not the only way of characterising our observations. For example, it is perfectly possible to model aspects of language – particularly, from our point of view here in the area covered by this book, in phonology and phonetics – using an artificial neural network approach. Other statistical methods are also possible, such as the use of Markov models, particularly if the model is to play the role of a learning machine as well. Because the majority of linguists in modern times have taken the rule based approach, this must not be taken as an indication that somehow or other cognitive processes *are* themselves rule based. The cognitive processes are what they are, and the model uses whatever is an *appropriate* approach or formalism depending on the researcher's purposes.

General theory related to phonetic theory

Theories are developed to account for the observed data. To this extent the exact (independent) nature of the data can condition the type and form of the theory; but in addition the observation process is necessarily influenced by any pre-existing theory. Thus a scientist expecting speech to be segmental in nature will tend to model the data as exhibiting segmental properties. Exemplification of a theory is by models illustrating areas of the underlying theory. The construction of models not only has this illustrative function, but readily points to gaps – and this is perhaps truest when the model is computational. An algorithm is expected to run to some recognisable termination, and if it does not it will reveal gaps which prevent this happening.

Theories, when correctly formulated, incorporate the means of their own destruction: that is, they indicate explicitly the kind of data which would prove a conclusive counter-example. Theories also generate predictive hypotheses about previously unobserved data, thereby serving to direct future observation of data. In order to be able to generate hypotheses and incorporate the means of their own refutation, theories must necessarily have predictive power. For example:

1. We can observe that /d/ – a planned [+voice] segment – may well be rendered by a speaker of English as lacking in vocal cord vibration from early in the time 'allocated' to the segment when it closes a syllable, particularly if that syllable is final in an utterance. Since vocal cord vibration is accepted as a fair correlate of the abstract [+voice] feature we can create a tentative first attempt model from this rather minimal data. That model can be expressed as a rule which tells us that, when rendered, /d/ has, for the most part, the vocal cord feature set to zero. Further inspection shows that /b/ does the same in English. We might look at several tens of examples of the rendering of each of these underlying segmental plans.
2. At this point, despite the sparseness of the data, we might generate the hypothesis that /g/ will also render with the vocal cord feature set to zero. This is a formal way of saying that there is another segment, /g/,

which can occur in a plan for rendering – and that we might as well take a look at the way it works – predicting that it behave in the same way as /d/ and /b/. And, of course, we find that it does: an underlying planned /b/ is rendered with the vocal cord parameter set to zero.
3. We are in a position to refine the model and formulate the observation that, since the three segments share the [stop] feature, it is possible to generate the hypothesis that underlying segments which are [+stop] and [+voice] are rendered without vocal cord vibration. There are no more stops in English, but if one were to be introduced the hypothesis would predict that it too would set the vocal cord vibration to zero on rendering.
4. Additional hypothesis is now possible: since [+stop] segments are members of consonantal class, perhaps all [+consonantal] segments behave in this way. Investigation directed by this hypothesis will show that it can be supported in the case of fricatives and affricates, but not in the case of continuant segments like [l] or [r]. The model now needs refining to exclude these segments.

However, whatever formalism might be used to characterise the phenomena we have just observed it is clear that the model does not have *explanatory* power. That the vocal cord parameter is set to zero is not a statement which of itself tells us *why* this happens. Too much of early phonetic theory was ready simply to assume that such things happened because this is the way speakers of this or that language do things, the implication being that they might well do otherwise. And in the case of our example we might observe that many speakers of French (particularly the metropolitan accents) behave differently: vocal cord vibration continues throughout the time slot allocated to final voiced plosives, fricatives and affricates. Hence the observation that English does one thing, but French does something else. And of course we could examine many languages and conclude that they were either like English or like French or like some compromise between the two. We shall see later that this model is naïve when it comes to trying to understand why the phenomenon occurs in English but not in French – no real explanation is being offered other than to imply that English speakers wish to behave one way and French speakers in some other way.

A theory of speech production must cover both phonology and phonetics

Speech production theories should really take account of both the phonological level and the phonetic rendering level. Apart from the obvious reason that no speech theory would be complete without an account of both the cognitive and physical aspects of speech production and perception, there is little doubt that there is interaction between the two levels which is more complex than a simple handing over of phonological objects for physical rendering. *How* that rendering is to take place is subject, sometimes in detail, to cognitive intervention.

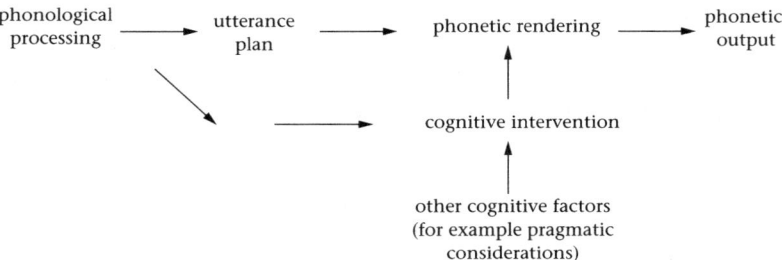

Mental representation of segments – speech planning and the CPA

It is easy to sustain the argument that there are representations of elements of speech and speech processes which are phonological in nature. Speech planning would not be possible without such representations – or at least this is the case if speech planning is considered to be a predominantly cognitive activity. Those researchers who espouse any kind of physiological target model must also hypothesise that there are physical representations of speech and its processes. Whether it is enough to say that objects such as coordinative structures are the repositories of the majority of this representation or information remains to be seen.

Do phonological or phonetic representations dominate the perceptual processes?

Some researchers have discussed whether phonological or phonetic representations dominate the perceptual processes. Evidence here suggests that the goal of speech perception is to work out the speaker's intended utterance plan, which, since it was derived entirely phonologically, must involve the perception in an association with phonological processes. Note, though, that the phonological processes themselves, their units and their representation are significantly constrained by subsequent rendering possibilities in the phonetics.

In general, phonetic processes – such as intrinsic coarticulation (though not such processes which might have been the recipients of cognitive intervention) – are not normally found within a listener's scope of awareness. Those researchers, however, who believe that one 'function' of coarticulation is to 'assist' perception must hypothesise that knowledge of coarticulatory processes would have to play a role in speech perception, even if there is no immediate awareness of such processes or their results.

It does seem that listeners can be, and sometimes *must* be, aware of the utterance plan and its underlying processes, but that it is unnecessary for them to be aware of processes logically coming later. The difficulty is that the evidence for awareness is clouded a little by the fact that speakers and listeners can be *made* aware of speech objects and processes which they might not normally be aware of. The obvious example here is of the trained phonetician who can 'hear' things lay speaker/listeners cannot – though it goes without saying that even the perception of the trained phonetician is subjectively based and itself subject to many constraints: the phonetician is also a normal listener and a user of language. Objectivity would be guaranteed only if the 'listening device' were neither human nor a user of language.

Part III
Areas of Focus, Modelling and Applications

Part II

9
Applications: Cognitive and Physical Modelling

Introduction

Humans learn to speak and understand language without apparent effort, barring a severe physical or cognitive deficit. The capacity, the potential, for language behaviour is said to be 'innate' (Chomsky 1965, Lorenz 1965, Givon 2001, Jackendoff 2002). Properties which are innate are seen as an essential feature of the mind and have not themselves been the result of some obvious learning processes. *Language* is the result of the exposure of this cognitive capacity to the individual's language environment. The term 'language' is sometimes seen as ambiguous: it can be the collective result of speaking or writing (a traditional use), or the set of processes by which that result is achieved (a more contemporary use).

Our ability to produce and understand language is seen as a feature of the mind; it is not seen by most researchers as arising solely in the transmission of neural signals in the grey matter of the brain. Language systems resulting from this human ability are described and to a limited extent explained by linguistics, with the assumption that language is essentially a cognitive, or mental activity.

The characterisation of language has proved complex in its detail (Chomsky 1965, Givon 2001, Jackendoff 2002); and the nature of both cognition and language itself is the subject of many model types and ongoing discussion among not only linguists but philosophers, cognitive neuroscientists, psychologists, neuro-linguists, language pathologists, cognitive scientists, language teachers, social psychologists, software engineers, anthropologists – even writers of fiction and advertising copy writers, among others.

The operation of the mind is revealed through cognitive behaviour, some of which is measurable, though some descriptions and reports are intuition based. In contrast, speaking is physically based. Since there are both cognitive and physical manifestations of language we need both cognitive and physical models in dealing language, especially in its spoken form.

Duality

Dividing the characterisation of spoken language activity into two types is referred to as a dualist approach because it incorporates two types of *processing*: cognitive and physical (Damasio 1994, Panksepp 1998). In fact, speaking is the major area of language production treated within linguistics that involves both the cognitive and the physical expression of the results of the underlying mental activity. (Writing also involves cognition and hand movements, but we will not be discussing this aspect.) *Neurolinguistics*, or language studies within the purview of neuroscience, also seeks to establish physical (neural) correlates of the cognitive processes characterised in linguistics (Chapter 12).

In modelling speech, two approaches have been taken:

1. characterise speech from two relatively separate points of view, the cognitive (phonology) and the physical (phonetics), without attempting to relate or even correlate the two types of activity (Chapter 1); or
2. suggest how an interrelation between these two areas might be modelled – illustrated, for example, by the direct mapping of Articulatory Phonology (Browman and Goldstein 1986), or by the direct mapping and linking supervisory scenario of Cognitive Phonetics (Tatham and Morton 2003, see also Chapters 3 and 6).

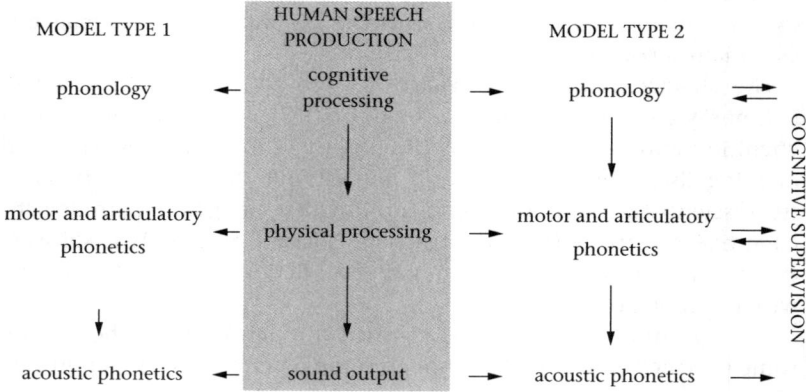

The diagram illustrates the two models and how they relate differently to human speech production. Model type 1 tends to keep the cognitive areas and physical areas separate – hence no linking arrow. An example might be the usual treatments of generative phonology and many phonetics models. Model type 2 models the relationship between cognitive processing explicitly and directly, sometimes using a linking cognitive supervisory process. In models incorporating a supervisory scenario the supervision depends on 'information' flow from and between both the cognitive and physical levels (Chapter 6 for details).

The phenomenon – what is being modelled

The use of language involves either speaking or writing (and other modalities like sign language). The meaning can be an intended or unintended message about thoughts, attitudes or feelings.

In speech, the waveform produced is a continuous physical event, which in the modelling process is often segmented and assigned sets of symbol-labels generally agreed upon by linguists and phoneticians. In Chapter 1 we saw that there is sometimes disagreement here since a largely subjective and impressionistic element is employed by the labeller. But no matter how assigned, the labels refer to different levels of representation, depending on what is being described: for example, sounds, words, phrases, etc. Because current strategies in modelling the speech waveform require *levels* of representation, the overall architecture is hierarchical. The hierarchy contains *two* types of phenomenon: cognitive and physical, as we saw in the above diagram illustrating just speech production. For difficult philosophical reasons these two types often sit uneasily together (Chapters 1 and 6).

Spoken language

There are two aspects to speech communication: production and perception. Within each of these two systems, there are two modes of activity: cognitive and physical. In linguistics, these two aspects of language behaviour are described by phonology (cognitive) and phonetics (primarily physical, although there are the sub-disciplines of auditory and perceptual phonetics). Perception studies deal with sensory detection (hearing) and perception.

In the general theory of speech production and perception, speech planning and the identification of the speech signal's content are described in cognitive terms *using a linguistic focus*. Speaking is seen primarily as physically based, but with the potential to modify on demand the cognitively determined phonological plan for an utterance (Chapter 6).

Speech and hearing/perceiving disorders

Occasionally the system works in a way that produces *disordered* speech (Chapter 12); and to address how we might understand or model what is happening there are several areas to look at for the source of such incomplete or abnormal production and/or perception. The list of possible sources of error is long, but includes:

- the acquisition of appropriate phonological units,
- details of phonological or other cognitive processing,
- the selection of biological structures and the associated motor patterns,
- timing relations in carrying out physical processing,
- the ability to detect the incoming signal,
- transmission of detected acoustic 'information' to the brain,
- neural and cognitive processing of the relevant information in order:
  - to assign appropriate patterns,
  - to plan the supervision, and adaptation of the entire speaking system
  - to changing dialogue contexts and other environmental contexts.

Disturbances in these systems can produce disordered speech (Chapter 12). The importance of appropriate modelling of such processes cannot be overemphasised when it comes to deciding how the clinician deals with assessed disorders.

Language teaching

In second language teaching (Chapter 11) examples of problem areas to be identified include:

- learning the right categories for the new language,
- retraining the motor system to render acceptable variants of phonological units,
- adequate perceptual processing of these units,
- overcoming possible interfering processing patterns developed in the first language.

Once again, language teaching demands the support of appropriate models.

Speech simulations

In simulations of speech production and perception – language technology (Chapter 10) – the choice is either

- to base engineering descriptions on what the human speaker/listener appears to do, or
- in synthesis – to produce an appropriate output (by whatever means) and hence provide an adequate input signal for the listener, and
- in recognition – to detect relevant acoustic patterns that correlate with speech produced by humans.

The speech technology engineer, again, needs the support of explicit models to produce an intelligible and appropriate signal for a human listener, or to recognise a speech-encoded language message from a human speaker.

Current modelling

The mind/brain distinction has been discussed in the speech literature in terms of two separate abstract units with a gap between them. Those aspects of spoken language production treated by phonology are one side of the gap, those treated by phonetics on the other side. The observation is often made that 'the output of the phonology is the input to the phonetics' (Wang and Fillmore 1961, Ladefoged 1965), but the situation is much more complex.

We accept that events in cognition and brain function correlate, without saying *how* or *why* they might be associated (Dennett 1996). Phonology does use *phonetic* features, a set of physical and perceptual characterisations, as evidence for positing some phonological rules (Hayes and Steriade 2004), but the reverse is not the case. Until further research produces plausible models which can show an explicit interconnection between areas which are currently designated either as either cognitive or physical (or mind/brain), we may be forced to continue to view spoken language activity as based in two separate 'units' linked by a *hypothetical* interface.

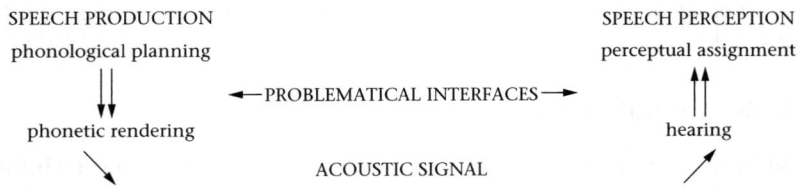

An old problem

The mind/brain division has been addressed historically by many, including, for example: Aristotle (see McKeon 2001) who divided organisms into matter, sensibility and form. These areas can be equated in broad terms to body (or brain), the sensory system (including awareness of the representations of the external object) and the cognitive functions currently associated with the construct 'mind'. Descartes (Descartes 1649, and see Cottingham 2000) addresses three areas: the corporal body, senses and perception, and the reasoning mind. Aquinas regarded the human as 'capable of supporting capacities of life, sense perception, and self conscious rational thought' (Eberl 2004, p. 364).

Today, cognitive neuroscience addresses the structure and function of the brain, the sensory system and awareness. The interconnection between areas is stated as an association between the results observed and measured. The experimental paradigm proceeds from an investigation into whether behaviour and brain function can be associated with an *acceptable probability rating* (Shanks 2005).

The basis for modelling mental activity arising from neural interaction is relevant for modelling speech production, which is concerned both with how to represent speech mental activity (the production of the utterance plan) and associated relevant brain activity, both together resulting in speech *behaviour*. Interpreting results is difficult. To quote and paraphrase Newsome (1977): 'performance of a specific cognitive task certainly consists of computations executed in parallel and in sequence within real neural pathways' (pp. 64–5), but restricting the description of mental phenomenon to a *specific* brain area may prove misleading. So in the case of spoken language there is brain activity *in parallel* associated with the plan to speak, and there is also brain activity *in sequence* for the resulting appropriate motor control. The complexity of identifying areas that may be directly correlated requires careful modelling.

We suggest that this framework may be useful for modelling speech production, but possibly may be useful in *applications*, for example, in identifying areas noted in language pathology from observations on disordered speaking, and leading to more focused treatment procedures (Chapter 12). Useful models of association between brain activity and cognitive activity may involve techniques such as functional magnetic resonance imaging (fMRI). The usefulness will depend on a well motivated, well designed, hypothesis driven language task and an understanding of the neural activity that might be associated with cognitive activity. A quotation from Raichle (2003) is relevant:

> The great strength of functional brain imaging is that it can contribute uniquely to such a task by providing a broad and detailed view of the processing architecture of cognitively engaged networks. (p. 3960)

However, we draw attention to the researchers in the field (for example, Raichle 1997, Ivry *et al.* 2001) who emphasise the need to take great care in rigorous experimental design. We raise this because there is currently a great deal of interest in associating linguistic activity with brain activity as revealed by fMRI work, and any conclusions that can be drawn from such work, especially as a foundation for applications modelling. Currently there are serious pitfalls for the unwary in such work, but there is little doubt that it will figure prominently in future modelling.

In the biopsychology research, what is not generally addressed but is essential for language production theory is the nature of the cognitive input to the motor system. The question here is: What activates the motor control of the articulators? There is very little modelling satisfactory for phonetic theory, and we emphasised earlier (Chapter 4) that we currently have the unfortunate situation where we are trying to model the phonetic rendering processes which lead to acoustic output *without* explicit knowledge of the nature of the input to these processes. We suggest that the brain activity accompanying the formulation of the phonological plan might be directly associated with the input to the motor control system, or to a component in the motor control system – itself an abstract concept when viewed as a *system*. Stored in the motor control area, or in memory accessible to motor control, is a set of default settings for producing rendered sound shapes. The two areas of brain activity could be mapped; and a cognitive phonetics agent (in TM, the CPA) with accompanying brain activity could modify the default settings on receipt of information from feedback, from linguistics, from areas that impinge on producing the appropriate language (Chapter 6).

244 *Areas of Focus, Modelling and Applications*

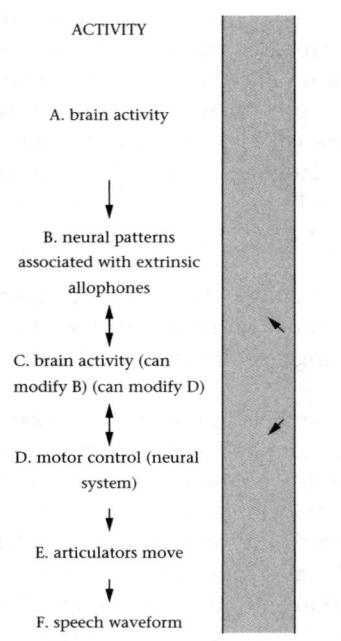

ACTIVITY	DESCRIPTIVE CHARACTERISATIONS
A. brain activity	a. general planning b. sound *pattern* processes leading to extrinsic allophone descriptions (the exemplar utterance plans – traditional phonology) c. dynamic module accesses static plane (TM)
B. neural patterns associated with extrinsic allophones	extrinsic allophones arranged as an actual utterance plan
C. brain activity (can modify B) (can modify D)	Cognitive Phonetics* (modifies B and/or D by supervisory process)
D. motor control (neural system)	no full description – models proposed: for example MacNeilage, Keating, Guenther, TM (Chapter 3)
E. articulators move	phonetics/phonology descriptions (Classical Phonetics)
F. speech waveform	acoustic phonetics descriptions (acoustic phonetics)

*Cognitive Phonetics, it is suggested, can modify rate and amplitude of speech in response to, say, changes as a dialogue unfolds. For example, the neural patterns associated with extrinsic allophones can change or the precursors to the motor control system can be modified so that different signals are transmitted; similarly an action that has begun might be interrupted.

Thus, neural patterns associated with the linguistic description 'extrinsic allophones' are either input to the motor control system, or mapped onto some precursor to actual activation – exciting or inhibiting the neurons in the general phenomenon called the 'motor control system'. But what we do not have at the moment is reliable information on the actual cognitive activity and neural representations that state the immediate precursors essential for input to the motor control system (Ivry *et al.* 2001 and Chapter 4). Cognitive phonetic processes are managed by an *agent*, accompanied by correlating brain activity that can change the specification of the immediate precursor to motor control (Chapter 6).

Cognitive and physical modelling

Much biopsychology research focuses on the processing of information from the external world, and the immediate effects on the individual (animal or human) or how this information relates to cognitive activity (Dickinson and Balleine 2000, Nobre *et al.* 2004, Wilkinson and Shanks 2004). For speech production, the modelling needs to know about the immediate stage before the neuronal activity in the motor cortex and how it might be organised. This model must take into account that speech is goal driven, that it is generally positive in that the speaker *wants* to say something.

An ideal model might incorporate findings such as whether the amygdala is involved in speech production; recent work (Baxter and Murray 2002) suggests the amygdala is involved in positive goal directed behaviour. The amygdala has access to memory, is involved in attention and in prediction (LeDoux 1996). Pathways connecting motor and cognitive areas have been investigated by Barinaga (1996). It is encouraging to believe that some brain activity related to *timing* may well be pulled together at some point just prior to motor activation, incorporating the results of plausible activity modelled from other areas. For example we might cite the role of the cerebellum (Ivry *et al.* 2001) in timing (Chapter 6). Such a nexus might help fill gaps in speech production models, so that we introduce hypotheses about the kind of activity that occurs just before the motor cortex becomes active.

Verification of brain activity accompanying planning would lend weight to the proposal of a CPA and other agents which are able to change any default settings constituting neural patterns in the motor cortex (Chapter 4). We need an *organisational principle* with which to view such data or other evidence. Unfortunately for speech production modelling, the evidence at this point is scarce, models are in the development stage (as far as speech production is concerned), and we ourselves cannot make defensible inferences from them for the module immediately preceding input to the motor cortex (see Bell-Berti *et al.* 1995, Damasio 1998).

Modelling the phenomenon – theory

A good theory will provide plausible explanations of why phenomena are the way they are. It will provide a framework within which it is possible to develop hypotheses enabling researchers to derive facts about the phenomena, and suggest ways of manipulating or modifying its *appearance* (Koch 1981, Feynman 1995). For example, if the theory posits that stuttering originates in brain dysfunction, different techniques to override some aspects of the speaking mechanism might be developed than if the theory suggests stuttering is a localised event occurring because the air pressure and rate of speaking are not synchronised. The goal could be adaptation to a brain system problem or to a retraining of the articulators to overcome a basic motor control system deficit. The techniques will be different, but will be *principled*, minimising guesswork. Applications models derived from theory might be more solidly based and thus more reliable and applicable to a wider range of instances. In speech synthesis, for example, if the goal is to simulate the human process and if the theory states that stored knowledge of speech as syllabic representations captures more generalisations than a segmental representation, the strategy for synthesis will be different. Again, strategies become principled in the theory driven paradigm of application.

Theories are not of course developed in a vacuum but rest on sets of general principles derived from experimental data (Feynman 1995). For example Darwin (1975) and Gould (2004) were able to famously generalise a descriptive system characterising animal life. A general principle, evolution, proved the linking factor for these descriptions. The principle involves hypothesising that features in the descriptions have a hierarchically organised derivational history. In this case, the class *human* is seen as the end product of a chain of animal classes related by specified features such as leg length, brain case size, circulatory systems, and so on.

Modelling the phenomenon – the empirical approach

The empirical approach is phenomenological – that is, the concept is based on the appearance of a phenomenon which exists in space and time (Eberl 2004). The term 'empirical' is used both broadly and narrowly:

- Used broadly, the term can refer to models based on experience, observation and with few formally stated generalisations about patterning in the phenomenon under study; a broad empirical approach is driven by events or phenomena, and observations.
- Used narrowly, the term can refer to hypothesis driven experimental work whose hypotheses are based on stand-alone observations but are not specifically within a standard model. The results can contribute to detailed model building as contributory evidence.

For example, observations about the inability of listeners to decode stops accurately in synthetic speech because their release frication is distributed wrongly across the spectrum contribute to a model of speech perception, although no experiment may have been designed specifically to test hypotheses about what frication bandwidths are acceptable.

Within theory development, the term 'empirical' refers to an interim modelling process necessary until there is enough data and modelling available to become fully formal. The broad meaning seems often to refer to the anecdotal, the accidental and random observations that display no apparent internal consistency, but may have practical value for the individual involved in dealing with an application. We refer to this type of approach as 'experiential'. It is important to keep clear the various meanings of empirical, and to decide which one is being used in any particular reference.

Application models within theory

Much applied work is empirical; that is, it not explicitly or formally theory based or theory bound. This is not the same as saying a particular application is *a*-theoretical which means there is no theory to apply, no perceived need to look for models or theories which might be useful in dealing with the phenomena under consideration, or even an explicit resistance to basing work on theory. Paradoxically, empirical work is often hypothesis driven where that hypothesis may not actually fit in to a particular theoretical framework (Koch 1981). For example, we observe that, as an everyday phenomenon, the sun comes up every morning though we have no need or interest in a model that provides a plausible explanation of how and why this occurs. Two more examples:

- We might notice that some children and adults have difficulty reading when no accompanying disability is observed: here models of reading might benefit from linguistic theory which might be able to invoke possible explanations (Studdert-Kennedy 1995, Blachman 1997).
- Speech synthesis software can be tweaked in an unprincipled way to enable an *experimenter*, repeatedly listening to his own work, to understand the speech output. Is it useful to understand *why* they can decode the speech in the laboratory, when a lay person can only understand the computer minimally, if at all?

Since spoken language is a phenomenon that is modelled within several different disciplines, their models might usefully, it could be argued, be invoked for specific applications. However this may *not* in fact be the most appropriate approach. Certainly, modelling based *outside* the discipline lends explanatory support to claims *within* a particular area, but the approach is not always guaranteed to be useful (Cook 1999 and 2003). So, empirically based work can give rise to own models worked out by people who need them and use them in their work. Empirically derived models, if they work well, are good models.

- Unfortunately, it is also possible to make relatively *casual* observations which are neither tested nor independently checked; and these can become part of the *folklore* of the discipline. In this case, these observations give rise to a rule-of-thumb approach and are not equivalent to actual modelling, empirically based or otherwise.

Usefulness of empirical work

Whilst accepting that models developed mainly from empirical work (and sometimes from experience only) are useful, we nevertheless suggest that

- working within frameworks derived from linguistic, psychological, and bio-psychological modelling and theory, and
- developing externally motivated, hypothesis driven approaches to understanding applications,

may be usefully productive: observations will be more constrained and focused – less random. For example, linguistic theory can describe the phonology of a language, compare it with English phonology and point out differences in the representations of the distinctive sound units of the language. Such a formality leads productively to pronunciation training within the articulatory boundaries defined by the representations, or to training by perception rather than articulation (Rosner and Pickering 1994, Kjellin 1999, Eskenazi 1999). A formal approach queries, and then establishes the *domain* of second language teaching or some aspect of second language teaching (Cook 2001 and 2003, Jordan 2004). We suggest that in all applications a theory based approach has value *simply because* it is ultimately more powerful than the experiential approach.

To ignore theory, to insist on the extreme version of empirical work, when that approach can lead to just a broadly defined collection of observations, can be very limiting. For example: in teaching English to a class of non-native speakers from different language backgrounds, formal knowledge of their phonological backgrounds (in their own languages) could be important. Japanese speakers sometimes have difficulty distinguishing *light* from *right*, Spanish speakers *doze* from *those*. If the attention of a speaker has never been directed to the differences between /l/ and /r/, or between /d/ and /ð/, the necessary contrasts may not be immediately made and the learning process will be prolonged. Consequently some language teaching techniques emphasise teaching perception rather than articulation (Chapter 11).

Testing models

The empirical approach and models derived from it are good if they have been developed properly. How do we know when we have done a good experiment? If the work was theory based, the theory itself tells us because it makes explicit what constitutes a good experiment and how to compare experiments, both in terms of their methodology and their results – and importantly how to *choose* between competing models. Feynman (1995) sums up the value of experimental work: 'The test of all knowledge is experiment. Experiment is the sole judge of scientific "truth"' (p. 2). Thus initially the generalisations are derived from experimental data, and based on an agreed methodology; the patterns are then checked again by experiment to see 'whether we have made the right guess'. In contrast, empirical models can be tested by looking for novel events and noting whether the premises seem to be borne out, but do not depend on a particular theoretical framework for interpretation of the results or evaluation with respect to *other* experiments.

A principal purpose of a theory is to explain relationships among a variety of descriptions, and to predict new instances. We suggest that a theory-based approach to building applications models is more powerful and gives more reliable results. We can ask:

- Why might this approach be useful?
- What do we have? and Is it adequate for our application?
- Why do we need a theory at all?
- What happens when more than one discipline is needed for the proper study of a particular phenomenon?

Note that theories and models can be called 'conceptual ordering devices' but they 'can never prove pre-emptive' (Koch 1981, p. 93).

Theories available for application – linguistically oriented models

a. *Models of language* – several models of language are currently implemented (Jackendoff 2002, Givon 2001). Many are based on the generative paradigm (Chomsky 1965) with explicit basic constructs, computational adequacy and encompassing the vast range of language behaviour (although in some cases sketchily); in phonetics, see Chapters 1 and 6.
b. *Cognitive and biological models* – many find various models in these areas useful. A number of models have been proposed about cognitive function (Eysenck and Keane 1999), and separately about brain processing (Toates 2001).
c. *Models from biopsychology* – this is a research area which attempts to relate cognitive and physical processing from several different points of view (Damasio 1998, Nobre et al. 2004, Blomert et al. 2004). An area of interest for speech perception is modelling how sensory input results in mappings to cognitive representations. For speech production, the relationship between brain function and speech output behaviour is relevant for speech modelling.

Limitations of current models in phonetic theory

Ideally, applications work involves taking from the constructs and models available, and fashioning some that work reasonably well for the particular application. However as far as speech production and perception is concerned there appears to be no single model for application which is adequate for all purposes. Current models of speech production and perception vary over the whole range from impressionistic assignment of symbols onto speech wave forms, to fully computational models. Within these extremes lie *experimentally* based models of some areas of production and perception and *concept* based models: mathematical descriptions, acoustic models, and those which attempt to integrate cognitive and physical processing with behaviour.

What do we know about cognitive and physical processes that will help in building a useful model?

a. We assume that there is cognition and *associated* brain activity although very little clear factual information is available, and that cognition and brain activity feed into the motor control system which in turn results in speech behaviour.

b. We have some information about what motor control is available, together with some measurable data about articulatory processes, and have a mass of data about speech output – the waveforms.

Linking with phonetic theory

We suggest that during phonetic processing there is a parallel CPA (Cognitive Phonetics Agent) supervising phonetic processing by monitoring the rendering processed in order to get the most appropriate speech output under the dialogue conditions (Chapter 6).

In TM, the action of the *cognitive* phonetics occurs in parallel with corresponding activated brain areas, but the CPA is an *abstract* agent with access not to its own parallel brain functioning but access to the phonetic processes occurring during dynamic phonetic rendering. The CPA can interact with and modify the motor control system operations, and receives generalised feedback from the biological stance of the speaker (for example, physically derived emotive features that may show up in the acoustic wave and trigger identification of the speaker's emotion state). What is needed is experimental research able to show brain activity *while* there is an adjustment to the articulatory system as a result of hypothesised feedback from ongoing speaking. This is analogous to current work in biopsychology that correlates activity from sensation and perception that is roughly in parallel, that is, with a small time delay (Kiefer 2005).

Cognitive and physical modelling

One specific question relevant to language processing concerns events which occur in parallel or sequentially. Parallel means that a physical process takes place (for example, brain activity) when performing cognitive activity, for example when constructing a sentence or utterance. In speaking (or writing) the cognitive processing in parallel with brain processing occurs logically prior to the movement of the motor control system for speaking or writing. The output of the planning process, the correlatable cognitive and brain activity is input to the motor control area (Chapter 6). In other words, planning what the speaker is going to say involves brain activity; carrying out the plan also involves brain activity but at a different time (Kiefer 2005) and in a different place in the brain (motor cortex). This may have implications in language pathology where it could be important to determine whether a disability in speech production is due to brain function accompanying planning, or arises during the process of motor control in rendering the plan. A separation of these two types of processing could be important in language pathology, providing supporting statements about aphasia and, say, dyspraxia: one is a cognitive brain-based impairment, the second is an inability to control the motor system – there are two different physical systems here.

Physical to physical – motor to acoustic

The final result of the cognitive/physical processing is the acoustic signal, which as a real world event is the result of composite sourcing. The acoustic event, as an information source, is basically a continuous information stream, occasionally showing discontinuities. But the physical system that produces it is not a single continuous 'vertically synchronised' event – it is made up of several sources (for example, vocal cord vibration, air pressure changes, movement of the articulators (all in varying time relationships) – more appropriately considered as a parametric system of quasi-synchronised events (Chapters 2 and 4).

It is central to model building that the distinction between the model and the real world event be maintained; they are *not* equivalent in status (Klahr and Simon 2001). In the case of voice onset time studies, for example, we see the vocal cords obeying the mechanical and aerodynamic physical laws under which they operate. We can take an engineering approach and describe how they move, enabling the construction of a model of vocal cord movement. Or another approach is possible: derive the essential features of the system, and describe the vocal cord output as a set of parameters – as for example the features of varying fundamental frequency and its overall range, the varying amplitude of the glottal pulse sound, the 'constituent' harmonics and associated amplitudes: in short, the features make up the glottal pulse. These features can be independently simulated outside the system, and when put together can simulate a glottal pulse shape. But the concept of parameter is the result of the descriptive system: it is a modelling 'device'. If it is considered that parameterisation of the speech system is plausible and can be consistently applied sufficiently well to be useful, then the method of building a parameterised model of speech is worth pursuing (Chapter 4).

Deficiencies of current theory

The range of applications that could be based on speech models is fairly wide, including teaching a new spoken language (language teaching/learning), or devising programs of therapy for relearning or correcting acquired errors (clinical language pathology), or building simulation systems of speech production and perception processes (synthesis and recognition in speech technology). However, current phonetic models, either classical and descriptive, or contemporary and explanatory, do not appear sufficiently robust to apply across the board. So we must consider why not.

The following are possible reasons:

a. the model is *incomplete*, or
b. it is *incorrect*, or
c. it is *not powerful enough* to deal with many instances facing the applications researcher, or
d. it *lacks a coherent underlying metatheory* to square it with the application, or
e. it cannot deal with *multiple areas needed* for a specific application.

Clearly, a model cannot be applied that is not coherent or about which there is a great deal of argument, or that does not go much beyond a collection of observations. It is in such circumstances that applications researchers are forced to fall back on less safe empirical modelling or on observations and experience. They must apply their individual knowledge and points of view to each instance (a person, a group, a software challenge) of the problem being tackled. They are hampered by masses of observations and very few templates to apply to the new event that confronts them. The range of variability of the presenting problems is so great that clear principles are needed or some robust taxonomy is needed. So far, neither exist in linguistics modelling designed within the core theory, yet extensible for the purposes of application.

Deficiencies in current theory about production (Chapters 6 and 8) seem to centre around the lack of an overall coherent model of speech production and perception. The components of such a model would probably incorporate sub-models of:

- *cognitive activity* – not directly observable or measurable (that is, data from behavioural experiments or subjective reporting);
- *parallel physical brain activity* – some is measurable;
- *predictable physical motor activity* (movement of the articulators, detection of the signal) – some measurable;
- *spoken language behaviour appropriate to dialog* (both speaking and understanding) – observable and describable.

When more than one model is needed

In applications such as language teaching, not only is a sound linguistics/phonetics model needed, but in addition a theory or model of *language acquisition*. Much has been written about theory and models of second language acquisition (SLA) (Graney 1995). Defining the domain, comparing and evaluating research models and methodology, the types of model most descriptive and possibly explanatory, and incorporating all this into the body of knowledge and experience needed for successful teaching – are thoroughly discussed in the literature (Ellis 2003, etc.). Particularly clear statements about similar problems that linguist/phoneticians *also* discuss is found in Gregg *et al.* (1997) and Long (1993). Neuroscience and speech technology are similarly engaged in defining areas of production research and formulating what constitutes the appropriate domain for proper model building (Chapter 6).

Metatheory

We have already indicated that an important reason why it is sometimes difficult to combine models from these different areas is that we do not have a convenient *metatheory* formally linking all these different aspects together.

We ourselves are primarily concerned with phonetic theory, but this is in the context of a much larger concern about spoken language production, perception and acquisition. We would like a coherent theory dealing with the ability of humans to produce speech and understand speech. This would require incorporating an overview system linking the capacity to plan utterances and the physical act of speaking in general and to move the articulators in such a way that the resulting specific acoustic waves can be detected and then recognised as meaningful speech by the listener. That overarching theory has not as yet been formulated – therefore we rely on building individual models each of limited domain.

Metatheory is needed to link these sub-domains of study; it does this by providing a common formal approach, which includes objects for manipulation by sets of rules or other mathematical devices. Put simplistically individual models of apples, plums and pears are relatively useless without a theory of fruit. The kind of domain overlap we mean is captured in a couple of examples:

- How do you teach a second language to someone who has a cognitive deficit, a peripheral disability or a motor dysfunction?
- How do you synthesise a deaf speaker's speech?

The only certain thing that might unite all these disciplines at the moment is a common mathematics.

Our proposal

We suggest two integrated types of model for characterising the relationship between phonological and phonetic processing: dynamic and static (see Tatham and Morton 2004, 2005). A *static model* characterises the knowledge base of objects and processes needed to speak. It is accessible on demand to a *dynamic model* which characterises when and how that knowledge needs to be accessed and how it is to be processed. We discuss the model in Chapter 6, and more can be found at www.morton-tatham.co.uk.

A computational approach

Klahr and Simon (2001) encapsulate the computational approach as modelling which 'enables us to express a theory rigorously and to simulate phenomena ... '; such models test 'the sufficiency of the proposed mechanisms to produce a given discovery and allow comparison between case studies, interpreting data in a common language to reveal both similarity and differences of processes' (p 75).

Computational modelling hypothesises *mechanisms*, and suggests *ways of functioning*. Each run through the system follows the same general path, though selection of different pathways is specified by enumerating changes in context. Basically models may be declarative (characterisation of data structures of the kind apparent in, say, traditional Generative syntax) or procedural (an enumeration of processes which operate on data structures apparent, in, say models of speech motor control). Cutting across these two approaches, procedures may be organised as sets of generalisations callable on demand at this or that stage in the overall behaviour being characterised, or they may be organised as specific to particular objects. This latter 'object-oriented' paradigm has been found particularly useful to us (Tatham and Morton 1988) when modelling articulatory structures such as the tongue, with its internal organisation of muscles, each 'knowing' how to behave (a formalisation of the coordinative structure model).

10
Speech Technology

Introduction

Speech technology – speech synthesis and automatic speech recognition by computer – is an important application of the theory of speech production and perception for two reasons:

- synthesis and automatic recognition constitute computational simulations of the human processes of production and perception;
- synthesis and recognition can be used as effective and productive test beds for models developed from the proposed theory: that is, they can be used to test *hypotheses* about speech – even pathological speech.

Speech synthesis – how natural?

Initially, researchers in synthetic speech were concerned with its intelligibility (Keller 1994, Holmes and Holmes 2001). This was almost always taken to mean *segmental intelligibility:* were the speech segments which make up words sufficiently well rendered to be correctly recognised? Usually tests for intelligibility were performed on isolated words or sentences, rather than on the total system's performance in, say, a dialogue environment. They did not take into account that intelligibility varies with context, and a dialogue simulation would today be a much more appropriate test environment for intelligibility.

Naturalness

Synthetic speech is now segmentally fully intelligible. However, researchers agree that the major remaining problem for synthetic speech is that it continues to be insufficiently natural, and for this reason they are examining areas for improvement of naturalness. Take, for example, *expressive content*. Unlike the segmental specification, there is no fixed prosodics for particular utterances, since there are many ways of speaking the same sentence; in turn these depend on features of expression (Chapter 6). Expressive content can vary over just a few words within an individual utterance. Currently it is unlikely that a speech synthesiser will reflect *any* expression adequately, let alone one which is varying continuously.

Expression is mostly conveyed by prosody (Morton *et al.* 1999, Tatham and Morton 2004). Therefore descriptions of the rendering of suprasegmental features – elements which span multiple segments – have become a focus of current research because failure here appears to be a primary source of unease for listeners. Prosody itself however is difficult to describe explicitly with respect to naturalness in speech because it is used as the vehicle for two different features of speech:

- the linguistic prosody associated with rendering utterances for their plain meaning,
- the prosody associated with rendering expressive content.

Adaptation and simulation

The voice output of current synthesis systems does not automatically adapt to changes that occur during the course of a dialogue with a human being. For example, currently a synthetic utterance which begins fast, ends fast; and one which begins sounding firm does not move to a gentler (or fiercer) style as the dialogue unfolds. Yet changes of this kind as a person speaks are a major source of the perception of naturalness in speech.

To simulate variable prosody a data structure characterisation sufficiently detailed to be able to handle *dynamic* changes of style or expression during the course of an utterance is needed (Tatham and Morton 2005). Also needed is the means to introduce *marking* into the utterance specification to reflect the style changes and provide the trigger for the appropriate procedures during synthetic rendering. The parameters of prosody in human speech – phonologically: stress, rhythm and intonation – are often characterised in a way which does not allow their use in human speech to be carried over to synthesis. For example, rate of delivery can vary considerably during the course of an utterance (a stretch of speech which might be characterised in linguistic terms as, say, a phrase or a sentence). Rate of delivery is a physical prosodic parameter which is used to render different speech styles which are characterised at an abstract level. For example, angry speech may be delivered at a higher than normal rate, bored speech at a lower than normal rate.

Take as an example the following utterance: 'Did he say *ethnologise?*' In the orthographic representation the word *ethnologise* has been italicised to indicate infrequent use. In speech the word might be

- preceded and/or followed by a pause,
- spoken at a slower rate than the surrounding words,
- marked by increased f0 change,
- given increased overall amplitude, and so on.

These attributes of the acoustic signal combine to draw attention to the word, in effect pointing out: *this is an unusual word*. In addition speaking the word slowly will usually mean that expected phenomena associated with fast delivery (increased coarticulation, vowel reduction, etc.) may not be minimised or reduced. To a great extent it is violation of the listener's *expectations* which signals that they must increase their attention level.

Speaker expectation

What a speaker expects is itself a variable. By this we mean that there is a norm or baseline expectation for the various parameters of speech, and that this expectation is relative. *Departure from expectation* is the point. In a sense the speaker works *with* the listener's expectations. We refer to the interplay between speaker and listener regularly in this book because it figures so prominently in speech communication.

Intelligibility – state of the art

A common belief among synthetic speech researchers is that intelligibility declines in a less than ideal environment. It has been observed that when listening conditions are adverse synthetic speech is perceived less well than human speech. This has given rise to the belief that human speech has more critical detail than synthetic speech. Initially the hypothesis was that by adding the missing detail we can improve intelligibility under adverse, more realistic listening conditions.

However, it is *not* self-evident that increased detail is actually what is needed. For example, possibly some of the systematic variation found in human speech is *not* actually used in the perception, and possibly some *non*-systematic detail *is* perceived, in the sense that if it is missing the result may be that the speech is not perceived as natural. What constitutes naturalness – essentially the humanness of human speech – is not entirely clear to anyone yet. Hence it becomes easy to equate naturalness with increased intelligibility and look to improved detail in the acoustic signal. If correct, then we go full circle on the observation that somehow or other human speech holds onto its intelligibility under adverse conditions where synthetic speech does not – even though both may be judged equally intelligible in the laboratory. Assertions of this kind are not helpful in telling us exactly what that detail of human speech might be; they simply inform us that human speech is perceptually more robust than synthetic speech.

We know that formant synthesis produces an incomplete sound wave. The parameters for formant synthesis were selected in the early days (for example, Holmes *et al.* 1964) based on their obvious presence in the acoustic signal and on the relevance to perception it was thought they had. Thus parameters like formant peak frequency, amplitude and bandwidth were seen to be important, and were incorporated. Later systems (for example, Klatt 1980) built on this model to include parameters which would deliver more of the acoustic detail while attempting to maintain the versatility of parametric synthesis. Fundamentally, it is quite true that however carefully formant synthesis models the acoustic production of speech the resultant signal lacks coherence and integrity. By definition a speech signal with 100 per cent integrity would require an *infinite* number of parameters to simulate it. What actually makes natural speech acoustically coherent is the robust correlation between vocal tract behaviour and the detail of the acoustic signal. This fine detail *reflects* the vocal tract behaviour and identifies the signal as *coming from a single talker*. Indeed, we go further: the correlation is not just robust, it is probably *absolute*. What this correlation does not do on its own, however, is guarantee *phonetic* coherence, since vocal tract behaviour has a non-linear relationship with phonetics and includes unpredictable cognitively sourced elements (Morton 1986, Tatham 1986a, 1986b).

In TM we are concerned with the integrity of the high-level parts of synthesis. Take, for example, our approach to prosody and expression which insists that *all* utterance plans be wrapped in prosodic containers which ultimately control the rendering of temporal and spectral features of the output signal whether this is derived in the human system or its simulation in synthetic speech.

Similar coherence problems also show up in concatenated waveform synthesis (Tatham and Morton 2005), even in those systems which attempt to optimise unit length. This leads us to believe that although a certain minimum level of acoustic detail is necessary in all synthetic speech, the robustness issue is not down solely to failure to replicate the greater spectral detail of human speech. What is left, of course, is prosodic detail and temporally governed variation of spectral detail. We are referring here to subtleties in fundamental frequency contours, and variations in intensity and rhythm for the prosodic detail *per se*; and also to the way spectral detail (for example, the variation in coarticulatory effects and the way they span more than just the immediately adjacent segments) is governed by features like rate variation. These features are very complex when considering prosody in general, but particularly complex when considering prosody as conveyor of expression (see Tatham and Morton 2005 for details).

Naturalness in human speech

The perceived feeling of naturalness about speech is clearly based on a complex of features which is difficult to enumerate. The reason for this is that listeners are unable to tell us precisely what contributes to naturalness. Several researchers have tried to introduce a metric for naturalness which goes beyond the simple marking of a scale, and introduces the notion of a parametric characterisation of what people *feel* as listeners. While not new in perceptual studies in general, such a method does go a long way toward enabling comparison between different systems by establishing the basis for a rough evaluation metric.

Sluijter *et al.* (1998) introduced a technique for naturalness scoring. Adapting this we could look for such factors as:

1. *general quality* – what general impression does the speech create?
2. *ease of comprehension* – a general consideration, eliciting an overall impression of ease of comprehension.
3. *intelligibility* – an overall ranking of general intelligibility.
4. *pronunciation / occurrence of deviating speech sounds* – does the listener feel that any particular sounds have been badly rendered and might be contributing to reduced naturalness or acceptability? Notice that errors in sounds *in certain combinations* will be less noticeable than in other combinations, such as the predictability of linear sound combinations in syllables.

5. *speaking rate* – is the speaking rate appropriate? One difficulty is the extent to which semantic and pragmatic factors enter into the appropriateness of speaking rate. Introducing variation of speaking rate may well introduce errors. This is one of the areas – along with other pragmatically sourced variations in prosody – which will benefit from additional mark-up of the input text or better prosody assignment algorithms within the synthesis system.
6. other features related to *pragmatic content* may also be important to the listener.
7. *friendliness* – this is a quality appropriate for limited domain synthesis systems – say, interactive enquiry systems. Appropriateness is again a consideration after determining that the default degree of friendliness is convincing.
8. *politeness* – again, a subjective evaluation of the default condition, degree of politeness in general, is called for.

Each of these evaluation parameters is subjective and defined only vaguely for that reason. And not enough provision is made for adaptation on the part of the listener. But the strength of such an approach is that notwithstanding the subjective nature of each parameter the evaluation of naturalness *as a whole* is made more robust, simply because it is based on the co-occurrence of a number of parameters. This stems partly from the way the model is put together in terms of identifiable features to which a *probability* might be attached, and in part from the possibility of indicating a *relationship* between the features. A parametric evaluation procedure gains over a non-parametric characterisation, and the approach may eventually lead to productive correlation between measured properties of the soundwave and naturalness.

Systems are now good enough for casual listeners to comment not so much on naturalness but on the *appropriateness* of style – as with the friendliness and politeness parameters above. This does not mean that style and so on are secondary to naturalness in terms of generating speech synthesis, but it does mean that *for some people* appropriateness and accuracy of style override some other aspects of naturalness.

Variability

One of the paradoxes of speech technology is the way in which variability in the speech waveform causes so many problems in the design of *automatic speech recognition systems* and at the same time *lack* of it causes a feeling of unnaturalness in *synthesised speech*.

We model variability in speech production in terms of a hierarchical arrangement of identifiably different types, modelled in different linguistic components. Thus:

TYPE OF VARIABLE	COMPONENT WHERE MODELLED
deliberately introduced and systematic	*phonology*
unavoidable, but systematic (coarticulation)	*phonetics*
systematically managed coarticulation	*Cognitive Phonetics*
random	*phonetics*

The variability introduced in phonology involves variants on the underlying segments or prosodic contours. So, for example, English chooses to have two non-distinctive variants of /l/ which can be heard in words like *leaf* and *feel* – Classical Phonetics called these clear [l] and dark [l] respectively. In the prosody of English, we could cite the variant turning up of the intonation contour before the end of statements as opposed to the usual turn down (Chapter 8). Neither of these variants alters the basic meaning of the utterance, though they can alter pragmatic interpretation. These are termed *extrinsic* variants (because they are extrinsic to the rendering processes, Chapter 1), and in the segment domain are called *extrinsic allophones*. Failure to reproduce extrinsic phonological variability correctly in synthetic speech results in a 'foreign accent' effect because different languages derive extrinsic allophones differently; the meaning of the utterance however is not changed, and it usually remains intelligible.

Segmental variants introduced unavoidably at the phonetic level are termed *intrinsic allophones* in most contemporary models of phonetics, and result from coarticulation. These effects are systematic, time governed, and are predictable. Examples from English might be the fronted [k] in a word like *key*, or the dentalised [t] in *eighth*; or vocal cord vibration might get interrupted by intrinsic aerodynamic effects during intervocalic underlying [+voice] stops or fricatives. Failure to replicate coarticulation correctly in speech synthesis reduces overall intelligibility and contributes very much to lack of naturalness. Normally listeners are not aware of coarticulatory effects, in the sense that they cannot report them: they are however extremely sensitive to their omission and to any errors.

Coarticulatory effects however *do* vary in a way related to the linguistics of the language. TM models this by borrowing the notion of *cognitive intervention* from bio-psychology to introduce the idea that within certain limits the mechanical constraints seen in coarticulation can be interfered with (Chapter 3). Moreover some effects intrinsic to the mechanism can be *enhanced* for linguistic purposes. Systematic cognitive intervention in the behaviour of the physical mechanism which produces the soundwave is covered by the theory of Cognitive Phonetics. Examples here might be the way coarticulation is reduced in any language when there is a high risk of ambiguity – the speaker slows down to reduce the time governed constraint – or the enhanced period of vocal cord vibration failure following some stops in a number of Indian and other languages (Ladefoged and Maddieson 1996). This cognitive intervention to control mechanical constraints enables the enlargement of either the language's extrinsic allophone inventory or sometimes even its underlying segment (phoneme) inventory (Morton and Tatham 1980). If the effects of cognitive intervention in phonetic rendering are not reproduced in synthetic speech simulation there can be perceptual problems with meaning, and frequently with the coherence of accents within a language. There is also a fair reduction in naturalness.

There is also some *random* variability in speech articulation. This is due to varying tolerances in the mechanical and aerodynamic systems: they are insufficiently tight to produce error-free rendering of the underlying segments (the extrinsic allophones) appearing in the utterance plan. While listeners are not at all sensitive to the detail of random variability in speech they do become uneasy if this type of variability is not present; so failure to introduce it results in a reduction of naturalness.

Style

Most synthesis systems can speak in only one particular style, and sometimes with only one voice. The usual style adopted, because it is considered to be the most general purpose, is a relatively neutral version of reading-style speech. What most researchers would like to see is the extension of systems to include a range of voices, and also to enable various global styles and local expressive content. All these things are possible – but not yet adopted successfully in systems outside the laboratory. There are two reasons for this: lack of sufficient data and a descriptive system for handling it, and lack of a basic model of expressive content in speech (but see Tatham and Morton 2004).

Prosody control is essential for achieving different styles within the same synthesis system. Speech rate control is a good place to start for most researchers because it *seems* relatively easy. However, the introduction of speech rate control in fact turns out to be far from simple. For example, a doubling of overall rate is not a halving of the time spent on each segment in an utterance – the distribution of the rate increase is not linear throughout the utterance. Focusing on the syllable as our unit we can see that a change in rate is more likely to affect the vowel nucleus than the surrounding consonants, but it is still hard to be consistent in predicting just how the relative distribution of rate change takes effect.

The usual model acknowledges the perceptually oriented idea of *isochrony* between rhythmic units, but though this is a useful concept in phonological prosody (that is, in the abstract) it is hard to find direct correlates in phonetic prosody (that is, in the actual soundwave). The isochrony approach would hypothesise that the perceived equal timing between stressed syllables is reflected in the physical signal. The hypothesis has been consistently refuted by researchers (but see Tatham and Morton 2001), largely because they have failed to factor out the effects of expressive and prosodic wrappers on the rendering process.

Data structures

In Tatham and Morton (2005) we discussed current work on high-level synthesis, and presented proposals for a unified approach to formal descriptions of high-level manipulation of the synthesis low-level systems, using a declarative XML-based formalism (Kim 2003). We feel XML is ideally suited to handling the necessary data structures for synthesis. There were a number of reasons for adopting XML; but mostly we feel that it is an appropriate *mark-up system* for

- characterising data structures,
- application on multiple platforms.

Modelling speech production in human beings or simulating human speech production using speech synthesis is fundamentally a problem of characterising the *data structures* involved. There are procedures to be applied to these declared data structures, of course – but there is much to be gained from making the data structures themselves the focus of the model, making any subsequent procedures *adjunct* to the focus. This is an approach often adopted for linguistics, and one which we ourselves have used in the SPRUCE computational model of speech production and elsewhere (Tatham and Morton 2003, 2004) with some success.

The multiple platform issue is not just that XML is interpretable across multiple operating systems or in-line within different programming languages, but more importantly that it can be used to manage the high-level aspects of speech synthesis in text-to-speech and other speech synthesis systems which hinge on high-level aspects of synthesis. Thus a high-level approach can be built which can logically precede multiple low-level systems. It is in this particular sense that we are concerned with the application across multiple platforms. As an example we can cite the SPRUCE system which is essentially a high-level simulation for testing TM – our computational model of speech production/perception – whose output is capable of being rendered on multiple low-level systems such as formant based or concatenated waveform based synthesisers.

Automatic speech recognition

Despite the progress made during the last two or three decades in automatic speech recognition (Young 2000, 2002), successes in enabling larger vocabularies and more speaker-independent applications have been at the expense of consideration of the human processes in speech perception. This has been disappointing to linguists or psychologists who tend to feel that automatic speech recognition which began as a promising simulation of speech perception has failed in this respect. However, the current model works rather well in terms of what speech technologists want it to do: recognise speech – not tell us how human beings perform the task.

There are three key factors responsible for most of the progress:

1. *Statistical modelling* One of the main problems with automatic speech recognition has been a feeling among researchers of the apparent *inappropriateness* of linguistic and phonetic models. The idea of statistical modelling is to provide representations of speech objects based on the general properties distributed among them. That is, the objects are not just speech segments but also processes such as the transitions or coarticulatory phenomena which appear to link them. This is important because the general approach used is based on the 'sequenced object' model of speech which regards speech on the surface as a linear string of juxtaposed speech segments, with rules governing how they abut. In phonetics this is Coarticulation Theory (Chapter 2).
2. *Learning* If statistical techniques enable us to approach the modelling of surface variation in speech by introducing uncertainty into the

equation, they can only be really successful if they are based on large scale evaluations of data. Since researchers do not know the statistical properties of speech and linguists have not modelled all the relevant details, it becomes necessary to scan and evaluate large quantities of data. This is impractical for doing by hand, but is a task very suited to devices capable of data-driven learning. At present most automatic speech recognition devices use the data-driven statistical learning approach by developing, for example, hidden Markov model (HMM) or artificial neural network (ANN) representations of speech during a learning or model building phase. The resultant *acquired* statistical model is then used to process novel data to output hypotheses as to the linguistic content of the incoming speech signal.
3. *Hypothesis development* Processing the waveforms to be recognised through the statistical models developed by learning results in a sequence of sets of hypotheses concerning the movement of the signal through the utterance(s). A contextually based evaluation system is usually able to narrow down the hypotheses to a plausible string of hits – solutions to the recognition task.

It is also possible to exploit various types of logic: approaches which incorporate *threshold logic* or *fuzzy logic* are useful because again they help us avoid an approach which is based on the certainties of linguistics. The point is that we need a means of representing both *data* and *processes* which are not fixed, but subject to variation. The problem with the *static* abstract approach common in phonetics (even in early models like Classical Phonetics) is that it tends to minimise the variability found in speech. Variability is known to be very important for speakers and listeners, which is why it is necessary to understand its different types and sources.

Advantages of the statistical approach to speech recognition

Statistical modelling has little to do with phonetic or phonological characterisations of speech as known in linguistics. At best it brings together a set of hypotheses concerning putative *output* from a knowledge based model, whereas linguistics is essentially a declarative, knowledge based approach to *characterising* language as a whole, rather than concentrating on *specific* outputs. Such an approach has been shown not only to provide good answers where the linguistics fails, but to supply useful and important hypotheses for linguistics research in the area of the detail of the soundwave and its systematic properties.

One of the ways in which contemporary linguistics has proved inadequate in both automatic speech recognition and speech synthesis has been its *static model* approach, which is essentially about constancy or certainty. In speech, certainly at the phonetic level, static modelling is clearly only part of the solution to understanding what is happening: dynamic modelling of the kind we use here (Chapter 6) and elsewhere (Tatham 1995, Tatham and Morton 2002, 2003, 2004, 2005) is more appropriate for modelling speech production and perception because it offers techniques for incorporating time, and uncertainty in the form of probability characterisations.

There was little or no attempt at dynamic modelling of speech in the early days of speech technology, and for automatic speech recognition the statistical approach offered the best solution for modelling both time and uncertainty.

The static modelling inherent in linguistics, exemplified in Chomsky's (1957, 1965) Transformational Generative Grammar approach, is very appropriate for capturing much of how language works in human beings. It is important to remember however that what is being modelled is the simultaneous underlying structure of the entire language. It cannot be overemphasised that linguistics, as approached by most contemporary theoretical linguists, does not come up with recipe models for creating this or that utterance (synthesis) or perceiving this or that utterance (recognition). It characterises simultaneously *all* the objects and processes which, when interacting, establish the structure of *all* utterances – and the number of utterances of course is infinite. What researchers in speech technology systems need to know is all this *and* in addition how to tap into the static model *dynamically* to produce or recognise this or that *particular* utterance – a specific instantiation from the generalised model. It would not be overstating the situation to say that most of what is needed is not in the characterisations provided by linguistics, because the dynamic processes involved in choice and selection which lead ultimately to instantiation are not included. This is *not* a problem in linguistics, but it is a serious problem in speech technology.

The success of the statistical approach in automatic speech recognition does not mean that the data-driven focus is inherently superior. It may simply mean that the earlier way of using rules and knowledge was inadequate because it was based on an understandable misconception of what linguistics is about. *'Illegally'* running a linguistics description – a grammar – does not produce individual sentences (for semantics and syntax) or utterances (for phonologically and phonetically processed sentences): it produces what linguists call *exemplar derivations*. These are static examples of the kind of *idealised surface object* the grammar characterises; they are *not* particular examples of anything dynamically produced by the grammar. They certainly are not like, and are not intended to be like, the highly variable utterances people speak or the kinds of data automatic speech recognition devices have to deal with.

Disadvantages of the statistical approach

Despite demonstrable advantages there are distinct disadvantages to the statistical approach. One of these is the tendency to ignore the *principle of plausibility* in the model in respect of what it is that human beings do. This does not matter usually in the engineering environment, but it matters considerably in the environment where speech technology is used to test models of human behaviour in producing and perceiving speech. But it can matter even if we are not really interested in finding out how human beings work. If speech technology is to be more than basically adequate in, say, dialogue systems it has to be sensitive to the *humanness* of speech. There is little doubt that modelling human speech production and perception as a statistically driven processes is ultimately *inappropriate*. This does not mean to say that some parts of the dynamic processing involved in speaking or perceiving particular utterances do not involve some statistical processing: it means that the processing is not statistically centred. After all, we do know that human beings sometimes proceed on a statistical basis.

The statistical models do not gel with the linguistics or psychology models because linguists have taken the line which emphasises representations which capture maximal generality and which *also* focus on symbolic characterisations. They are right to do this because clearly part of the way in which human beings work is in terms of symbolic representations; these tend to factor out variability. Linguistics and psychology tend to neglect modelling the relationship between these abstract representations which play down variability and the data itself which is exhibiting the variability. It was this problem which undermined Classical Phonetics (Chapter 1). At the moment we cannot do much about this – but at least the nature of the problem can be explored and some tentative proposals for future directions made. Levinson (2005) sums it up:

> Since using the present state of the art requires a serious diminution of our natural abilities and since we presently cannot leap the performance chasm between humans and machines, it seems only

prudent that we should invest more in fundamental science in the expectation that it will eventually lead not only to a mature speech technology but also to many other things as yet unimagined. (p. 242)

For a more complete account of how things might proceed in the future, see Tatham and Morton (2005).

11
Second Language Acquisition

Introduction

Language acquisition and second (or more) language learning cover quite large academic and practical areas of research and application. We cannot begin to discuss these areas, but only comment in a very limited way as to whether the model incorporating the idea of static and dynamic planes (Chapter 6) might be useful.

Models of second language acquisition (SLA) have been proposed by many researchers, but for examples see Cook (2003) and Gregg (1993). Some of these are empirically based, and some derive from the standard theory and model building framework outlined in Part I. These theorists are concerned primarily with *language* acquisition and not specifically with speech, although exposure to language initially is most often through detecting and perceiving speech: second language acquisition, other than for reading knowledge only, includes understanding and producing speech.

There is no overall model of acquisition or of possible interference or enhancement from a first language, and both research and teaching methods proceed from different points of view. Graney (1995) in a Review of Tarone *et al.* (1994) points out the wide range of problems and solutions that they address. We cannot evaluate applied linguistics and SLA work, but it is quite clear that for the near future, there is scope for developing empirical models and testing them rigorously with the expectation that at some point a generalised theory of SLA might be developed. In fact the basis for generalised modelling for SLA is being established currently, with researchers beginning to ask questions such as (Gregg 2005):

- What is the *domain* of a theory of SLA?, and
- What counts as a good *explanation* of the phenomena in that domain?

These two questions are fundamental to model building, and when answered go some way toward establishing a sound basis for further research. We suggest the proposed static and dynamic model might be useful since the phonological knowledge bases will be largely different for each language.

In this model the phonetic dynamic model is drawn from a universal set of possible gestures in each language. We suggest a set of parameterised co-produced gestures for these, and a set of articulatory/phonological units preferably of syllable size. The details of the prosodic wrapper are largely language specific; so the learner must adapt the physical mechanisms available for speaking to the demands of the phonological pattern and other constraints of prosody such as stress patterning and timing. It seems safe to assume that new speaking patterns can be learned, and that these are related to the phonotactics of the language. Training both perception and production has become more explicit in recent times, and strategies for doing this might well contribute evidence for modelling 'core' production and perception in linguistics/phonetics. There is more emphasis also on exactly what needs training, since basic theory is becoming more explicit on just how languages might differ. For example assimilation and coarticulation will perhaps need different treatments since coarticulatory effects are assumed to be constant because of their universal origins (Chapter 2), and can be clearly defined and separated from assimilatory effects. Assimilatory effects themselves will be different in each language.

One of the main claims made in TM and in this book in general is the considerable interdependence of speech production and perception. And a question theorists might address is whether there is unambiguous evidence from language learning concerning the nature of this interdependence. As with so many areas of application there are findings and ideas to be exchanged:

- Do ideas arising as a result of the core theory assist or influence theory or practices in the applications?
- Do empirical findings in the areas of application feed back to the underlying theory?

We need reliable data using standardised methods to provide evidence for phonetic claims in both directions. The diagram shows the relationship, as we see it, between general research in the area of speech production/perception and applied research – and how they both feed into the development of the underlying theory and the associated applied theory.

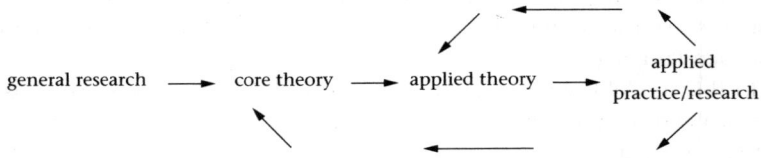

The relationship between production and perception in SLA

However, the question of the relationship between production and perception in SLA is not clear. In practice, two ways have been proposed. The first is to train pronunciation by producing the appropriate articulatory setting. The second is to listen to targeted differences between minimal pairs and the claim is that both perception and production improved (Eskenazi 1999). Along these lines, a method has been suggested for training pronunciation by training initially the perception of prosodic patterns (Kjellin 1999) – this accords well with our wrapper hypothesis (Chapter 6), since we would predict improved results if segmental pronunciation is trained *within* prosody. Chun (2002) examines specifically the function of intonation and rhythm in L2 acquisition. These patterns are difficult to master, and Chun suggests exploring methods of training perception. We suggest, with respect to the model we propose, that training perception results in training the acquisition of specific patterns on the dynamic plane generalisable to patterns to be stored on the static plane. Units in phonology and gestures in phonetics will initially conflict with L1 patterns on the static plane. Presenting visual patterns may help some learners, since it is well known that some people respond well to graphical representations.

Hancock (2003) emphasises the importance of pronunciation training for perception (meaning here: listening to speech) as well as training the articulators (our 'articulatory groupings' or 'coordinative groupings') to produce appropriate speech sounds. Training for both production and perception is divided into two categories: segmental, for example consonants opening and closing syllables, and prosodic, for example the correct syllable stressing, important in English. The initial stage for the listener is recognising the sound pattern, having learned what that pattern is. The approach is not new (Gimson 1989, Jones 1956). Both emphasise the necessity of training both phonological and phonetic levels, and also prosody – though usually separately, neglecting any possible advantages from the wrapper approach.

Several researchers ask what happens when the perception and production abilities are not equivalent. Many people report that they cannot *speak* a language but they can *understand* it. Researchers in this area ask, in our terms, a number of linked questions (see, for example, Cook 2003):

- What resources is the speaker drawing on?
- What resources is the listener drawing on?
  – Are they the same resources?

If the resources for listening and speaking are the same, or fairly similar:

- Why are the results different?
- Are the results due to different abilities?
  – What needs training – perception, production or some underlying representation common to both?

And finally:

- It is plausible that we might hypothesise a monolingual or bilingual *mind* in language production and perception?

We look at these questions in terms of establishing a different phonological static sound and prosodic patterns, and different retrieval patterns for perception and production. Dynamic phonology provides strings of input units to phonetics for production. For production, the recognition of the patterns may be filtered through a different system, bypassing phonetic articulatory representations for retrieval (in contradiction to the Motor Theory of Speech Production (Liberman *et al*. 1958 – Chapters 4 and 7), and identifying the wrapping prosodic patterns. Understanding the nature of such a filter is essential in modelling perception, and would make the rule set different from the production rules on the dynamic planes of speech production.

Production unit size and feedback

A hierarchal method of teaching is proposed by Mortimer (1985) among others, in which the teaching separates phrases by inserted pauses, thus focusing attention on smaller units within larger utterances, emphasising a rudimentary hierarchy. In our terms, this suggests that speakers retrieve units from the static planes, and can provide feedback to themselves to correct strategies for repairing the plan as part of perceptual processing. For example, repairing incorrect rendering of assimilation rules in phonology would contribute to more native sounding speech. In a kind of iterative procedure, the speaker, by focusing on small details, can also train articulatory strategies for rendering at the phonetic level.

Another area of interest to language teachers and learners involves feedback using an additional modality: 'visible speech'. There is a long history associated with the development of useful visual speech patterns and attempts to transfer some visual information to auditory processing, beginning with Potter *et al.* (1947). Recently Massaro and Light (2004) have investigated the effectiveness of training production and perception of deaf speakers using visual feedback. As with dyslexia, there is a conflicting body of opinion about whether two modalities can interact productively. The question as to the possible existence of a common phonological static plane, which we propose for speech, with *both* visual and audio representations remains, we think, an open question. Again, a metatheory relating the two modalities with a general language theory would be valuable, and experiments specifically related to speech, addressing fine detail, might be useful.

Application of an application

An 'application of an application' can be seen in computer aided language training. For example, a combination of phonetic theory and automatic speech recognition (ASR – Chapter 10) techniques can be applied to computer aided language teaching/learning (CALL). Eskenazi (1999, among others) has developed a system which uses an ASR system and guided linguistic/phonetic based training for second language learning. The combination of technology allied with cognitive, biological, linguistic and phonetic models for a practical purpose such as training is an interesting area in the development of applications modelling.

Theoretically motivated pronunciation training techniques

Classical Phonetics seems to be the most common base for pronunciation training. A *linear* model of this type appears to work well even with the inconsistencies introduced by idiosyncratic application of symbols inherent in the IPA system (Chapter 1). Celce-Murcia *et al.* (1996) present a fairly traditional method of speech description, detailed labelling and contrastive analysis. Again, the task for the learner is to incorporate a new system either within or accompanying that already acquired. The modelling problems are typical of this kind of approach, and can be summarised as:

- How are two or more phonologies to be specified?
- Is their representation to be on two static planes, or within one general static plane?
- Are dynamic search strategies modified from L1 to L2, or are two separate dynamic planes required?
- If interference between the two languages is noted, can this be modelled as interference in retrieval of correct units, as *crosstalk* between two separate planes for two separate languages, or inadequate training resulting in inadequate dynamic phonetic retrieval?

We ask these questions, not as criticism but as a way of testing the *applicational robustness* of the computationally oriented model outlined in Chapter 6. We ourselves would like to understand how the non-applied model can contribute to and learn from the applied models, and to what extent either can benefit from strengthening.

If we can assume that capacity to learn language is *unchanged*, can we also assume that the static phonological and phonetic databases change in a second language? Perhaps we should say here that in our view the Critical Age Hypothesis (Singleton and Lengyel 1995) does not indicate that the learning capacity is at all diminished – there certainly seems to be no sustainable argument from bio-psychology to support this idea. Phonological theory specifies that phonological representations are language specific, so the knowledge repository associated with L2 needed for the static plane has to be different from what is needed for L1. The capacity to *access* this plane is presumably *unchanged* for L2, as are the rules, but the retrieval processes specified by the rules must be learned. Hence for production:

- Is there interference in retrieval?
- Do new strategies replace old ones, or are they in addition and more complex than what has been established in the first language?
- As far as speech production is concerned, do languages differ only in their phonological/phonetic static specifications?
- More practically, how effective are pronunciation drills in training retrieval from the static phonetic plane of *how* to pronounce? Does

the Cognitive Phonetics Agent (the CPA) need to be trained to recognise inappropriate pronunciation and modify it?
- If necessary, how could the CPA be trained?

And for how production and perception are perhaps mutually dependent:

- Is training *perception* a useful route, assuming that the correct units will be inferred from what is perceived, and become entered into a new static plane?
- How can perception training facilitate retrieval strategies?

The question of the relationship between production and perception in language learning is not clear. (Rosner and Pickering 1994, Eskenazi 1999, Chun 2002, Hancock 2003, among others.) Two main possibilities have been proposed.

1. The first is to train pronunciation by producing the appropriate articulatory setting.
2. The second is to listen to targeted differences between minimal pairs and the claim is that both perception and production improved.

This is an area which is bound to be of interest to speech theory based in linguistics, since the relationship between production and perception is fundamental to spoken language.

Accent and dialect studies

We define dialect as a variant of a language, including syntax, semantics, and phonology. Accent refers to variant phonology/phonetics (Wells 1982). Thus a speaker has an accent within a dialect within an overall description of a language class such as English, French, Chinese, and so on. A way of modelling accent within the generative framework is to conceive of accents within a hierarchal relationship (Chapter 6). The description is a typical phonological one where what we describe on the surface is related to an underlying sound pattern. Thus the underlying representation will be virtually, if not *the* same for all dialects and accents – that is the sound pattern of the *class* of language. This is the standard modelling technique for comparing variants – they are related *via* the common ancestry – *not* in any linear fashion.

The derivational history of the differing surface phenomena, what we speak and observe when hearing relates back to this underlying representation. It cannot, of course, be pronounced without rendering because it is an *abstract representation*, and within the theory constitutes a set of *hypotheses* about language. For example, a /t/ in the English word *metal* is rendered by some speakers as a voiceless alveolar plosive and laterally released into the following syllabic /l/. Another speaker might render the underlying form as a voiceless glottal stop.

A linear model cannot properly relate such surface objects, but what may seem dissimilar, say in the case of the different renderings of /t/, may in fact be meaningful to speakers and hearers as an English /T/ (the upper case T is used here to represent a deep accent-free abstract underlying object). Thus this model allows comparison between the two renderings, cognitively relating them as the *same* by reference to the underlying representation they have in common, but also describing their differences physically using articulatory terms.

Implications for language teaching are that learner/perceivers can map accents to a common representation, and can become accustomed to a *range* of renderings of the underlying phonology. This approach has wide repercussions: for example, in language pathology (Chapter 12), a formal distinction between what the patient has always rendered and what he is now rendering pathologically may help in treatment of language disorders. There perhaps is no point in trying to retrain a speaker from East Anglia in the accent usually found in Somerset; it may also be difficult to determine whether someone has a language/speech disorder or whether they simply have an unfamiliar but typical speech from a small region of the country. A simple example of this would be a typical Cockney rendering of the word *nothing*: [ˈnʌfiŋk] – there is no implication at all that Cockney speakers are suffering from an inability (quite common and temporary among very young children) to discriminate [f] and [θ]!

In our terms, the contents of the phonological static plane remain constant across speakers of a language, but the contents of the static model of phonetics vary. The dynamic planes access their respective static planes (Chapter 6).

12
Speech Disorders

Introduction

In this chapter we look at some features of the TM model presented in Chapter 6, and consider whether some aspects can be easily applied to areas of language pathology and the speech production/perception areas of neurolinguistics in general. We comment on work that might be interpreted in the terms of our model with a view to improving its robustness and potential development for applicability.

Underlying this approach is the generalised paradigm framework, which considers that in speech production there exist abstract cognitive processes and physical processes which are to be treated as a pair of models related within a hierarchical architecture:

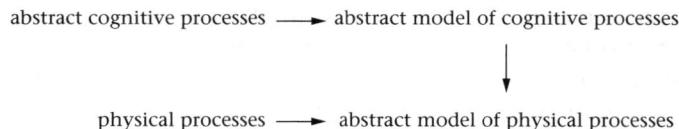

The abstract models constitute two sets of hypotheses based on different types of object. It is important not to confuse the abstract model of physical processes with the abstract cognitive processes underlying their own abstract model.

We look at coarticulation as an example of the possible application of this construct to this area of applied work. Coarticulation effects are sometimes invoked when a speaker seems not to be precise in their phonetic rendering. The assumption is made that the clinician can detect and assign a label at the point at which the speech is imprecise (or slurred). Assuming that this is possible, what coarticulation or co-production processes might be operating? The reason why we say 'assuming that this is possible' is that it is by no means clear that anyone can be objective enough to make such an assessment. The clinical assessment paradigm is illustrated in this diagram:

speaker's utterance ⟶ clinician's subjective perception ⟶ clinical assessment
⇡
theory of speech production/perception

What the diagram shows is that a clinical assessment is based on the way the clinician interprets their perception of the speaker's utterance in terms of a *particular theory of speech*. As a simple example, the assessment may identify an error in the speaker's rendering of a particular consonant – if the underlying theory hypotheses that speech is rendered in terms of the serial motor control of coherent individual segments; this is a largely discredited theory (Chapter 2). But if the underlying theory hypotheses motor control in terms of a parametric gesture rendering model based on syllables – as in TM, for example, and perhaps in Browman and Goldstein's (1986) Articulatory Phonology – then the 'conclusion' will be that the speaker has failed in the rendering of such-and-such a parameter over such-and-such a stretch of gesture. It might well be worth an empirical investigation of the hypothesis that the proposed treatment of the condition, or indeed an assessment of its cause, will depend on this underlying model. This is not a criticism of speech clinicians; it is a general remark – which is true – that scientific observation involves perceiving the object of study from a theoretical stance: a position which is unavoidable. The duty of the scientist is to make sure that the underlying theory is the best available for the job.

A model based on the biology of concurrent or parallel operating systems, moving the vocal tract into different ongoing configurations could help pinpoint what is creating the effect of imprecise speech. Those muscle systems could be targeted in a planned way. These are two of the main questions to be addressed:

- Is the lack of perceived accurate coarticulatory effects meaningful when retraining speech judged to be inadequate after neural damage?
- How can this concept be fitted into applications modelling?

Coarticulation is the result of overlapping parameters – the co-production explanation. Defective coarticulation effects, in our terms, are the result of imperfect phonetic retrieval, mis-stored units or inappropriate cognitive intervention in the process.

Neuroscience applications

Neuroscience, as applied to language, is a broad area including neuropsychological (language pathology) errors in the acquisition of spoken language (for example, deafness and dyslexia). We look at some recent work to suggest ways that the theoretical construct of a model structure involving dynamic and static planes might be useful, bearing in mind the basic problem is how to correlate two types of activity – the results of cognition and physical expression. We feel that the basis of all applications work in speech would appropriately be a reliable model of cognitive and physical processing, an understanding of the relationship between these components and a plausible link between the modalities of audition and *vision*.

The neuropsychology of speech

This term currently usually refers to some specific aspects of language pathology, and should not be confused with cognitive neuroscience which refers to the biological basis of those abilities that are assigned to cognition.

The production disorder, aphasia, is concerned with the identification of disorders ascribed to aphasia, and is a large area of research. Recent interest has centred on characterising the relationship between aphasia, a production disorder, and syllable structure units. In our TM terms, syllables are stored on the phonological plane – they are basic phonological units.

Some researchers suggest, however, that aphasia might be a *production* deficiency. This would suggest either an incomplete or imperfect storage on the *static* phonetic plane, or a retrieval malfunction on the phonetic *dynamic* plane. Romani and Galluzzi (2005) following on from a paper by Nickels and Howard (2004) report a set of experiments relating cognition and speech output in terms of complexity. Is the complexity noted a matter of syllable *structure*, which would indicate an inaccurate storage and retrieval on the static and dynamic phonological planes? We wonder if a narrowing of the focus of interest in the relationship between cognition and speech production by modelling storage, access and retrieval of speech units on both the cognitive and physical levels (planes) would be a useful follow-up to these researchers' work.

An experiment examining a clearly defined speech effect, set in a larger context (with implications for that larger context) is reported by Kurowski *et al.* (2003). Appropriate speech output is the result of precise articulatory timing control and/or correct selection of phonological segments to be rendered. This paper reports an experiment designed to eliminate some phonological and phonetic variables:

> More specifically, the deficits displayed by these patients could be the result of either higher order impairments in the selection and planning of speech output or a low level impairment in the articulatory implementation of selected and planned speech segments. (p. 354)

A 'pervasive timing effect' was eliminated, as were possible coarticulatory effects. The inability was narrowed down to laryngeal control. The result of the experiment

> ... suggests that the deficits observed in these subjects are not due to the selection of inappropriate speech segments, but rather to lower level impairments in articulatory implementation. (p. 369)

We wonder, using our TM terms again, if the model could be stated as a query whether the dysfunction might be down to

- the failure of the correct retrieval of information from the static phonetic plane, assuming the patient had stored the appropriate information before the problem arose, or
- whether the circuitry which allowed retrieval at all was disturbed.

Or whether it might, in fact, be the experimenters' own conclusion that the difficulty was the inability of the motor system to carry out any function involving laryngeal control. In this case, further work could examine this last hypothesis in more detail. We suggest applying the dynamic and static plane model, because it is a more precise and explicit model for locating potential sites of imperfect processing – even it turns out to be inadequate in this case. Such an experiment so detailed in description lends itself to the transfer of the hypotheses to other models in this way. Not all experiments are so transparent and detailed or could be said to offer definite contributions to the development not only of the local model but of the underlying theoretical position.

An acquisition disorder – deafness as error

It is commonly observed that deaf speakers have an apparent coarticulatory difficulty and a reduced fundamental frequency range or variation in comparison with non-deaf speakers. This is sometimes reported as 'slurred' speech. The obvious question to ask is whether the effect arises

- because the underlying phonological representations are inadequate, and *appear* to be coarticulated incorrectly simply because the wrong phonological unit (or rule, or constraint) has been retrieved, or
- because the motor control system is not operating with the required degree of precision despite having access to the *correct* underlying units?

In terms of the planes model we can ask whether the output is inadequate because

- the knowledge on the phonetic static plane is incomplete, or because the wrong information is being accessed by the dynamic phonetics? Or
- has the wrong phonological unit been accessed by dynamic phonology? Or
- have incorrect phonological processing rules been stored on the static phonological plane?

TM can go further, and introduce a new element to the research. In our model all rendering (phonetic) processes are supervised or managed. Management is performed by the Cognitive Phonetics Agent (CPA) which takes in, among other things, information derived from feedback. This enables us to introduce a new hypothesis:

- Despite the fact that the phonological units and processing have been correctly accessed and applied dynamically, and the phonetic units have been correctly retrieved and processed, the supervision of these processes has failed – resulting in relatively unmanaged motor control with predictable errors in controlling coarticulation and rhythm.

We suggest there is some advantage in being as precise as possible in narrowing the broad terms 'cognitive' and 'physical' down to more precise types of processing: phonological *vs.* phonetic, static *vs.* dynamic, and, importantly, basic control *vs.* control *management*.

Some researchers hypothesise that for deaf speakers there is a relationship between reading and spelling for deaf individuals. Olson and Caramazza (2004) discuss the relationship between spelling and reading in language users who cannot reference full hearing. They conclude that linguistic knowledge may not be dependent on an intact hearing system. This suggests that a plan for articulation, on the static phonetic plane, is dependent on the ability to hear, but that the cognitive based units are independent of the retrieval rules and the units. The Olson and Caramazza conclusions support the static/dynamic and phonology/phonetics perspectives on the planning then rendering of speech.

Cognitive approaches to understanding emotive content

Cognitive constructs involving behaviour and extending to incorporate biological models fall under the general heading 'cognitive neuroscience' (Gazzaniga *et al.* 1998). The term means that there is an association between brain and mind, and this concept enables, for example, a comprehensive modelling of the emotive content of speech. Looking at the example of emotive speech, linguistic phonetic theory that adopts the cognitive neuroscience approach is able to contribute significantly to characterising emotive content in a formal or computational way (Tatham and Morton 2005).

The change from classical phonetics to contemporary phonetics is characterised by underlying principles such as a requirement for explanation of the described phenomena, and the preference, if not requirement for a computationally adequate description (Chapter 6). Studies of cognitive neuroscience have been oriented toward examining possible underlying systems which appear to present at the surface. Thus a methodology of mapping from deep to surface structure is common to both general cognitive neuroscience and contemporary speech production theory (Ivry *et al.* 2001). Expressive/emotive content of speech is rooted in such mappings (Tatham and Morton 2004). We suggest that future work relating subsystems that might be related to the surface representation of emotive content of speech can be correlated with cognitive neuroscience models and related to common mapping methods and common approaches to computational adequacy.

Perception

In Chapter 8 we discuss the relationship between hearing and perception and the degree of active participation in the perceptual process. We ask a number of questions based on various models of perception that researchers have offered. As with all applications work the research paradigm involves a two-way exchange between the underlying general theory and specific derived applicational theories, based on a two-way exchange of empirical investigation. So, having identified various areas of processing (Chapter 7) we can investigate, with a combined linguistics/neuroscience approach the degree and nature, for example, of active processing of the heard acoustic signal. This processing involves, importantly, repairing defective content (either errors in the original signal, or errors due to failure of the peripheral hearing systems) and assignment of known elements to the heard signal to output a cognitive representation which matches the speaker's original utterance plan. Thus there is scope for detailed research using the combined approaches of linguistics and neuroscience with a view to discovering the relative balance of effects of hearing errors, cognitive processing errors, linguistic assignment errors and managerial errors in explaining an apparently *mis-perceived* signal. Once again, we stress the importance of the transparency afforded by a multi-planed, hierarchically organised underlying model in pointing toward clearer more precise research questions. These questions additionally form the basis of unravelling potential sources of error in the perceptual processes.

Cross-modal linking

Researchers have been building independent models of vision and audition, but now are moving toward across-modal linking. The results of such modelling might be of interest to researchers in the areas of dyslexia and pronunciation teaching for deaf users of the language. Evidence comes from studying brain function, attention, memory, and presenting both auditory and visual stimuli to a speaker of the language. Results are ambiguous for the moment, and point to either independent modes of operation, or to plausible models of integrated processing (Critchley, M. and Critchley, E. 1978, Eimer 1999, Macaluso *et al.* 2001, Pourtois and de Gelder 2002, Guttman *et al.* 2005). We cannot discuss here either their findings or the hypotheses upon which their work is based, but we can observe that it seems early days to posit robust spoken language modelling and applications deriving from these models without a firm cognitive and biological basis. However, such a basis seems to be some way in the future, and there are questions to address until such time; but we suggest caution. The association between modalities is not clear; there is no metatheory describing a procedure for linking models of different senses. Some of the observations made are about phenomena occurring *outside* language, such as synaesthesia (Sacks 1996, Ramachandran and Hubbard 2003).

Two modalities – audition and vision

Dyslexia is an area of research activity which combines two modalities – one of which involves *speech* modelling. Researchers have observed over many years (Studdert-Kennedy and Mody 1995) that some people seem to have difficulty in linking the visual representation of speech sounds – that is the 'letters of the alphabet' (which in English do not correspond in a one-to-one relationship with pronunciation) – and the visual representation of written words drawn from the pool of the same letters of the alphabet. The link between what is heard and what is read is said to be either missing or incomplete. A number of observations and suggestions have been made, focussing on the difficulty of relating shapes of letters with sound shapes and a consequent ability to spell, read aloud, and speak. There are difficulties in recognising sounds (within words), and in processing rapid visual information. Some researchers suggest brain impairment (Fawcett and Nicholson 2001) as a cause, and some suggest genetically based differences (Frith 1997). The two modalities, *speaking* and *reading*, may be interrelated, implying two different descriptions and two different methodologies.

In addition to the presence or absence of perceived categories of the sound system of the language, there are questions to be raised about

- access and subsequent processing in general,
- the conduits for processing,
- possible cognitive and biological bases for positing these units,
- their usefulness in contributing to descriptions of reading and speaking problems, and
- establishing a common base for discussion of dyslexia as a problem involving both reading and speaking.

There is currently much interest in the concepts of *phonological awareness* (PA) and *phonological deficit*. The term PA seems to have been derived from early work by Liberman *et al.* (1967). Kavanaugh and Mattingly (1972), elaborated in Bertelson and de Gelder (1991), among others). The suggestion is that reading, as well as speaking, needs retrieval of the *phonological* representation of the structure of what is being read. Furthermore, there is an interrelationship, it is hypothesised, between reading, speaking and writing (Fawcett and Nicolson 2001). The construction, PA, is used in investigations into the nature of dyslexia and treated as a focus for potential deficit in phonological categorisation and representation (Studdert-Kennedy and Mody 1995), or in the perception of auditory events (Tallal *et al.* 1993).

However some studies suggest that the errors noted arise in phonological processing (Blomert *et al.* 2004, among others). They looked at the effect of acoustic, phonetic, and phonological contexts and present results that suggest 'the phonological core deficits in developmental dyslexia may be attributed to deviances in online phonological processing' – a result which would not contradict the model of dynamic phonological and phonetic processing presented in Chapter 6. Others (Purcell-Gates 2001) suggest written, not oral, development is basic to literacy.

Some researchers (Farmer and Klein 1995, Studdert-Kennedy and Mody 1995, Ivry *et al.* 2001, among others) suggest that there may be an association between two or more of the following areas: speech processing, audition, vision, perception and brain systems. If two or more apparently different difficulties are noted, such as speech problems and dyslexia, both types of event need to be precisely described, and if even a simple relationship is suggested, for example a similar computational approach, those relationships can be modelled more explicitly. A computational model, by definition a model than runs algorithmically from initial to final stages, can reveal deficiencies in the description, and suggest formal similarities and differences in processes being characterised.

- The value of computational models is considerable, in our view: they describe how to do something, not what to do. Though the algorithms describe how to do something, the something itself must, of course, be specified within the data structure. The substance of the formal properties is characterised by the researchers in the respective contributing fields. When expectations are not realised – that is, the computational model does not predict the data correctly – then the hypothesis can be changed and an iterative process entered into that gradually converges the model's predictions with the observed data. In the case of dyslexia, phonological awareness as a construct may be an interim hypothesis – but it may turn out that a typical *brain* function may provide a sounder basis for relating dyslexia and speech. Or some other hypothesis might be appropriate, which might be suggested by re-specifying contexts and redoing algorithms, thus enabling the researcher to think of other plausible constructs than current approach allows.

If the phonological awareness hypothesis is equivalent to proposing knowledge of a phonological database, then we ask:

- Does *reading* access the *same* static database as speaking and are the same access strategies used?

- Since vision and hearing are different modalities, should there be different ways of representing sound shapes and visual objects?
- How relevant could phonetic theory be to reading since by definition it focuses on speaking?
- Reading requires *visual* input; so is it appropriate to converge these two models of production and perception involving both speaking and vision without a revision of the two currently different *metatheories* – should a common metatheory be devised to make the 'combined' model more plausible?

Some researchers are pursuing the line that speaking and reading problems may have a common base in similar brain functions. In that case, since reading and speaking appear to be quite different, questions arise concerning the mapping from the common area to the specific areas, in order to result in the appropriate motor activity. Researchers have posited brain-level mechanisms which might be *associated* with some aspects of language, but how that activity might *support* language is not clear. In short, claims about locating areas of the brain which might be associated with reading and speaking difficulties are not sufficiently strong as yet to provide a satisfactorily robust model (Frith 1997). An approach which links speech sound processing, vision processing, and language brain systems with written and spoken languages seems to be not yet properly formalised.

The relationship between reading and spelling, and methods of teaching are discussed by Fletcher-Flinn *et al.* (2004) with respect to whether skills in the one might transfer to the other. They point out a number of sources of variability in the experimental conditions which need to be taken into account, such as early teaching methods, irregularity in grapheme to phoneme mapping, and phoneme to grapheme mapping to recognised words; strategies for dealing with new words, non-words, phonologically simple and complex words, simple and complex spellings and the age of the children being tested. They point out that reading is a recognition activity, spelling is a production activity. It seems that assuming transfer of orthographic knowledge to spelling, and the reverse, needs more careful justification. Are teaching methods and model building which are based on this assumption resting on an adequately firm foundation?

Klima (1991) pointed out that 'it has come to be self-evident that phonological representations are involved in reading and learning to read' (p. 414). And that 'interpretation and production of language can include orthographic information' (p. 414). He points out, however, that what is not clear is under what circumstances such orthographic instances occur or even when they *could* occur. His comment suggests that incorporating reading as a cognitive activity within a language processing model which also models speech production and perception cannot be assumed to be a straightforward matter. And there is no evidence so far to suggest that he exaggerates.

fMRI evidence

Evidence put forward based on fMRI scans needs careful interpretation *within* the theory or model which generates the hypotheses for gathering this type of data. There is currently some focus on fMRI data, but we should introduce such evidence with great caution: it still is not clear what precise activity occurs in a scan process (Raichle 2003), and interpretations must be done with care (Nichols and Newsome 1999). For example, one commonly used technique is to look at oxidative metabolism during activation within the brain. 'Does every area of the cerebral cortex behave in this manner? Is this true for both excitatory and inhibitory energy-requiring processes?' (Raichle 1977, p. 30). We might add: Are these markers always reliable for making inferences for spoken language modelling? We are not being critical of using such data for speech production phenomena, but strongly suggesting that we are aware of the importance of keeping 'the limits of our knowledge in mind when it comes to the interpretation of our data' (Raichle 1977, p. 30). And to paraphrase Ivry *et al.* (2001): because a brain structure is activated during 'retrieval tasks does not mean this structure contributes in a causal manner to the retrieval process' (p. 197).

We suggest that a metatheory developed to encompass understanding brain *and* cognitive function in speech, even in outline, might be useful, since the relationship between spoken language production and perception, and cognitive and brain function is giving rise to much experimental work and data gathering from many points of view. For example Ivry *et al.* (2001) have looked at brain, language, and implications for dyslexia. They state: 'One might ask whether the cerebellum supports an essential cognitive function that, when impaired, can lead to very different disorders if combined with other neural insults and/or environmental contexts' (p. 189). They further suggest a way of describing and linking both cognitive and brain function in language use: 'In suggesting this connection between the cerebellum, verbal rehearsal, phonological representation, and reading, we do not mean to suggest this particular etiology as the potential *explanation* for dyslexia'

(p. 205 – authors' italics). Given the extensive descriptions of the many systems hypothesised to be involved in speaking, reading, writing, and understanding language, the *source* of problems with language related systems is difficult to determine. Again, there seems to be no *metatheory* of language linking the many models under one set of principles which will provide not only descriptions but perhaps explanation. For the development of a robust and integrated theory along these lines, such a metatheory is a *sine qua non*.

A basic assumption – phonological awareness

The phonological awareness hypothesis is worth revisiting, since it forms a basic *assumption* for many researchers. The speaker's phonological model of the language is derived from heard speech; and knowledge about the sound structure developed from infancy is derived from the speech heard from infancy. Can this knowledge of the sound structure be applied to reading, which is not production based?

There is some disagreement about how to define PA, other than to say the construct refers to the knowledge about the phonological segments in speech (for a segmentally based approach – but what of other phonological objects like prosodic features?). Whatever, the observations and experiments, they seem to point to the need for a strong model of phonological representations. The problem lies in characterising how to *access* the knowledge base, how units and rules interact with, say, a *phonetic* database, and the nature of the subsequent processing of any retrieved data. Models of perception and underlying brain function might contribute to developing *processing* models, but very little work has been done in this area. Hypothesis driven research could possibly provide a firmer basis for continuing model building so that applications could more reliably be made based on the idea of PA. What seems to be needed is a move toward hypotheses developed to provide an explanatory basis for the observations made by researchers.

For example, teachers need to apply such constructs as PA to their practical problems in the classroom. There is an awareness of the need for definitions of constructs on which teaching methods can be based. Blachman (1997) tells us: 'The challenge remains to translate the research in phonological awareness into appropriate education practices that remain *grounded in theory* and that are flexible enough to *absorb new research* as it becomes available' (p. 425 – authors' italics).

We ask how the model of static and dynamic processing might be useful in discussing phonological awareness and speaking/reading problems. This model takes into account facts of speaking (the knowledge bases and the accessing and processing strategies) and the resulting acoustic waveform. It suggests a common base for accessing and retrieving phonological units. If a model relating speaking, reading, and writing is seen to be appropriate, perhaps a dynamic model relating access to the same phonological knowledge base might provide some justification for the construct of phonological awareness. Otherwise phonological processes described for reading and speaking would be separate – which of course may be the case. In this case, reading and speaking might only be described in the future with representations that could be mapped onto a larger set within a proper integrating *metatheory*.

Levels of representation and the metatheory

Among the main advantages of a metatheory for production and perception are

- ease of matching levels of representation and arriving at similar symbol assignments in the different levels,
- arriving at correlations between differing sets of symbolic representations and processes – perhaps through common model types – such as dynamic *vs.* static paradigm.

At the moment, although it is only assumed that appropriate biological structures exist for cross-modal interaction, the hypothesis is that PA, a cognitive activity, converges on both reading and speech errors (though *how* is usually not specified). Phonological awareness, it is hypothesised, relates brain and cognitive activity, and its failure to do so properly will result in both brain and cognitively generated reading and speech errors:

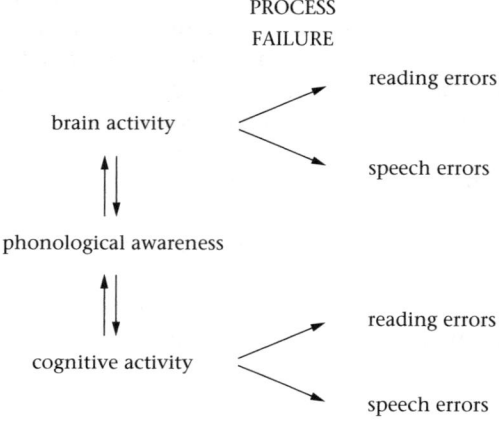

If reading errors *are* bound up with speech errors, not only might it be useful to find brain areas in common, it might also be useful to have model types in common so that it would be possible to relate one model with another – to relate them, of course (and we repeat) *via* an explicitly developed common underlying metatheory. Then both the substrate (brain) and the models of the result of the activity of the substrate would be similar and easier to compare when hypothesising about the cognitive processing (and its failure) involved in reading and speaking. They might not only have features in common, but arise from a common source.

Phonetics related to other areas of linguistic description

Relating speech production models and phonetic data is accepted for developing phonological theory, since this utilises phonetic information as evidence for modelling phonological processes (Hayes 1995). However, implications from speech modelling can be drawn for higher level language processing, detailing plausible lexical–semantic relationships. Blumstein (2004) and others have modelled the structure of phonetic *categories* of speech, associating perception with features of the phonetic *structure*.

Blumstein, discussing the perceptual effects of acoustic variability, questions 'whether this acoustic variability that influences the perception of the phonetic categories of speech also influences higher levels of language processing' (p. 18). The assumption of this research is that phonetic structure affects lexical access, which specifies the sound shape of the word, and which in turn accesses and 'ultimately activates a lexical semantic network' (p. 19) – that is, not only the semantic representation of the word itself but 'words that may be semantically related to it' (p. 20). The results of this experimental approach suggest that phonetic structure representations contribute to phonological representations, which in turn influences the lexical-semantic network, but 'do not speak to the nature of the representation of lexical form itself' (p. 23). Thus although we cannot transform phonetic features into cognitive features, it *is* possible to relate abstractions at different levels.

Odell and Shriberg (2001) also discuss the relationship between speaking and higher levels of representation involving phrasing, rate and stress. They discuss apraxia – a disorder of speech production which involves motor planning, programming and subsequent movement of the articulators. In our terms, the investigation can be seen as addressing two types of event: accessing and then retrieving the correct phonological units for phrasing, and the subsequent storage and retrieval of correct parametric gestures for programming the articulators. If it could be shown that during development *incorrect* gestures or units had been established, then in later development those erroneous units and gestures would be retrieved (unless they had been modified during development). Relating the cognitive level to the physical level can take many forms; and this is perhaps one of the basic problems in language production modelling: for the moment no one approach seems to have more value than another. We again point to the advantage of a strict computational approach, since at the very least it can formally separate objects and processes. Real world theory hypothesis driven results such as reported in this paper can provide confirmation or refutation of the model's features (Shriberg *et al.* 2004)

Diagnostic applications

Phonetic constructs derived from experimental data are being used as a diagnostic in practical work. For example, speech onset delay studies such as Shriberg *et al.* (2003) of children with *otitis media* and a possible deficit in intelligibility show that studies which are model based can reinforce the strength of the model itself. That is, hypothesis driven experiments can, by an iterative process, reinforce the model from which they are derived – in this case phonetic theory and how it deals with timing constraints. An example involving phonology can be seen in Edmonds and Marquardt (2004) where the experiment was based on investigation of syllable shape and occurrence. Differences were found in the type of syllable, and explanations (preliminary, the researchers state) are given in terms of syllable based features such as stress, fundamental frequency change and speech rate changes. Syllable based work can capture generalisations which may be more relevant to spoken language than segment based work, and provides some evidence that spoken language might be better described as syllable based rather than conjoined segment based.

Harel *et al.* (2004) applied a well documented (Lisker and Abramson 1964) speaking phenomenon, voice onset time (VOT), as a marker for variability in Parkinsonian speech. Observations have been made that speech motor control progressively deteriorates, but there are few techniques for quantifying these changes. In this case, the acoustic wave was measured with a view to correlating VOT changes with the deterioration. The VOT literature suggests that it is possible to identify and assign labels to segments, so we would expect to be able to assign progressive misidentifications. However there is some possibility of error, since such assignment is somewhat impressionistic. Assignment of labels by the researchers assumes a coherent symbol set and that the assigner has knowledge of acoustics, the symbol set and can make a reasonable guess as to how the segment in a deteriorating state relates to the symbols. This experiment also assumes that Parkinsonian speech output can be described accurately according to an agreed system, and that the Parkinson's speaking features and the assigned segmental labels on the waveform can reliably be correlated.

The information from the acoustic analysis was used to confirm the medical hypothesis (based on other indicators) that Parkinson's disease existed. The researchers point out that just because an event is measurable it is not in itself a definitive indication of its own cause. It is essential in speech work to realise that the second stage, interpreting the measurements, gives rise to some error, since there is room for error in both the measurements and in their interpretation (the assignment of symbols).

Finding a stretch of speech where a segment can be marked, and the assignment of the symbol identifying it would ideally be a reliable task, but unfortunately in speech research this is seldom the case because of serious mismatches (explained in Chapter 1) between the acoustic signal and its symbolic representation. In the case of VOT, the obvious question is: Where precisely does the vowel begin following the initial voiceless stops? The particular work we are reporting was well done and has produced interesting results, but many researchers fail to realise that vowels and stops are abstract objects and that the acoustic wave can only correlate in some ill-defined way with such objects.

Other factors which must also be taken into account when dealing with the acoustic signal are:

- How much detail is recorded – that is, what are the sampling rates and bit density (the number of bits used to encode amplitude)?
- If fine detail is noted, is this a characteristic of the speaker (the idiolect), the dialect, or the testing environment; or do some of the details arise from some temporary physical state such as being tired or anxious?

However, such sources of experimental error may be small (with the exception of where the vowel begins), and the overall pattern may well be a useful early indicator or diagnostic of a deterioration which could lead to further medical investigation.

These examples suggest that well founded observations, experience, and linguistic/phonetic based hypotheses can be applied to practical problems. Relating linguistic phonetic descriptions to underlying cognitive and biological processes contributes to an overall speech production and perception metatheory. In application work, we suggest the more theory based the approach is, the more likely the procedures developed will be reliable and predictive in the long term. Essentially 'experiential' work is unable to provide the robust conclusions we associate with theoretically driven empirical investigation.

Clinical Phonetics – procedures and expert systems: modelling clinical assessment

To provide an illustration of the computational approach to model building we begin with the suggestion that a statement of standard procedures couched in computationally oriented terms might be useful as an aid to identifying a patient's error or difficulty. Clinicians often have to work with incomplete descriptions, and the intention here is to illustrate how formal procedures interact with such descriptions. To resolve the practical problem facing therapists, they must *de facto* filter information from the patient through their knowledge and experience. It is this information which will often be incomplete, but provided the clinician's viewpoint is robust useful progress is made.

The following assessment procedure is described by Schriberg and Kent (1982), who seem to have coined the term 'clinical phonetics'. The procedure is clearly laid out, presenting a scoring method in assessing patients who appear to have speech difficulties. The initial step is to judge whether the speech is right/wrong, acceptable/non-acceptable, correct/incorrect, and so on. The procedure is based on informed judgement by the clinician. By 'informed', we mean that the judgement is arrived at through a knowledge of linguistics, phonetics, psychology, biology and self awareness, as determined to be essential by the professional accrediting body to which the clinician belongs. Broken down into stages, the following *procedures* can be identified:

IF the speech is right/correct
    THEN EXIT;
IF the speech is wrong/incorrect
        THEN the following is a possible description of what is happening [judgement]
            STATE the problem;

requires:
> a descriptive system which the clinician can use to assign labels to waveform
> an understanding of the symbols used in the descriptive system [phonology, phonetics]
> an understanding of how the waveform derives from the production process [phonetics]
> a descriptive system to account for speech production in general [knowledge from phonetics]
> an understanding of how to assign labels to the stages of production [phonetics, training/experience]

HYPOTHESISE which production processes are producing the wrong waveform; [theory, empirical model, observation/experience]
CONSULT or DEVELOP exercises to change the production process;
ASSIGN labels to sound wave;
COMPARE new labels with original labels;
> IF labels match, problem solved
> IF labels don't match
>> THEN reiterate procedure
> IF labels converge, problem solved

IF problem is *not* solved after a number of iterations THEN look for source of error.

Based strictly on the model, and without editing from experience, some sources of error might be:

a. the descriptive system is inadequate [phonetics knowledge]
b. the assignment of labels is faulty [phonetics knowledge and interpretation]
c. any prior exercises to produce correct waveform have been inadequate or inappropriate [phonetics]
d. the patient cannot produce required sound because of
   - physical impairment – impediment or motor control problem: can this be fixed?
   - cognitive inability – unaware of distinctions to be made, poor attention span: language training required?

The general idea is to formalise the procedures followed by the clinician/expert in assessment, diagnosis and prescribing treatment. The above methodology can be interpreted or restated as a Bayesian expert system which works on *probability assessments* at each stage of the unfolding procedure. In the actual system *prior* probabilities are assigned to each solution or sub-solution before any investigation (call these the *prior intrinsic probabilities*); these prior probabilities on their own would provide decisions (leading to a diagnosis and treatment prescription) which reflect the average, 'all things being equal' situation.

The strategy of an expert system is to take these prior probabilities with their expected 'normal' outcome and proceed through a series of diagnostic queries. Each query leads to decision, and with each informed decision the *balance* of probabilities is modified by adjusting the probability weightings on each decision parameter as appropriate. After all processes are complete an outcome decision is made according to the concluding probability balance (a judgement based on the *final probabilities*). The diagram shows the general format of a simple expert system. Note that the final decision *could* be automatic, but because many of the answers along the way will be based on *experiential judgement* it is appropriate in clinical assessment for the final decision also the be performed with an injection of experiential judgement.

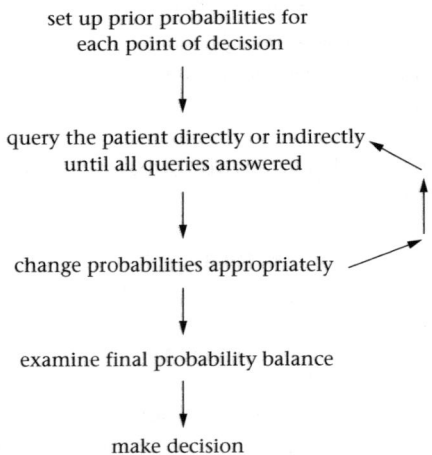

Areas that need further specification

The above example may seem to be a simple example of stating a procedure in computational terms which could in fact be perfectly clearly stated verbally. The point of a computational statement is that sources of error can be easily noticed and areas of vagueness can be identified simply because the entire assessment procedure is broken down into explicit queries. But in addition because the same procedures are applied to each patient the diagnoses are directly comparable. This is of considerable help in building a coherent body of knowledge, either for the applied discipline or for feeding back into the underlying theory. For example,

a. judging perceived sound to be *either* in the category phonology *or* phonetics (but cannot be *both*);
b. assignment of the appropriate label systematically within each category;
c. assigning labels consistently to perceived sounds judged to be identical;
d. assigning labels consistently in agreement with *other* clinicians' labels;
e. reliable and *repeatable* judgement of errors, for example those due to assimilation (phonological) or co-articulation (phonetic);
f. reliable mapping from e. to probable cognitive or physical origins (if the perceived error judged not to be dialect bound);
g. perceived error judged not to be a result of non-native speaking ability or an idiolect or acquired (but otherwise normal) characteristic of the speaker.

And finally

1. Is it possible to determine features of the perceptual range of the clinician and how finely tuned this might be to range of variability?
2. Are the problems residing in the patient capable of being perceived by the clinician? or detected by the tests?
3. Is the problem one of articulation or something else?

From the phonetic theory point of view, perhaps the most basic question is whether the variation is phonological or phonetic; and secondly, what is an appropriate theory-based exercise to help in dealing with the error. That is: Is the theory capable of providing both the information and the characterisation of the underlying system that the clinician needs, hence provide pointers toward clinical decisions?

Scrutiny of these queries perhaps leads to the conclusion that

- the linguistic/phonetic descriptive system is not fully adequate yet,
- feedback from applications does not appear to be adequately incorporated into the available descriptions,

- the gaps between theory, model descriptions, prediction, application models and practical procedures need careful bridging.

These observations prompt the suggestion of the critical need for a coherent unifying metatheory.

Some of the distance between the crucial areas is created by the basic cognitive/physical gap, some by no agreed reliable modelling of phonology/ phonetics for application in the neuroscience environment, and perhaps a lack of common ground in, say, computational terms which can reveal procedural errors and reveal those areas which need a human mind to interpret consequences – and some by lack of theory. Halliday (2005) states the view clearly 'that in the diagnosis and treatment of speech and language disorders there is a similar need for a theory-based engagement with language, in place of piecemeal observations of isolated (and hence liable to be rather superficially interpreted) linguistic features' (p. 133).

When dealing with humans, the usefulness of the constructs of *cognitive* and *physical* processing may be limited in diagnosis. But it may be useful to ask a question: Can a cognitively based therapy designed to correct linguistic knowledge (such as phonological awareness) be distinguished from physical therapy designed to get muscles functioning smoothly again under command of whatever cognitively sourced intention?

We wonder whether the static/dynamic modelling approach would be helpful. Sources of error could include: a non-standard phonological system (dialect or idiolect variation), deletions or distortion of units on the phonological plane, inability to retrieve the correct unit (dynamic phonology), deletion of correct command on rendering (static phonetic), inability to access either plane (physical), inability to retrieve correct rendering, inability to carry out correct rendering (physical), inability to monitor internally (cognitive phonetic), lessened capacity to be aware of the situation because of medication (cognitive and physical effects), anxiety, or lack of understanding of the task.

Conclusion

In this book we have treated speech production and perception as part of a general theory of speech. We have also included an applicational focus toward the end. Our objective has been to identify key areas of speech production and perception where we believe theoretical work needs to concentrate. Classical Phonetics provided a foundation for moving toward truly explanatory modelling. But speech is an area where several disciplines intersect, and we have warned against piecemeal interaction between these – interaction and cross fertilisation need to proceed with a common metatheory if true explanation of observations is to be achieved. Important areas of application (and we have mentioned just one or two) need a better speech theory than has so far been available, and we have made suggestions to this end. With Cognitive Phonetics and its central Supervisory Agent we develop a clearer, more dynamic and explanatory model to speech. Whatever models may be developed, the theory needs to link the main areas being investigated as we try to understand speech production and perception as special characteristics of human beings which extend out into all areas of our lives.

References

Abercrombie, D. (1967). *Elements of General Phonetics*. Edinburgh: Edinburgh University Press.

Adolphs, R. and Damasio, A. (2000). 'Neurobiology of Emotion at a Systems Level', in J. Borod (ed.), *The Neuropsychology of Emotion*. Oxford: Oxford University Press 194–213.

Baringa, M. (1996). 'The Cerebellum: Movement Control or Much More?', *Science* 272: 482–3.

Baxter, M. and Murray, E. (2000). 'Reinterpreting the Behavioural effects of Amygdala Lesions in Nonhuman Primates', in J. Aggleton (ed.), *The Amygdala; a Functional Analysis*. Oxford: Oxford University Press 545–68.

Baxter, M. and Murray, E. (2002). 'The Amygdala and Reward', *Nature Reviews; Neuroscience* 3: 563–80.

Bell-Berti, F., Karakow, R., Gelfer, C. and Boyce, S. (1995). 'Anticipatory and Carryover Implications for Models of Speech Production', in F. Bell-Berti and L. Raphael (eds), *Producing Speech: Contemporary Issues*. New York: American Institute of Physics 77–97.

Bertelson, P. and de Gelder, B. (1991). 'The Emergence of Phonological Awareness: Comparative Approaches', in I. Mattingly and M. Studdert-Kennedy (eds), *Modularity and the Motor Theory of Speech Perception: Proceedings of a Conference to Honor Alvin M. Liberman*. New Jersey: Lawrence Erlbaum 393–412.

Blachman, B. (1997). 'Early Intervention and Phonological Awareness; A Cautionary Tale', in B. Blachman (ed.), *Foundations of Reading Acquisition and Dyslexia; Implications for Early Intervention*. New Jersey: Lawrence Erlbaum 409–30.

Bladon, R. and Al-Bamerni, A. (1976). 'Coarticulation Resistance in English /l/', *Journal of Phonetics* 4: 137–50.

Blomert, L., Mitterer, H. and Paggen, C. (2004). 'In Search of the Auditory, Phonetic, and/or Phonological Problems in Dyslexia; Context Effects in Speech Perception', *Journal of Speech, Language, and Hearing Research* 47: 1030–47.

Blumstein, S. and Stevens, K. (1979). 'Acoustic Variance in Speech Production: Evidence from Measurements of the Spectral Characteristics of Stop Consonants', *Journal of the Acoustical Society of America* 66(4): 1001–17.

Blumstein, S. (2004). 'Phonetic Category Structure and Its Influence on Lexical Processing', in A. Agwuele, W. Warren and S-H Park (eds), *Proceedings of the 2003 Texas Linguistics Society Conference*. Somerville MA: Cascadilla Proceedings Project 17–25.

Borden, G. and Harris, K. (1980). *Speech Science Primer: Physiology, Acoustics, and Perception of Speech*. Baltimore: Williams and Wilkins.

Browman, K. and Goldstein, L. (1986). 'Towards an Articulatory Phonology', in C. Ewan and J. Anderson (eds), *Phonology Yearbook 3*. Cambridge: Cambridge University Press 219–53.

Carmichael, L. (2003). 'Intonation: Categories and Continua', in *Proceedings 19th Northwest Linguistics Conference*. Victoria, BC.

Celce-Murcia, M., Brinton, D. and Goodwin, J. (1996). *Teaching Pronunciation: A Reference for Teachers of English to Speakers of Other Languages*. Cambridge: Cambridge University Press.
Chen, M. and Wang, W. (1975). 'Sound Change: Activation and Implementation', *Language* 51: 255–81.
Cho, T. (2002). *The Effects of Prosody on Articulation in English*. New York: Routledge.
Chomsky, N. (1957). *Syntactic Structures*. The Hague: Mouton.
Chomsky, N. (1965). *Aspects of the Theory of Syntax*. Cambridge MA: MIT Press.
Chomsky, N. and Halle, M. (1968). *The Sound Pattern of English*. New York: Harper & Row.
Chun, D. (2002). *Discourse Intonation in L2*. Amsterdam: Benjamins.
Cook, V. (1999). 'Using SLA Research in Language Teaching', *International Journal of Applied Linguistics* 9(2): 267–84.
Cook, V. (2001). *Second Language Learning and Language Teaching*. London: Arnold.
Cook, V. (2003). 'The Changing L1 in the L2 User's Mind', in V. Cook (ed.), *Effects of the Second Language on the First*. Clevedon: Multilingual Matters 1–18.
Cooper, F. (1966). 'Describing the Speech Process in Motor Command Terms', *Status Reports on Speech Research*, Haskins Laboratories, SR 515, 2.1–2.7
Cottingham, J. (2000). 'Intentionality or Phenomenology? Descartes and the Objects of Thought', in T. Crane and S. Patterson (eds), *History of the Mind–Body Problem*. London and New York: Routledge 131–48.
Critchley, M. and Critchley, E. (1978). *Dyslexia Defined*. Springfield, Illinois: Charles C. Thomas.
Cruttenden, A. (2001). *Gimson's Pronunciation of English*. London: Hodder Arnold.
Damasio, A. (1994). *Descartes' Error: Emotion, Reason, and the Human Brain*. New York: Penguin Putnam.
Damasio, H. (1998). 'Neuroanatomical Correlates of the Aphasias', in M. Sarno (ed.), *Acquired Aphasia*. New York: Academic Press 43–70.
Daniloff, R. and Hammarberg, R. (1973). 'On Defining Co-articulation', *Journal of Phonetics* 1: 239–48.
Daniloff, R., Schuckers, G. and Feth, L. (1980). *The Physiological of Speech and Hearing: An Introduction*. New Jersey: Prentice-Hall.
Darwin, C. (1975). *The Origin of Species*, Introduction by L. Matthews. London: Dent.
De Courtenay, B. (1875). *Opyt fonetiki rez' janskix govorov*. Warsaw, cited in Trubetskoy.
Dennett, D. (1996). *Darwin's Dangerous Idea; Evolution and the Meanings of Life*. London: Penguin.
Descartes, R. (1649). *The Philosophical Writings of Descartes*, trans. J. Cottingham, R. Stoothoff and D. Murdoch (1984–91). Cambridge: Cambridge University Press.
Dickinson, A. and Balleine, B. (2000). 'Causal Cognition and Goal-directed Action', in C. Heyes and L. Huber (eds), *Evolution of Cognition*. Cambridge MA: MIT Press.
Eberl, J. (2004). 'Acquinas on the Nature of Human Beings', *The Review of Metaphysics* 58: 333–65.
Edmonds, L. and Marquardt, T. (2004). 'Syllable Use in Apraxia of Speech: Preliminary Findings', *Aphasiology* 18(2): 1121–34.

Eimer, M. (1999). 'Can Attention be Directed to Opposite Locations in Different Modalities: An ERP Study', *Clinical Neurophysiology* 110:1252–9.

Ellis, N. (2003). 'Constructions, Chunking and Connectionism: the Emergence of Second Language Structure', in C. Doughty and M. Long (eds), *Handbook of Second Language Acquisition*. Malden: Blackwell.

Eskenazi, M. (1999). 'Using Automatic Speech Processing for Foreign Language Pronunciation Tutoring: Some Issues and a Prototype', *Language Learning and Technology* 2: 62–76.

Eysenck, M. and Keane, M. (1999). *Cognitive Psychology*. Hove: Taylor and Francis.

Fant, G. (1960). *Acoustic Theory of Speech Production*. The Hague: Mouton.

Fant, G. (1973). *Speech Sounds and Features*. Cambridge MA: MIT Press.

Farmer, M. and Klein, R. (1995). 'The Evidence for a Temporal Processing Deficit Linked to Dyslexia', *Psychonomic Bulletin and Review* 2: 460–93.

Farnetani, E. and Racasens, D. (1999). 'Coarticulation Models in Recent Speech Production Theories', in W. Hardcastle and N. Hewlett (eds), *Coarticulation: Theory, Data and Techniques*. Cambridge: Cambridge University Press 31–65.

Fawcett, A. and Nicolson, R. (2001). 'Dyslexia: the Role of the Cerebellum', in A. Fawcett (ed.), *Dyslexia: Theory and Good Practice*. London: Whurr.

Feynman, R. (1995). *Six Easy Pieces: the Fundamentals of Physics Explained*. Penguin: London.

Firth, J. (1948). 'Sounds and Prosodies', *Transactions of the Philological Society* 127–152. Reprinted in W. Jones and J. Laver (eds), *Phonetics in Linguistics: A Book of Readings*. London: Longman.

Fletcher-Flinn, C., Shankweiler, D. and Frost, S. (2004). 'Coordination of Reading and Spelling in Early Literacy, Development: An Examination of the Discrepancy Hypothesis. *Reading and Writing: An Interdisciplinary Journal* 17, 617–44.

Fougeron, C. and Keating, P. (1997). 'Articulatory Strengthening at Edges of Prosodic Domains', *Journal of the Acoustical Society of America* 106(6): 3728–40.

Fowler, C. (1980). 'Coarticulation and Theories of Extrinsic Timing', *Journal of Phonetics* 8: 113–33.

Fowler, C. (1986). 'An Event Approach to the Study of Speech Perception From a Direct–Realist Perspective', *Journal of Phonetics* 14: 3–28.

Frijda, N. (1993). 'Moods, Emotion Episodes, and Emotions', in M. Lewis and J. Haviland-Jones (eds), *Handbook of Emotions*. New York: Guilford Press 381–403.

Frijda, N. (2000). 'The Psychologists' Point of View', in M. Lewis and J. Haviland-Jones (eds), *Handbook of Emotions*. New York: Guilford Press 59–74.

Frith, U. (1997). 'Brain, Mind and Behavior in Dyslexia', *Dyslexia* 5(4): 192–214

Fry, D. (1955). 'Duration and Intensity as Physical Correlates of Linguistic Stress', *Journal of the Acoustical Society of America* 27, 765–8.

Fry, D. (1958). 'Experiments in the Perception of Stress', *Language and Speech* 1: 126–52.

Garland, A. and Alterman, R. (2004). 'Autonomous Agents Learn to Better Coordinate', *Autonomous Agents and Multi-Agent Systems* 8(3): 267–301.

Gazzaniga, M., Ivry, R. and Mangum, G. (1998). *Cognitive Neuroscience: the Biology of the Mind*. New York: Norton.

Gibson, J. (1954). 'A Theory of Pictorial Perception', *Audio Visual Communication Review* 1: 3–23.

Gimson, A. (1989). 4th edition. *An Introduction to the Pronunciation of English*. London: Edward Arnold.
Givon, T. (2001). *Syntax: An Introduction*. Amsterdam: Benjamins.
Goldsmith, J. (1990). *Autosegmental and Metrical Phonology: An Introduction*. Oxford: Blackwell.
Gould, S. (2004). *The Hedgehog, the Fox, and the Magister's Pox*. London: Random House.
Graney, J. (1995). Review of *'Research Methodology in Second-Language Acquisition'* E. Tarone, S. Gass and A. Cohen (eds), (1994). Hillsdale New Jersey: Lawrence Erlbaum. *TESL-EJ*: 1(3) R 23.
Gregg, K. (1993). 'Taking Explanation Seriously: or, Let a Couple of Flowers Bloom', *Applied Linguistics* 14:(3): 276–94.
Gregg, K. (2005). 'A Response to Jordan's (2004) "Explanatory Adequacy and Theories of Second Language Acquisition"', *Applied Linguistics* 26(1): 121–24.
Gregg, K., M. Long, G. Jordan and A. Beretta (1997). Rationality and Its Discontents in SLA', *Applied Linguistics* 18(4): 538–58.
Grundy, P. (2000). *Doing Pragmatics*. London: Arnold.
Guenther, F. (1995). 'Speech Sound Acquisition, Coarticulaton, and Rate Effects in a Neural Network Model of Speech Production'. *Psychological Review* 102: 594–621.
Guttman, S., Gilroy, L. and Blake, R. (2005). 'Hearing What the Eyes See: Auditory Encoding of Visual Temporal Sequences'. *Psychological Science* 16(3): 228–35.
Halliday, M. (2005). 'A Note on Systemic Functional Linguistics and the Study of Language Disorders', *Clinical Linguistics and Phonetics* 19(3): 133–5.
Hammarberg, R. (1976). 'The Metaphysics of Coarticulation', *Journal of Phonetics*, 4: 353–63.
Hancock, M. (2003). *English Pronunication in Use*. Cambridge: Cambridge University Press.
Handbook of the International Phonetic Association. Cambridge: Cambridge University Press.
Hardcastle, W. and Hewlett, N. (1999). *Coarticulation: Theory, Data, and Techniques*. Cambridge: Cambridge University Press.
Harel, B., Cannizzaro, M., Cohen, H., Reilly, N. and Snyder, P. (2004). 'Acoustic Characteristics of Parkinsonian Speech: a Potential Biomarker of Early Disease Progression and Treatment', *Journal of Neurolinguistics* 17: 439–53.
Hayes, B. (1995). *Metrical Stress Theory: Principles and Case Studies*. Chicago: University of Chicago Press.
Hayes, B. and Steriade, D. (2004). 'Introduction: The Phonetic Basis of Phonological Markedness', in B. Hayes, R. Kirchner and D. Steriade (eds), *Phonetically Based Phonology*. Cambridge, MA: MIT Press, 1–34.
Henke, W. (1966). 'Dynamic Articulatory Model of Speech Production Using Computer Simulation' Unpublished doctoral dissertation. Cambridge, MA: MIT.
Holmes, J. (1988). *Speech Synthesis and Recognition*. London: Taylor and Francis.
Holmes, J. and Holmes, W. (2001). *Speech Synthesis and Recognition*. London: Taylor & Francis.
Holmes, J., Mattingly, I. and Shearme, J. (1964). 'Speech Synthesis by Rule', *Language and Speech* 7: 127–43.

Ivry, R., Justus, T. and Middleton, C. (2001). 'The Cerebellum, Timing, and Language: Implications for the Study of Dyslexia', in M. Wolf (ed.), *Dyslexia, Fluency, and the Brain*. Timonium MD: York Press 189–211.
Jackendoff, R. (2002). *Foundations of Language: Brain, Meaning, Grammar, Evolution*. Oxford: Oxford University Press.
Jakobson, R. (1960). 'Linguistics and Poetics', in T. Sebeok (ed.), *Style in Language*. Cambridge MA: MIT Press.
Jakobson, R., Fant, C. and Halle, M. (1952). *Preliminaries to Speech Analysis*. Technical Report B. Acoustics Laboratory, MIT. Reprinted (1963) Cambridge, MA: MIT Press.
Johnstone, T., Van Reekum, C. and Scherer, K. (2001). 'Vocal Expression Correlates of Appraisal Processes', in K. Scherer, A. Schorr and T. Johnstone (eds), *Appraisal Processes in Emotion*. Oxford: Oxford University Press, 271–81.
Jones, D. (1956). *The Pronunciation of English*. Cambridge: Cambridge University Press.
Jones, D. (1918 and 1962: 9th edition) *An Outline of English Phonetics*. Cambridge: Heffer.
Jordan, G. (2004). 'Explanatory Adequacy and Theories of SLA', *Applied Linguistics* 25(4): 539–43.
Kavanaugh, J. and Mattingly, I. (1972). *Language by Ear and by Eye*. Cambridge, MA: MIT Press.
Kearns, K. (2000). *Semantics*. New York: Macmillan.
Keating, P. (1988). Underspecification in phonetics. *Phonology* 5, 275–92.
Keating, P. (1990). 'The Window Model of Coarticulation: Articulatory Evidence', in J. Kingston and M. Beckman (eds), *Papers in Laboratory Phonology I*. Cambridge: Cambridge University Press 451–70.
Keller, E. (ed.) (1994). *Fundamentals of Speech Synthesis and Speech Recognition*. Chichester: John Wiley.
Kiefer, M. (2005). 'Repetition Priming Modulates Category-related Effects on Event-related Potentials: Further Evidence for Multiple Cortical Semantic Systems', *Journal of Cognitive Neuroscience* 17: 199–211.
Kim, C. (1966). *The Linguistic Specification of Speech*. Working Papers in Phonetics 5: University of California at Los Angeles.
Kim, L. (2003). *The Official XMLSPY Handbook*. Indianapolis: Wiley & Son.
Kjellin, O. (1999). 'Accent Addition: Prosody and Perception Facilitate Second Language Learning', in O. Fujimura, B. Joseph, and B. Palek (eds), *Proceedings of LP'98, 2*. Prague: The Korolinum Press 373–98.
Klahr, D. and H. Simon (2001). 'What Have Psychologists (and Others) Discovered About the Process of Scientific Discovery?', in *Current Directions in Psychological Science* 10(3): 75–9.
Klatt, D. (1979). 'Synthesis by Rule of Segmental Durations in English Sentences', in B. Lindblom and S. Öhman (eds), *Frontiers of Speech Communication*. New York: Academic Press 287–99.
Klatt, D. (1980). 'Software for a Cascade/Parallel Formant Synthesizer', *Journal of the Acoustical Society of America* 67: 911–950.
Klima, E. (1991). 'Comment: Linguistic Awareness and Metalinguistic Control', in I. Mattingly and M. Studdert-Kennedy (eds), *Modularity and the Motor Theory*

of Speech Perception: Proceedings of a Conference to Honor Alvin M. Liberman. New Jersey: Lawrence Erlbaum 413–21.
Koch, S. (1981). 'The Nature and Limits of Psychological Knowledge' in S. Koch and D. Leary (eds), *A Century of Psychology as Science*. New York: McGraw-Hill.
Kurowski, K., Haxen, E. and Blumstein, S. (2003). 'The Nature of Speech Production Impairments in Anterior Aphasics: An Acoustic Analysis of Voicing in Fricative Consonants', *Brain and Language* 84: 353–71.
Ladd, D. (1984). 'Declination: A Review and Some Hypotheses', *Phonology Yearbook* 1: 53–74.
Ladefoged, P. (1965). *The Nature of General Phonetic Theories*. Georgetown University Monograph on Languages and Linguistics (18). Washington, DC: Georgetown University.
Ladefoged, P. (1993). 3rd edition. *A Course in Phonetics*. Orlando: Harcourt Brace Jovanovich.
Ladefoged, P. (2005). 2nd edition. *Vowels and Consonants*. Oxford: Blackwell.
Ladefoged, P. and Maddieson, I. (1996). *Sounds of the World's Languages*. Oxford: Blackwell.
Lakoff, G. and Johnson, M. (1999). *Philosophy in the Flesh: The Embodied Mind and Its Challenge to Western Thought*. New York: Basic Books.
Lashley, K. (1951). 'The Problem of Serial Order in Behavior', in L. Jeffress (ed.), *Cerebral Mechanisms in Behavior*. New York: Wiley.
Laver, J. (1994). *Principles of Phonetics*. Cambridge: Cambridge University Press.
Lazarus, R. (2001). 'Relational Meaning and Discrete Emotions', in K. Scherer, A. Schorr and T. Johnstone (eds), *Appraisal Processes in Emotion*. Oxford: Oxford University Press 37–69.
LeDoux, J. (1996). *The Emotional Brain*. New York: Simon & Schuster.
Lehiste, I. (1970). *Suprasegmentals*. Cambridge MA: MIT Press.
Levinson, S. (1985). *Pragmatics*. Cambridge: Cambridge University Press.
Levinson, S. E. (2005). *Mathematical Models for Speech Technology*. Chichester: Wiley & Sons.
Liberman, A. and Mattingly, I. (1985). 'The Motor Theory of Speech Perception Revised,' *Cognition* 21: 1–36.
Liberman, A. Delattre, P. and Cooper, F. (1958). 'Some Cues for the Distinction between Voiced and Voiceless Stops in Initial Position', *Language and Speech* 1: 153–67.
Liberman, A., Cooper, F., Shankweiler, D. and Studdert-Kennedy, M. (1967). 'Perception of the Speech Code', *Psychological Review* 74(6): 431–61.
Lindblom, B. (1963). 'Spectrographic Study of Vowel Reduction', *Journal of the Acoustical Society of America* 35: 1171–81.
Lindblom, B. (1964). 'Articulatory and Acoustic Studies of Human Speech Production', *Quarterly Progress and Status Report: Speech Transmission Laboratory*. Stockholm: Royal Institute of Technology.
Lindblom, B. (1983). 'Economy of Speech Gestures', in P. MacNeilage (ed.), *The Production of Speech*. New York: Springer-Verlag 217–46.
Lindblom, B. (1990). 'Explaining Phonetic Variation: a Sketch of the H and H Theory', in W. Hardcastle and A. Marchal (eds), *Speech Production and Speech Modelling*. Dordrecht: Kluwer 403–39.

Lindblom, B. and MacNeilage, P. (1986). 'Action Theory: Problems and Alternative Approaches'. *Journal of Phonetics* 14, 117–32.

Lisker, L. and Abramson, A. (1964). 'A Cross- language Study of Voicing in Initial Stops: Acoustical Measurements', *Word* 20: 384–422.

Long, M. (1993). 'Assessment Strategies for Second Language Acquisition Theories', *Applied Linguistics* 14(3): 225–49.

Lorenz, K. (1965). *Über Tierisches und Menschliches Verhalten*. München: R. Piper. Trans. R. Martin (1970). *Studies in Animal and Human Behavior*. London: Methuen.

Lubker, J. and Parris, P. (1970). 'Simultaneous Measurements of Intraoral Air Pressure, Force of Labial Contact, and Labial Electromyographic Activity During Production of the Stop Consonant Cognates /p/ and /b/', *Journal of the Acoustical Society of America* 47: 625–33.

Luck, M., McBurney, P. and Priest, C. (2004). 'A Manifesto for Agent Technology: Towards Next-Generation Computing', *Autonomous Agents and Multi-Agent Systems* 9: 203–52.

Macaluso, E., Frith, C. and Driver, J. (2001). 'Multisensory Integration and Crossmodal Attention Effects in the Human Brain: Response', *Science* 292: 1791.

MacNeilage, P. (1970). 'Motor Control of Serial Ordering of Speech', *Psychological Review* 77: 182–96.

MacNeilage, P. and De Clerk, J. (1969). 'On the Motor Control of Coarticulation in CVC Monosyllables', *Journal of the Acoustical Society of America* 45: 1217–33.

Massoro, D. and Light, J. (2004). 'Using Visible Speech for Training Perception and Production of Speech for Hard of Hearing Individuals, *Journal of Speech, Hearing, Language, and Hearing Research* 47(2), 304–20.

Matthews, P. (1964) 'Muscle Spindles and Their Motor Control'. *Physiological Review* 44, 219–88.

McKeon, R. (ed.) (2001). *The Basic Works of Aristotle*. New York: Modern Library.

Mortimer, C. (1985). *Elements of Pronunciation*. Cambridge: Cambridge University Press.

Morton, K. (1986). 'Cognitive Phonetics: Some of the Evidence', in R. Channon and L. Shockey (eds), *In Honor of Ilse Lehiste*. Dordrecht: Foris 191–4.

Morton, K. (1992). 'Pragmatic Phonetics' in W. Ainsworth (ed.), *Advances in Speech Hearing and Language Processing 2*. London: JAI Press 17–53.

Morton, K. (1996). 'Spoken Language and Speech Synthesis in CSCW', in J. Connolly, and L. Pemberton (eds), *Linguistics Concepts and Methods in CSCW*, 23–33. London: Springer-Verlag.

Morton, K. and Tatham, M. (1980). 'Production Instructions'. *Occasional Papers 23*. Colchester: University of Essex 14–16.

Morton, K. and Tatham, M. (1995). 'Pragmatic Effects in Speech Synthesis', *Proceedings of Eurospeech*, Madrid 1819–22.

Morton, K., Tatham, M. and Lewis, E. (1999). 'A New Intonation Model for Text-to-Speech Synthesis', *Proceedings of the 14th International Congress of Phonetic Sciences*, Berkeley: University of California 85–8.

Murray, I. and Arnott, J. (1993). 'Toward the Simulation of Emotion in Synthetic Speech: A Review of the Literature on Human Vocal Emotion', *Journal of the Acoustical Society of America* 93: 1097–108.

Newsome, W. (1977). 'Perceptual Processes', in M. Gazzaniga (ed.), *Conversations in the Cognitive Neurosciences*. Cambridge, MA: MIT Press 53–68.

Nichols, M. and Newsome, W. (1999). 'The Neurobiology of Cognition', *Nature* 402: C35–38.
Nickels, L. and Howard, D. (2004). 'Correct Responses, Error Analyses, and Theories of Word Production', *Cognitive Neuropsychology* 21(5): 531–6.
Nobre, A., Coull, J., Vandeberghe R., Maquet P., Frith, C. and Mesulam, M. (2004). 'Directing Attention to Locations in Perceptual versus Mental Representations', *Journal of Cognitive Neuroscience* 16 (3): 363–73.
Nooteboom, S. (1975). 'On the Internal Auditory Representation of Syllable Nucleus Durations', in G. Fant and M. Tatham (eds), *Auditory Analysis and Perception of Speech*. Academic Press: London 413–30.
Nooteboom, S. (1983). 'Is Speech Production Controlled by Speech Perception?', in M. van den Broecke, V. van Heuven, W. Zonneveld (eds), *Studies for Antonie Cohen. Sound Structures*. Dordrecht: Foris Publications 183–94.
Oatley, K. and Johnson-Laird, P. (1998). 'The Communicative Theory of Emotions', in J. Jenkins, K. Oatley and N. Stein (eds), *Human Emotions: A Reader*. Oxford: Blackwell, 84–97. Originally pub. In L. Martin and A. Tesser (eds), *Striving and Feeling: Interactions Among Goals, Affect, and Self-Regulation*, Hillsdale, NJ: Erlbaum (1996) 363–6, 372–80.
Odell, K. and Shriberg, L. (2001). 'Prosody-voice Characteristics of Children and Adults with Apraxia of Speech', *Clinical Linguistics and Phonetics* 15(4): 275–307.
Öhman, S. (1966). 'Coarticulation in VCV Utterances: Spectrographic Measurements', *Journal of the Acoustical Society of America* 39: 151–68.
Öhman, S. (1967) 'Numerical Model of Coarticulation', *Journal of the Acoustical Society of America* 41: 310–20.
Olson, A. and Caramazza, A. (2004). 'Orthographic Structure and Deaf Spelling Errors: Syllables, Letter Frequency, and Speech', *The Quarterly Journal of Experimental Psychology: Section A* 57 (3): 385–417.
Panksepp, J. (1998). *Affective Neuroscience: The Foundations of Human and Animal Emotions*. Oxford: Oxford University Press.
Panksepp, J. (2000). 'Emotions as Natural Kinds within the Mammalian Brain', in M. Lewis and J. Haviland-Jones (eds), *Handbook of Emotions*. New York: Guilford Press 137–56.
Pierrehumbert, J. (1981). 'Synthesizing Intonation', *Journal of the Acoustical Society of America* 70: 985–95.
Plutchik, R. (1994). *The Psychology and Biology of Emotion*. New York: Harper Collins.
Potter, R., Kopp, G. and Green, H. (1947). *Visible Speech*. New York: Van Nostrand.
Pourtois, G. and de Gelder, B. (2002). 'Semantic Factors Influence Multisensory Pairing: A Transcranial Magnetic Stimulation Study', *Neuroreport* 13(12): 1567–73.
Prince, A. and Smolensky, P. (2004). *Optimality Theory: Constraint Interaction in Generative Grammar*. Malden: Blackwell.
Purcell-Gates, V. (2001). 'Emergent Literacy is Emerging Knowledge of Written, not Oral, Language', *New Directions for Child and Adolescent Development* 92: 7–22.
Raichle. M. (1997). 'Brain Imaging', in M. Gazzaniga (ed.), *Conversations in the Cognitive Neurosciences*. Cambridge, MA: MIT Press 15–33.
Raichle, M. (2003). 'Functional Brain Imaging and Human Brain Function', *Journal Neuroscience* 23(10): 3959–62.
Ramachandran, V. and Hubbard, E. (2003). 'Hearing Colors, Tasting Shapes', *Scientific American*, May.

Repp, B. (1984). 'Categorical Perception: Issues, Methods, and Findings', in N. Lass (ed.), *Speech and Language 10, Advances in Basic Research and Practice*. Orlando: Academic Press 244–335.

Rolls, E. (1999). *The Brain and Emotion*. Oxford: Oxford University Press.

Romani, C. and Galluzzi, C. (2005). 'Effects of Syllabic Complexity in Predicting Accuracy of Repetition and Direction of Errors in Patients with Articulatory and Phonological Difficulties', *Cognitive Neuropsychology* 22: 34–52.

Rosen, R. (1985). *Anticipatory Systems: Philosophical, Mathematical and Methodological Foundations*. Oxford: Pergamon.

Rosner, B. and Pickering J. (1994). *Vowel Perception and Production*. Psychology Series. Oxford: Oxford University Press.

Sacks, O. (1996). *An Anthropologist on Mars*. New York: Random House.

Saltzman, E. and Munhall, K. (1989). 'A Dynamic Approach to Gestural Patterning in Speech Production', *Ecological Psychology* 1, 333–82.

Scherer, K. (1993). 'Neuroscience Projects to Current Debates in Emotion Psychology', *Cognition and Emotion* 7: 1–41.

Shanks, D. (2005). 'Implicit Learning', in K. Lamberts and R. Goldstone (eds), *Handbook of Cognition*. London: Sage 202–20.

Sharma, C. and Kunins, J. (2002). *Voice XML: Strategies and Techniques for Effective Voice Application Development with Voice XML 2.0*. New York: Wiley & Sons.

Shriberg, L. and Kent, R. (1982). *Clinical Phonetics*. USA: Wiley & Sons.

Shriberg, L., Flipsen Jr, P., Kwiakowski, J. and Mcsweeny, J. (2003). 'A Diagnostic Marker for Speech Delay Associated with Otitis Media with Effusion; the Intelligibility–Speech Gap', *Clinical Linguistics and Phonetics* 17(7): 507–28.

Shriberg, L., Aram, D. and Kwaitkowski, J. (2004). 'Developmental Apraxia of Speech:II Toward a Diagnostic Marker', *Journal of Speech and Hearing Research* 40(2): 254–72.

Silverman, K., Beckman, M., Pitrelli, J., Ostendorff, M., Wrightman, C., Price, P., Pierrehumbert, J. and Hirschberg, J. (1992). 'ToBI: a Standard for Labelling English Prosody', in *Proceedings of the 2nd International Conference on Spoken Language Processing* 2: 867–70.

Singleton, D. and Lengyel, Z. (1995) (eds.). *The Age Factor in Second Language Acquisition: A Critical Look at the Critical Period Hypothesis*. Clevedon: Multilingual Matters.

Sluijter, A., Bosgoel, E., Kerkhoff, J., Meier, E., Rietveld, T., Swerts, M. and Terken, J. (1998). 'Evaluation of Speech Synthesis Systems for Dutch in Telecommunication Applications', *Proceedings of the 3rd ESCA/COCOSDA Workshop of Speech Synthesis*. Jenolan Cowles, Australia: CD-ROM.

Spencer, A. (1996). *Phonology: Theory and Description*. Oxford: Blackwell.

Stampe, D. (1979). *A Dissertation on Natural Phonology*. New York: Garland.

Stevens, K. (1989). 'On the Quantal Nature of Speech', *Journal of Phonetics* 17: 3–46.

Stevens, K. and Halle, M. (1967). 'Remarks on Analysis by Synthesis and Distinctive Features', in W. Wathen-Dunn (ed.), *Models for the Perception of Speech and Visual Form*. Cambridge, MA: MIT Press 88–102.

Studdert-Kennedy, M. and Mody, M. (1995). 'Auditory Temporal Perception Deficits in the Reading-impaired: A Critical Review of the Evidence', *Psychonomic Bulletin and Review* 2: 508–14.

Sweet, H. (1877). *Handbook of Phonetics*. Oxford: Clarendon Press.

Tallal, P., Miller, S. and Fitch, R. (1993). 'Neurobiological Basis of Speech; A Case for the Preeminence of Temporal Processing', in P. Tallal, A. Galaburda, R. Linas and C. van Euler (eds), *Temporal Information Processing in the Nervous System; Special Reference to Dyslexia and Dysphasia*. New York: Annals of the New York Academy of Sciences 682: 27–47.

Tarone, E., Gass, S. and Cohen, A. (1994). *Research Methodology in Second-Language Acquisition*. New Jersey: Lawrence Erlbaum.

Tatham, M. (1970). 'Coarticulation and Phonetic Competence', *Occasional Papers 8*. Colchester: University of Essex.

Tatham, M. (1971). 'Classifying Allophones', *Language and Speech* 14: 140–5.

Tatham, M. (1986a). 'Cognitive Phonetics: Some of the Theory', in R. Channon and L. Shockey (eds), *In Honor of Ilse Lehiste*. Dordrecht: Foris 271–6.

Tatham, M. (1986b). 'Towards a Cognitive Phonetics', *Journal of Phonetics* 12: 37–47.

Tatham, M. (1990). 'Cognitive Phonetics', in W. Ainsworth (ed.), *Advances in Speech, Hearing and Language Processing 1*, London: JAI Press 193–218.

Tatham, M. (1995). 'The Supervision of Speech Production', in C. Sorin, J. Mariani, H. Meloni and J. Schoentgen (eds), *Levels in Speech Communication: Relations and Interactions*. Amsterdam: Elsevier 115–25.

Tatham, M. and Lewis, E. (1992). 'Prosodics in a Syllable-based Text-to-speech Synthesis System', in *Proceedings of the 1992 International Conference on Spoken Language Processing*. Banff: CSCP.

Tatham, M. and Morton, K. (1969). 'Some Electromyography Data towards a Model of Speech Production', *Language and Speech* 12(1).

Tatham, M. and Morton K. (1980). 'Precision', *Occasional Papers 23*. Colchester: University of Essex 104–13.

Tatham, M. and Morton, K. (1988) 'Knowledge Representation and Speech Production/Perception Modelling in an Artificial Intelligence Environment', in W. Ainsworth and J.N. Holmes (eds), *Proceedings of Speech '88* (7th FASE Symposium), Edinburgh: Institute of Acoustics 1053–60.

Tatham, M. and Morton, K. (2000). 'Intrinsic and Adjusted Unit Length in English Rhythm'. *Proceedings of the Institute of Acoustics-WISP 2001*, 189–2000. St Albans: Institute of Acoustics.

Tatham, M. and Morton, K. (2002). 'Computational Modelling of Speech Production: English Rhythm', in A. Braun and H. Masthoff (eds), *Phonetics and Its Applications: Festschrift for Jens-Peter Köster on the Occasion of his 60th Birthday*. Stuttgart: Franz Steiner Verlag 383–405.

Tatham, M. and Morton, K. (2003). 'Data Structures in Speech Production', *Journal of the International Phonetics Association* 33: 17–49.

Tatham, M. and Morton, K. (2004). *Expression in Speech: Analysis and Synthesis*. New York: Oxford University Press.

Tatham, M. and Morton, K. (2005). *Developments in Speech Synthesis*. Chichester: Wiley & Sons.

Tatham, M., Morton, K. and Lewis, E. (1998). 'Assignment of Intonation in a High-level Speech Synthesiser', *Proceedings of the Institute of Acoustics*, St Albans: Institute of Acoustics, 255–62.

Tatham, M., Morton, K. and Lewis, E. (2000). 'SPRUCE: Speech Synthesis for Dialogue Systems', in M. M. Taylor, F. Néel and D. G. Bouwhuis (eds), *The Structure of Multimodal Dialogue* 2, 271–92. Amsterdam: John Benjamins.

Toates, F. (2001). *Biological Psychology: An Integrative Approach*. Harlow: Pearson.

Trubetskoy, N. (1939). *Grundzüge der Phonologie* (TCLP VII): Prague. Trans. from 3rd edition Göttingen: Ruprecht. C. Baltaxe (1971). *Principles of Phonology*. Los Angeles: University of California Press.
Verschueren, J. (2003). *Understanding Pragmatics*. London: Arnold.
Wang, W. and Fillmore, C. (1961). 'Intrinsic Cues and Consonant Perception', *Journal of Speech and Hearing Research* 4: 130–6.
Wells, J. (1982). *Accents of English*. Cambridge: Cambridge University Press.
Westbury, J. (1994). *X-ray Microbeam Speech Production Database Users Handbook*. Madison: Waisman Center, University of Wisconsin.
Wickelgren, W. (1969). 'Context-Sensitive Coding, Associative Memory, and Serial Order in (speech) Behavior', *Psychological Review* 76: 1–15.
Wilkinson, L. and Shanks, D. (2004). 'Intentional Control and Implicit Sequence Learning', *Journal of Experimental Psychology: Learning Memory and Cognition* 30: 354–69. www.morton-tatham.co.uk
Young, S. (2000). 'Probabilistic Methods in Spoken Dialogue Systems', *Philosophical Transactions of the Royal Society (Series A)* 358 (1769): 1389–402.
Young, S. (2002). 'Talking to Machines (Statistically Speaking)', *International Conference on Spoken Language Processing*. Denver: CD-ROM.
Yule, G. (1996). *Pragmatics*. Oxford: Oxford University Press.

Name Index

Abercrombie, D., 67, 224
Abramson, A., 292
Adolphs, R., 184
Al-Bamerni, A., 25
Alterman, R., 175
Aram, D., 292
Aristotle, 242
Arnott, J., 180

Balleine, B., 245
Barinaga, M., 245
Baxter, M., 245
Beckman, M., 159
Bell-Berti, F., 245
Beretta, A., 254
Bertelson, P., 285
Blachman, B., 247, 289
Bladon, R., 25
Blake, R., 284
Blomert, L., 250
Blumstein, S., 213, 291
Borden, G., 31
Bosgoel, E., 260
Boyce, S., 245
Brinton, D, 275.
Browman, K., 22, 120, 238

Cannizzaro, M., 292
Caramazza, A., 282
Carmichael, L., 156
Celce-Murcia, M., 275
Chen, M., 229
Cho, T., 83, 89
Chomsky, N., 9, 59, 267
Chun, D., 272
Cohen, A., 270
Cohen, H., 292
Cook, V., 248,
Cooper, F., 107, 167, 285
Cottingham, J., 242
Coull J., 245, 250
Critchley, E., 284

Critchley, M., 284
Cruttenden, A., 3

Damasio, A., 184
Daniloff, R., 31, 75
Darwin, C., 246
DeClerk, J., 44
DeCourtenay, B., 15
de Gelder, B., 284, 285
Delattre, P., 211
Dennett, D., 241
Descartes, R., 242
Dickinson, A., 245
Driver, J., 284

Eberl, J., 242
Edmonds, L., 292
Eimer, M., 284
Ellis, N., 254
Eskenazi, M., 248
Eysenck, M., 250

Fant, C., 107, 150, 206
Farmer, M., 286
Farnetani, E., 91
Fawcett, A., 285
Feth, L., 31
Feynman, R., 167, 249
Fillmore, C., 17, 70
Firth, J., 22, 120, 175
Fitch, R., 285
Fletcher-Flinn, C., 287
Flipsen Jr, P., 292
Fougeron, C., 154
Fowler, C., 22, 29, 91, 112, 118
Frijda, N., 184
Frith, U., 245, 250, 285
Frost, S., 287
Fry, D., 134

Galluzzi, C., 280
Garland, A., 175

Gass, S., 270
Gazzaniga, M., 283
Gelfer, C., 245
Gibson, J., 206
Gilroy, L., 284
Gimson, A., 3, 10, 272
Givon, T., 237
Goldsmith, J., 76, 120
Goldstein, L., 22, 120, 238
Goodwin, J., 275
Gould, S., 246
Graney, J., 254, 270
Green, H., 274
Gregg, K., 254, 270
Grundy, P., 190
Guenther, F., 87, 89
Guttman, S., 284

Halle, M., 9, 150
Halliday, M., 298
Hammarberg, R., 75
Hancock, M., 272
Hardcastle, W., 57
Harel, B., 292
Harris, K., 31
Haxen, E., 280
Hayes, B., 220, 291
Henke, W., 67, 70
Hewlett, N., 57
Hirschberg, J., 159
Holmes, J., 62, 70, 256
Holmes, W., 256
Howard, D., 280
Hubbard, E., 284

Ivry, R., 177, 283, 286, 288

Jackendoff, R., 237
Jakobson, R., 55, 150
Johnson, M., 227
Johnson-Laird, P., 186
Johnstone, T., 184
Jones, D., 15, 272
Jordan, G., 248
Justus, T., 177, 143, 283, 286, 288

Karakow, R., 245
Kavanaugh, J., 285
Keane, M., 250

Kearns, K., 190
Keating, P., 26, 55, 76, 154, 220
Keller, E. 256
Kent, R., 294
Kiefer, M., 251
Kim, C., 70, 74, 105
Kim, L., 264
Kjellin, D., 248
Klahr, D., 252, 255
Klatt, D., 145, 259
Klein, R., 286
Klima, E., 287
Koch, S., 246, 249
Kopp, G., 274
Kunins, J., 121
Kurowski, K., 280
Kwiakowski, J., 292

Ladd, D., 149
Ladefoged, P., 17, 25, 71, 103, 130, 148, 220, 263
Lakoff, G., 227
Lashley, K., 60, 108
Laver, J., 12, 18, 27
Lazarus, R., 184
LeDoux, J., 184, 245
Lehiste, I., 129
Lengyel, Z., 275
Levinson, S., 194
Levinson, S. E., 213, 268
Lewis, E., 158
Liberman, A., 107, 208, 211, 285
Light, J., 274
Lindblom, B., 60, 64, 78, 112, 216
Lisker, L., 292
Long, M., 254
Lorenz, K., 237
Lubker, J., 36
Luck, M., 175.

Macaluso, E., 284
MacNeilage, P., 35, 78, 108, 112, 218
Maddieson, I., 263
Mangum, G., 283
Maquet P., 245, 250
Marquardt, T., 292
Massoro, D., 274
Matthews, P., 37, 62
Mattingly, I., 62, 208, 283, 288

McBurney, P., 175
McKeon, R., 242
Mcsweeny, J., 292
Meier, E. 260
Mesulam M., 245, 250
Middleton, C., 177, 283, 288
Miller, S., 285
Mody, M., 285
Mortimer, C., 272
Morton, K., 18, 26, 118, 189, 238, 257, 259, 264, 267
Munhall, K., 113
Murray, E., 245
Murray, I., 180

Newsome, W., 242, 288
Nichols, M., 288
Nickels, L., 280
Nicolson, R., 285
Nobre, A., 250
Nooteboom, S., 218

Oatley, K., 186
Odell, K., 291
Öhman, S., 61, 64, 74, 96
Olson, A., 282
Ostendorff, M., 159

Panksepp, J., 184, 238
Parris, P., 36
Pickering, J., 248
Pierrehumbert, J., 157, 159
Pitrelli, J., 159
Plutchik, R., 186
Potter, R., 274
Pourtois, G., 284
Price, P., 159
Priest, C., 175
Prince, A., 175
Purcell-Gates, V., 286

Racasens, D., 91
Raichle. M., 243, 268, 288
Ramachandran, V., 284
Reilly, N., 292
Repp, B., 211
Rietreld, T., 260
Rolls, E., 184

Romani, C., 280
Rosen, R., 179, 217
Rosner, B., 248

Sacks, O., 284
Saltzman, E., 113
Scherer, K., 184
Schuckers, G., 31
Shanks, D., 242, 245
Shankweiler, D.,107, 285, 287
Sharma, C., 121
Shearme, J., 62, 259
Shriberg, L., 291, 294
Silverman, K., 159
Simon, H., 252, 255
Singleton, D., 275
Sluijter, A., 260
Smolensky, P., 220
Snyder, P., 292
Spencer, A., 97
Stampe, D., 104
Steriade, D., 220
Stevens, K., 213, 209
Studdert-Kennedy, M., 107, 247, 285
Sweet, H., 220
Swerts, M. 260

Tallal, P., 285
Tarone, E., 270
Tatham, M., 18, 26, 43, 80, 90, 111, 118, 149, 158, 238, 259, 264, 267
Terken, J., 260
Toates, F., 250
Trubetskoy, N., 15,152

Vandeberghe R., 245, 250
Van Reekum, C., 184
Verschueren, J., 191

Wang, W., 3, 17, 70, 229
Wells, J., 10, 276
Westbury, J., 11
Wickelgren, W., 58
Wilkinson, L., 245
Wrightman, C., 159

Young, S., 265
Yule, G., 190

Subject Index

abstract, 8, 13, 21, 49, 53, 107
abstraction, 14, 35, 58, 291
   levels, 105
accent, 11, 99, 212, 276
accommodation, 29, 33
   contextual, 27
acoustic
   domain, 20, 147, 157, 205
   object, 18, 133, 168, 240
   phonetic, 244
   signal, 119–20, 122, 139, 188, 201, 206
   target, 10, 32, 112
   variability, 14, 158, 204, 258, 291
   waveform, 126, 198, 285
acquisition, 118
   disorder, 281
   phonological units, 240
   second language, 254, 270
Action Theory, 36, 112, 207, 229
   time, 114–15
adaptation, 28, 246, 260
   articulation, 28
   simulation, 258
   supervision, 239
adaptive variability, 222
adjustment, 37, 58, 89, 110, 170, 251
agent, 37, 111, 176, 244, 276, *see* CPA
algorithm, 138, 162
   reading, 286
   synthesis, 261
allophone, 70
   classifying, 71, 103
   coarticulation, 262
   extrinsic, 35, 49, 56, 204, 244, 262
   intrinsic, 17, 49, 71–2, 103
allophonic variation, 5, 80
   intrinsic, 94, 126
ambiguity, 155
ambisyllabic, 129
amplitude, 86, 122, 139, 194, 258
amygdala, 245
analogue, 223

analytic, *see descriptive*
anticipatory
   coarticulation, 22–6
   cognitive phonetics, 181
   cognitive processing, 179
   models, speech production, 217
   systems, 179, 217
aoristic, 6, 49
aphasia, 252, 280
apraxia, 291
application
   models, 247, 297
   see speech technology
   see speech disorders
   see second language learning
articulation, 37, 53
   constraint, *see* coarticulation
   control, 106
   ease, 220
   managed, 154, 171, 212
   precision, 44–6, 154, 183
   prosodic effects, 153
   targets, 35, 92, 109
articulatory
   control, 75, 106
   domain, 19
   economy, 64
   parameters, 23, 64
   phonology, 115, 120, 151, 208, 238
   response, 223
   spatial position, 87
   unit, 32
assignment, 163, 202, 206, 214–16
   dialect, 90
   feature, 10, 124, 131
   segment, 124, 194, 204, 293
   articulatory representation, 220, 290
   listener, 219
   perceptual representation, 20, 41, 65, 138
   prosody, 152–5
   representations, *see* speech representations

assignment – *continued*
  stress, 138–9
  waveform, 195, 204, 212, 250
assimilation, 23, 40, 72, 77, 152
  coarticulation, 53, 56, 72–5, 83, 271
asynchrony, 228
a-theoretical, 247
attitude, 26, 121, 176, 189
  concealed, 179
  revealed, 179
auditory, 285
  cortex, 169, 194, 200
  feedback, 169
  nerve, 170, 194
  phonetics, 6
  space, 218
automatic speech recognition (ASR), 265, *see* speech technology
awareness, *see* phonological

Bayesian, 296
bi-directional, 28
biopsychology, *see* cognitive neuroscience
black box, 92, 143
brain, 109, 171, 194, 226, 244
  mind, 238–40, 250, 282, 288

categorical perception, 211
category, 12, 141, 212, 296
central processor, 28
cerebellum, 177, 244, 289
Classical Phonetics, 3–20, 224, 244
  pronunciation training, 273
  variability, 265
classification and description, 103
clinical neuroscience, 192
  clinical phonetics, 293
  coarticulation, 278, 281
  deafness, 281
  phonetics, 232, 282, 291, 295
  precision, 191
  TM model, 197, 221, 223, 262, 278
coarticulation,
  adaptation, 28
  aggression, 86, *see* enhancement
  anticipatory, 25
  application, 278,

assimilation, 23, 271
blocking, 30
'blurring' effect, 4, 198
boundaries, 33, 227
co-production, 29, 132, 278
cognitive phonetics, 18, 30
constraint, *see* resistance
defective, 279
definition, 22
enhancement, 32, 87, 91, 222
involuntary, 29, 35, *see* processes
left to right, 23, 28, 30, 36
managed, 18, 261, 271
models, 57–98, 206, 221, 234
overlap, 26
perception, 44, 220
resistance, 53, 78, 83, 86
right to left, 23, 24, 30
rhythm, 281
target, 25, 32, 40, 221
theory, 13, 18, Ch. 2, Ch. 3, 34, 49–56, 181
voluntary, 21, 23, 29, 35, *see* processes
wrapper, 26
cognition
  brain activity, 226, 240, 250
  discrete linguistic units, 42, 117, 226
  phonology, 73, 82, 119
  speech production models, 29, 172, Ch. 3, Ch. 4, *see* CPA
cognitive
  emotive content, 283
  interpretation, 172, 184
  intervention, 26, 46, 67, 184, 200, 227
  neuroscience, 240, 279, 282
  parameters, 33, *see* parameter
  planning, 54
  processes, 55, 119, 172, 217, 227
  psychology, 13
  sourced, 44, 48, 160, 184, 258, 297
Cognitive Phonetics, 9, 18, 21, 26, 37, 69, Ch. 3, Ch. 6
  anticipatory, 179, 181, 217
  articulation, 86

Subject Index

Cognitive Phonetics – *continued*
  constraint, enhance, 94
  cognitive intervention, 26, 31, 44, 73, 159, 184, 201
  processing, 150, 159
  production and perception, 158, 216, 238, 244
cognitive phonetic agent CPA, 128, 176, 221, 281, 233
  brain activity, 242
  expressive content, 181–3
  listener's behavior, 176, 217
  monitoring, 30, 70, 217
    see supervision
  planes, *see* planes
  rendering, 7, 22, 27, 32, 50, 87, 89, 157, 282, *see* rendering
  supervision, 89, 143, 159, 176–83, 250, 281
collaboration
  production and perception, 96
  speaker and listener, 212, 217
comparator, 204, 215
computational modelling, 104, 255, 296
computational models, 111, 137, 250, 286, *see* speech production, TM intonation
configuration
  articulatory, 55, 107
  muscles, 28
  spatial, 109
  vocal tract, 119, 214
consonant, 7, 126, 141,
  classification, 103, 110, 127, 149–54
  stops, 10, 29, 66, 115, 128, 141, 293
  syllable, 27, 272
  vs. vowels, 194, 293
constraints, 46, 83, 89, 96, 100, 178, 261
  cognitive, 30, 148, 222
  phonetic, 10, 30, 58, 126, 143, 183
  phonological, 5, 183, 222
  pragmatic, 173, 175
  prosodic, 148, 270
  temporal, 65
  wrapper, 176
control models, 229
coordinative structure, 114–16

co-production, 14, 22, 27, 278
coarticulation, 29, 49, 72–5, 91–118
  cognitive phonetic, 76
continuant, 127, 233
continuum, 100, 110, 230
CPA *see* cognitive phonetics agent
cross-modal, 284, 290
cross-talk, 275

data structures, 255, 257, 264
declination, 148–9
description and classification, 103
descriptions, 7, 240, 242, 289
  phonetic, 21, 100, 188, 293
  phonological, 21, 183, 256
descriptive adequacy, 64, 188
derivation, derivational history, 32, 49, 99, 183, 192, 204, 242, 266, 275
diagnostic applications, 292
dialect, 75, 101, 119, 276, 297
digital, 223
diphone, 169
direct perception, *see* perception
disordered speech, 240, 278, 281
Distinctive Feature Theory, 46, 150
duality, 173, 237, 240, *see* mind–body
duration, timing, 105, 114, 125, 145, 177, 223
  isochrony, 147
  length, 109, 140, 143
  perception, 134
  plan, 222
dynamic, 255, 257
  models, 176, 265
  phonetic, 144, 222, 274
  phonological, 280, 285
  planes, Ch. 6, *see* planes
  processing, 266
  waveform, 181
dyslexia, 285–287, 289

ease of articulation, 221
electromyography, 28, 30, 227
emotion
  anger exemplar, 181, 185
  basic, 185
  biological, 178, 184
  mapping, 187
  perception, 139, 189
  secondary, 186

emotion – *continued*
  static plane, 173
  vector representation, 185
  wrapper, 121, 184
emotive content, 177, 179, 182
  cognitive approaches, 283
empirical, 84, 146, 169, 248–9, 250,
    see model building
  observations, 248, 252
  theory, 246, 271,293
enhancement, 31, 69, 86, 87, 91, 222
exemplar, 57, 88, 112, 128, 173, 176,
    242, 266
experiential, 247, 274
explanation, 47, 93, 270, 279
  cognitive phonetic, 149
  co-production, 118
  phonetic, 104, 119, 140, 156
  phonological, 104, 143, 156
  scientific, 20, 44, 46, 246
explanatory adequacy, 64, 84, 104
expression space, 184
expressive content, 178–85, 194
  lack of, 210, 263
  perception, 184
  prosody, 257
expressive/emotive content,
    179–84, 282
  linguistically motivated, 180
  biologically motivated, 181
  sources, 184
  supervision, *see* CPA, supervision
extrinsic allophone, 17, 63, 74,
    244, 262
  intrinsic, 71, *see* allophone intrinsic
  planning, 40, *see* CPA
  rendering the plan, 133, 244,
    see plan
  underlying form, 56, 71, 167, 205

feature spreading rules, 76
feature transfer, 125
feedback, 36, 62, 169–171, 273
  auditory, 169
  CPA, 177
  intramuscular, 170
  speaker/listener, 178, 187, 215,
    250, 272
feed-forward anticipatory model, 217
fMRI, 243, 288

formalism, 68, 230, 264
formants, 63
French, 95, 99, 122, 147, 234, 275
functional brain imaging, 243
functional definitions, 225
fundamental frequency, 158, 160, 179
  expression, 187
  intonation, 148
  laryngeal activity, 138
  stressed syllable, 134

gamma loop, 171, 218
gestural
  context, 208
  score, 120
gesture, 23, 29, 80, 192, 291
  articulatory, 51, 55, 93, 113
  muscle pattern, 206, 240
  phonetic, 208
  phonological, 115

[h], 225
hidden Markov, 56, 266
hierarchy (tier), 26, 31, 112, 148, 152,
    160, 182, 227
  accent, 99
  duration, 143
  production, 58, 112
  representations, 57, 160, 239
  wrapper, 134
hypothesis, 50, 54, 143, 200, 263, 278,
    289, *see* model building
  allophone, 19, 27
  cerebellum, 177
  coarticulation, 30, 97
  emotion, 185
  experiment, 247, 255, 264
  fiction, 19
  perception, 201, 209, 216
  phonology, 167, 205, 281
  plan, 144, 234
  prosody, 152
  speaker, 217
  wrapper, 121, 182, 271

identification, vs. assignment, 202, 211
independent, 131–3, 144
inertia, 43, 47, 70, 72, 96, 94
  aerodynamic, 27, 96
  mechanical, 27, 65, 96, 143

inference, 191
information processing, 113
innate, 237
input, 55, 72, 87, 115, 143, 167, 216, 200, 251
   CPA, 177
   perception, 139
   plan, 230
instantiation, 129, 173, 185, 265
   utterance, 20, *see* utterance
intelligibility, 99, 256, 258
interaction, 51, 79, 132, 172
   cognitive/physical, 223, 232, 290
   co-production, 92
   cross-modal, 290
   speaker/listener, 33, 200, 217
interface, *see* mapping
International Phonetic Alphabet (IPA), 8, 163, 274
   symbolic representation, 17
interpretation, 44, 57, 77, 114, 157
   active, 208
   assigning labels, 16, 20
   cognitive, 20, 162, 170, 183, 194
   fMRI, 288
   theory, 249
intonation, 152, 205, 261, *see* declination
   assigning labels,
   expression, 182
   ToBI, 160
   TM, 157–8
   wrapper, 182
intrinsic
   allophone, 70, *see* allophone
   duration, 124, 145
invariance, 36, 79, 109, 124, 182, 213
isochrony, 124, 147, 264

juncture (syllable), 129

knowledge, 54, 121, 160, 174, 204
   articulators, 209
   base, 198, 204, 214, 255, 270, *see* plane
   CPA, 221
   Interpretation, 162, 296
   perception, 75, 149, 183

phonological awareness, 286, *see* phonological awareness
representation, 143, 173, 221, 249

language pathology, *see* clinical neuroscience, disordered speech
language specific, 49, 71, 75, 80, 118, 274
language teaching/learning, 192, 240
   accent, 261, 275
   articulation, 279
   assimilation, 271
   capacity, 274
   critical age hypothesis, 275
   feedback, 281, 296
   interference, 36, 275
   modelling, 270
   perception, 272
   production, 237, 272
   second language acquisition (SLA), 270, 272
   TM model, 278
   training, 192, 249, 274
laryngeal, 137
length, *see* phonology
   cognition, 125
   perception, 135
   rhythm, 124
   segment, 125
   stress, 134
linear, 3, 9, 11, 25, 32, *see* model
linguistic, 97, 124, 180, 237, 291
   characterisation, 266
   constraint, 48, 83, 220
   context, 84, 143
   focus, 100, 239
   grammar, 75, 112, 173, 265
   model, 162, 226, 250–253
   rule-based, 230
lip
   closure, 28, 172, 229
   rounding, 22, 68, 91
   spreading, 29
listener, 124, 128, 187
   active, 187
   attitude/emotion, 189, 192
   Cognitive Phonetics, 69, 217
   goal, 196, 234
   isochrony, 124

listener – *continued*
  knowledge, 190, 201, 272,
    see knowledge
  mapping, 205, 208
  naturalness, 259
  perceptual goal, 12, 93, 196, 218,
    see perception
  perceptual separation, 197
  perceptual task, 198
  plan, 3, 11, 198
  speech waveform, 18, 54, 122, 209,
    216
look-up tables, *see* mapping
lossy, 162

management, 36, 51, 61
  CPA, 281
  interpretation, 178
  rendering, 69, 73
mapping, 70, 183, 212, 238, 282, 288
  cognitive/physical, 24, 70, 212
  emotion, 187
  perceptual space, 8, 187
  phonetic, 8
  speaker/listener, 205
  supervision, 238
marking, 9, 55, 224, 257
meaning, 18, 53, 72, 101, 261, 272, 279
metatheory, 50, 189, 252, 254, 286–8, 290–3
metrical organisation, 144
mind/body, 116, 238
mind/brain, 242
model building, 168, 237
  computationally adequate, 55, 286, 297
  empirical, 14, 93, 247–9, 270, 279, 293, 167
  experiment, 143, 169, 210, 240, 242, 246, 249, 280
  guess, 143, 167
  hypothesis, 54, 18, 27, 201, 209, 216, 218, 221, 232, 247, 255, 280, *see* hypothesis
  metatheory, 189, 254, *see* metatheory
  representations, *see* speech representations
  scientific, 12, 38, 44, 210, 226, 279

  testing, 249, 250, 264, 274, 293
  theory, 245, 250, 252, *see* theory
models, *see* speech production
  models, speech perception models
  acoustic, 107
  action, 112, *see* action theory
  active (perception), 203
  adaptive variability, 222
  analysis by synthesis, 209
  anatomical, 106
  anticipatory, 25, 179, *see* coarticulation, cognitive phonetics
  application, 237
  articulation, 172
  articulatory phonology, 117, 151
  associative store, 213
  categorical perception, 211
  coarticulatory, 64
  cognitive, 172
  cognitive phonetics, 210, 216, *see* cognitive phonetics
  computational, 111, 231, 250
  coordinative structure, 109
  co-production, 80, 91
  direct perception, 206
  direct realism, 212
  distinctive feature, 107
  duality, 238
  dynamic, 87, 255, Ch. 6
  feature spreading, 75
  filter, 205
  hierarchal, 273
  hybrid, 163, 209
  linear, conjoined, 31, 35, 62
  look-ahead, 67
  motor control, 99, 170
  motor theory, 107, 207, *see* motor theory
  neural network, 266
  numerical, 110
  parametric, 9, 152, 224
  passive (perception), 202
  physical, 8, 12
  physical world, 168
  positional, 36
  predictive, 54, 179
  production for perception, 218
  prosodic analysis, 150

models – *continued*
  quantal, 213
  serial ordering, 60, 109
  spatial target, 61, 109
  static, Ch. 6
  systematic synthesis, 74, 105
  target, 219, 221, 229
  task dynamic, 116
  template, 204
  tiered, 221
  translation, 207
  vowel carrier, 61
  window, 6, *see* window
monitoring, 177
  supervision, 176, 181, 250
motor
  control, 99, 109, 143, 171, 218, 229, 244
  command, 12, 63, 109, 223
  precision, 86, 154, *see* precision
  uniqueness, 34, 229
Motor Theory,
  perception, 184, 207–10

nasality, 4, 44
naturalness, 256–60
  expressive/emotive speech, 192
  simulation, 193
neural network, 57, 230, 264
neurolinguistics, 227, 237
neuromuscular control, 27
neuropsychology, *see* clinical neuroscience
neuroscience, 237, 284, 298
  applications, 280
  clinical, 192
  cognitive, 240, 288
  speech technology, 254
node, 100, 126,

objectivity, 234, 279
ordering, 249
  serial, 61, 108
  temporal, 111
output, 54, 65, 71, 89, 140, 143, 218
  listener, 177, *see* listener
  plan, 32, 80, 167, 251, *see* plan
  plane, 173
  speech, 184, 238, 279
  waveform, 54

overlap, 91–2
  coarticulation, 26
  motor commands, 108

paradigm, 104, 169,
  generic, 202–4
  shift, 22, 104, 118
  wrapper, 26
parameter, 9, 13, 29, 36, 132, 204
  acoustic, 140, 187
  articulatory, 9, 62, 91, 114, 137, 221, 229, 295
  cognitive, 33
  evaluation, 261
  Firth, 22, 152
  overlapping, 48, 92
  physical, 33, 94, 107
  perception, 44, 205, 270
  prosodic, 152, 181, 257
  segment, 132
  synchronicity, 151
  synthesis, 61, 187
  vocal tract, 116, 232
pattern seeking, 196
perception, 199, 233
  active models, speech, 202, 210
  articulator response, 223
  direct, 206
  hearing, 240
  hybrid, 209
  motor theory, 207
  passive models, filtering, 205
  passive, template, 204
  perceptual goal, 196
  perceptual task, 198
  phonology, 12, 20, 75
  production for perception, Ch. 8
  prosody, Ch. 7
  segments, 12, *see* segment
  separation, 177, 197, 221
  space, 8, 187, 218
  speech production, Ch. 8
  speaker collaboration, 200, 216
  task, 198
perceptual separation, 221
phonation, 10, 221
phone, 18
phoneme, 4, 15, 40, 58, 61, 110, 127
  accent, 140

phoneme – *continued*
  defining, 15, 105
  label, 5, 13, 15, 103
phonetic segments, 6, 23, 72, 176
phonetics
  articulatory, 6
  auditory, 6
  categories, 291
  classical, *see* classical phonetics
  cognitive, *see* cognitive phonetics
  descriptions, 21, 104, 293
  dynamic, *see* planes
  inventory, 99, 292
  modern, 22, 66, 107, 110, 152
  plane, *see* planes
  speech perception, *see* speech perception
  speech production, *see* speech production
  static, *see* planes
  structure, 291
  theory, 231
  transcription, 17
phonological
  awareness, 259, 289–90
  units, 26, 45, 58, 208, 270, 291
phonology
  articulatory, 115
  autosegmental, 161
  coda, 126
  constraints, 5
  dynamic, *see* planes
  knowledge, 203
  label, 212
  length, 140
  metrical stress, 144
  onset, 126
  optimality theory, 220
  plane, *see* planes
  static, *see* planes
  stress, 133, *see* stress
  syllable, 128, 132, *see* syllable
pitch, 161
plan, 4
  expression, 179
  isochrony, 147
  neural, 57, 240, 251
  perception, 18, 138
  phonetic, 58, 87
  phonology, 56, 118, 230

pragmatics, 189
prosodic, 148
speaker, 12, 66, 134
rendering, 68, 87, 104, 128, 217
timing, 144, 222
utterance, 40, 68, 107, 136, 167, 263
wrapper, 149, *see* wrapper
planes, 173–6, 255, *see* speech production, TM model
  dynamic–procedural, 173, 188, 275
  expression, 183
  static–declarative, 275
  supervision, 176
planning, 54, 233, 242
  brain activity, 245
  cognitive, 16, 37
  CPA, 38, 233
  motor, 291
  phonetic, 134, 282
  phonological, 134, 240, 282
  output, 251
  rendering, 136, 282
  segmentally based, 131, 133
plasticity, 27, 223
plosives, 5, 79, 91, 119, 126, 233
post-Classical, 107
posture vs. gesture, 224
pragmatics, 189
  Inference, 190
  presupposition, 190
Prague School, 107, 155
precision, 154–5
  articulation, 78, 155, 220
  blur, 24
  control, 23, 86
  CPA, 155
  distance, 154
  perception, 43
  predictability, 26
  target, 24
  variability, 182, 197
predictive modelling, 179, *see* models
  anticipatory reasoning, 219
  feed-forward, 219
  perception, 178
preference, 102, 128
presupposition, *see* pragmatics
principle of least effort, 23
probability, 201, 261, 266, 296
  rating, 242

processes
  cognitive, 172, 212
  involuntary, 29, 33, 36, 40, 91, 156, 178
  phonetic, 40, 159, *see* rendering
  phonological, 41, 49, 73, 90,104, 119, 159, 202, 233
  rule-governed, 230
  voluntary, 29, 36, 40, 178
processing, *see* input, output
production for perception, 184, 216, 218–20
programming
  articulators, 93, 292
  coordinative structures, 29
prominence, 136, *see* stress
pronunciation, 99, 192, 248,
  teaching, 271, 274, 284, Ch. 11
prosodic
  domain-final lengthening, 154
  framework, 6, Ch. 5, Ch. 8
  intonation, 124, *see* wrapper, TM model
  production, Ch. 5
  perception, 194, Ch. 8
  precision improvement, 154
  rhythm, 122, *see* time, duration, isochrony
  suprasegmental, 256
  strengthening, 156
  syllable, 131, 188, 191, 272
  TM model, 149, 157
  wrapper, 133, 150, 156, 174, 188, 270
prosody
  acoustics, 124
  contour, 89, 132
  expression, 257
  information bearing, 183
  intonation, 148, 152, 160, *see* declination
  hypotheses, 133, 152
  stress, *see* stress
psychological reality, 12, 33, 94, 126, 226
psychology, *see* perception, planning linguistics

reading, 247, 270, 282
  database, 285, *see* phonological awareness
  speaking, 286, 290–1
  spelling, 288
  writing, 290
recognition
  computer, 193, 253, 256, 265–7
  human, 196, 287, *see* perception
reflex, 53, 109
rendering, 34, 86, 174, 183, 202, 276
  cognitive intervention, 26, 118, 140
  constraints, 70
  management (supervision), 52, 69, 89, 176, 217, 230
  phonetic, 78, 233
  physical, 72, 145, 157, 229
  plan, 44, 104, 111, 139, 148, 174
  perception, 196
  prosodic, 128, 133, 159, 177, 256
  segmental, 125, 142, 152, 232
repair
  error, 96, 178
  misperceived signal, 284
  plan, 273
  signal, 178, 283
representations
  accent, 275
  acoustic, 109, 167, 188
  articulatory, 167, 272, 276
  assigning, 189
  computational, 182
  expression, 185, 282
  levels of, 167, 290
  matrices, 7, 9, 56
  neuro-digital, 194
  perception, 20, 138, 157, 187, 192
  phonological, 168
  prosodic, 183
  reconciling types, 34, 56
  speech *see* speech representation
  surface, 56, 185, 282
  symbolic, 16, 178
  underlying, 104, 167, 185, 272
  vector, 185
researchers (speech model building)
  Browman, 238, *see* Task dynamics
  Chomsky and Halle, 106
  Daniloff and Hammarberg, 75
  Fant, 107
  Firth, 120, *see* prosodics
  Fowler, 112, *see* Action Theory
  Fry, 134
  Gibson, 206

researchers – *continued*
  Goldstein, 238, *see* Task dynamics
  Henke, 70
  Holmes, 62
  Jakobson, 149
  Jones, 272
  Keating, 76, *see* Window model
  Kim, 70, 105
  Ladefoged, 71, *see* positional model
  Lashley, 60, 108
  Liberman and Mattingly, 207
  Lindblom, 64
  MacNeilage, 61, 109, *see*, target
  Öhman, 61, 110
  Stevens, 213
  Tatham and Morton (TM), Ch. 6, *see* cognitive phonetics
  Tatham, 218
  Trubetskoy, 230
retrieval tasks, *see* fMRI
rhythm, 257
  pattern, 111, 145
  prosody, 261
  stress patterns, *see* stress
  structure, 50
  temporal ordering, 111, 122
rule-governed, 230
rules, 173, 202, 254, 273, 281
  linguistic, 112, 169
  phonetic, 76, 78, 108, 264
  phonological, 77, 80, 202, 240
  window width, 82

scalar, 223
second language acquisition, 240, 270
  research, 270
segment
  abstract, 13, 16, 200, 205, 224, 240
  adjacent, 22, 44, 132, 259
  classes, 3, 61, 84, 151, 185
  definition, 61, 62, 71, *see* allophone
  label, 14, 18, *see* vowel, consonant
  physical, 21, 76
  spanned, 132
  string of discrete, 22, 23, 54, 92
segmental
  boundaries, 114, 126, 227
  classification, 7, 10, 103, 201
  psychological reality, 225, 233

segmentation, 13, 21, 119, 224
self-organising, 29, 38, 83, 113, 171, 212
serial ordering, 60, 108, 111
simulation, 193, *see* speech technology
smoothing, 42, 51, 66
sounds, sound, 7
  continuous, 11, 57
  discrete, 3–4, 21
  pattern, 105, 119, 242
  sequence, 7
span, 6, 122, 132, 152
speaker, 13,
  acoustic, 70
  attitude, emotion, 121
  effort, 217
  expectation, 258
  goal, 70, 181, 192, 218, 234, 244
  isochrony, 123
  motor command, 108
  plan, 40, *see* plan
spectrogram, 11, 46, 57, 206
speech, general
  acoustic, 20, Ch.10, 230, *see* acoustic
  articulation, 35–6, *see* articulation
  continuum, 230
  disorders, 40, 240, 278
  dynamic, 173, 255, *see* planes
  expressionless, 147
  framework, 7, 270, 278
  models, *see* models, model building
  naturalness, 257
  parameters, 258
  representations, 18, 57, 214, 55, 86, 220, 292, *see* allophones, phonemes
  segments, 11, 122, 126, *see*, segment
  signal, 197, 239, 258
  sounds, 57, 242
  style, 257, 261, 263
speech, general – *continued*
  syllables, 128, *see* syllables
  theory, domain, 19, *see* theory
  units, 14
speech perception, 44, 201, 240, 264, *see* Part II
  coarticulation, 54
  mapping, 199

speech perception – *continued*
  models, 172, 184, 194, 199, 200, 201–18
  plan, 233, *see* plan
  predictive , 179, 197
  processing, 233
  prosody, 194
  simulation, 162, 241, 264, *see* speech recognition
  task, 198
speech production, 44, 89 *see* Part I
  application, 247, 250, 256
  coarticulation, 55, 96, *see* coarticulation
  CPA, 176,216, *see* CPA
  constraints, 96, *see* constraints
  control, 229
  data structures, 264
  disorders, 240
  inertia, 72
  input, 37, 167, 246, 282
  linguistic, 134
  mechanism, 12, 44, 70, 201, 250
  models, 16, 23, 71, 104, 171, 174, 233, 264, *see* models
  perception, 201, 264, *see* perception
  phonetic, 20, 233, 291
  phonology, 233, 291
  plan, 199, *see* plan
  planes, 173,
  plasticity, 223
  precision, 155, *see* precision
  processing, 22, 78, 92, 104, 227
  rendering, 69, 176
  simulation, 241, 259, *see* speech technology
  theory, 14, 99, 239, 245, 275, *see* theory
  variability, 261
  wrapper, 174, 178, *see*, wrapper
speech simulations, 241, 261, *see* speech technology
speech technology, Ch.10
  allophone, *see* allophone
  data structure, 264
  expression, 259
  intelligibility, 256, 258, 261
  multiple platform, 265
  naturalness, 256, 259, 260
  parametric, 187
  perception, 198
  simulation, 198, 241, 259
  speech model, 138, 265
  speech synthesis, 63, 104, 138, 174, 230, 256
  speech recognition, 256, 265
  statistical modelling, 264, 265
  variability, 264
statistics, statistically, 100, 266
stress, 111, 129, 132, 133, 159
  contrastive, 134, 182
  intonation, 124, 152
  pattern, 145
  perceptual assignment, 138–40
  prominence, 136
  rhythm, 123, 145
  sentence, 149, 158
  syllables, 133
  timed, 147
  trigger, 138
style, 26, 263–4
subjective
  interpretation, 162, 239, 260
  judgement, 6, 234
subjectivity, 7, 89
supervision, 143, 176, 250, *see* monitoring
  cognitive phonetics, 73, 240, 281
  CPA, Ch. 3, 176
  rendering, 71, *see* rendering
suprasegmentals, 129, 130
surface effects, 143, 183, 223
syllable
  constituents, 126
  definitions, 128, 224
  boundary, 14–15, 26, 32, 67, 211, 228
  CPA, 181
  juncture, 129
  perception, 139
  phonetic, 48, 128, 137
  phonological, 68, 89, 98, 128, 135, 279
  prosody, 131, 154, 181, 205, 272
  rhythm, 145
  segment, 224
  stress, *see* stress
  structure, 126
  timing, 145
  unstressed, 146
  XML, 182

symbol, 214, 239, 242
  assignment, 8, 16, 214, 290
  labels, 238
  object-symbol, 150
  symbol-object, 56
symbolic representation, 16–20, 58, 72, 157, 161, 177, 194, 201, 211, 290, see representations
  abstract, 211, 290
  allophones, 126
  assignment, 13, 53, 167, 177, 212
  CPA, 157, 216
  definition, 16
  IPA, 9, 18
  nature of, 16
  segments, 12, 70
syntagmatic, 127
synthetic, see explanatory

target
  acoustic, 112
  articulator, 23, 35, 70, 218
  canonical, 23
  cognitive, 76
  internalised, 139
  management, 36, 229
  missed, 25, 65
  representations, 34, 55, 86, 93, 221
  response, 223
  segments, 28, 229
  sequence, 32
  size, 35
  spatial, 35, 37, 63
  specification, 32, 35, 42, 70, 87, 143, 154
  structures, 223
  theory, 32, 37, 115, 221
  unique, 229
Task Dynamics, 81, 116
  articulation, 115, 238
  phonology, 117
Tatham–Morton (TM) model, Ch. 6
  coarticulation, 220, see coarticulation
  cognitive intervention, 160
  constraint, 82, 222, see constraint, enhancement
  coordinative structure, 37, 113
  CPA, cognitive Phonetics, 80, 88, 154, 176, 243, see CPA

data structure, 257, 264
expression, 185, 189, see pragmatics
intonation, 158, 160, see intonation
labels, 14, 222
management, supervision, 114, 119, 281
phonetics, 69
phonology, 69
plan, 50, 56, 218, see utterance
planes, 150, 220, 244, see planes
perception, 138, 158, 197, 210, 214, 219, 271, see perception
precision, 155, see precision
processes, 73, 159
production, see speech production
prosody, 149
rendering, 70, 92, 221
representations, 34, 72
speaker's goal, 135
supervision, 176
target, 82, 221
wrapper, see wrapper
template, 204, 253
temporal feature, 50
testing, 249
theory, 245, 250, 252, see models, model building, metatheory
  applications, see applications, Part 3
  coarticulation, chapter 2, see coarticulation
  framework, 249
  speech production, see Part 1
  speech perception, see Part 2
threshold logic, 266
time, timing, 50, 114, 105, see duration, cerebellum
  constraints, 292
  control, 111, 114, 170, 239, 280
  plan, 144, 222
  stress pattern, 270
  wrapper, 144
ToBI, 159–62, 175
tone, 130
tongue, 8, 21, 33, 51, 62, 98, 107
transcription, 17, 127, 140, 162, see IPA
  phonetic, 4, 9, 143
  phonemic, 6, 16, 143

transcription – *continued*
  symbolic representation, 17–20
  ToBI, 175
  variation, 18
transformation, *see* speech
  representations
trigger, 111, 182, 187, 195, 216, 222, 225
tuning, 114

underspecification (phonetics), 26
universal sets
  allophones, 74, *see* allophones
  Classical Phonetics, 7, 125
  coarticulation, 22, 86, 139
  declination, 148
  gestures, 270–1
  processing, 76
  window, 79
utterance, 3, 40, 68, 137, 167, 196–8, 204, 263
  exemplar, 16, 50, 112, 173, 267
  coarticulation, 25
  constraints, 176
  expression, 182
  metrical organisation, 144
  plan, 12, 26, 33–7, 70, 96, 147
  production, 145, 174, 220, 242
  rendering, 107, 111, 133, 181
  representation, 18
  syllabic structure, 102, 128
  wrapper, 102, 133, 182

variability, 16, 87, 89, 218, 260–4
  assignment, 34, 196
  acoustic, 182, 291
  cognitive phonetics, 73
  expression, 160, 182
  perception, 52, 156
  phonetic, 16, 34, 78
  pragmatics, 189
  random, 156, 263
  sources of, 87, 187, 189, 192, 209, 261, 288
  systematic, 156
vector, 68, 86–8
  expressive/emotive content, 185
  perception, 211
vision, 280
vocal cords

laryngeal activity, 137
  vibration, 72, 86, 137, 141, 194, 225, 232
vocal tract, 12, 37, 107, 182–2
  articulation, 9, 25, 51
  configuration, 182, 214, 259
  gestures, 206, 115, 206
voice onset time (VOT), 68
  diagnostic, 292
vowel
  classification, 8–12, 128, 103–5
  coarticulation, 110–14
  consonants, 194
  duration, 125
  formants, 205
  length, 140
  precision, 154
  reduction, 257
  stressed, 134, 196

waveform
  dynamic nature, 181–5
website, www.Morton-Tatham.co.uk, 255
window, see Ch. 3, model
  coarticulation, 78
  production process, 78
  rules, 81
  segments, 221
  targets, 78, 89
  value ranges, 79, 85, 87
wrapper, 102
  coarticulation, 26
  declination, 148
  expression, 133, 182
  Firth, 150
  hypothesis, 26, 271, *see* model building
  metrical organisation, 144
  paradigm, 26
  perception, 188
  processes, 159
  prosody, 133, Ch. 6, 157, 159
  rendering, 129, 174, 176, 263, *see* rendering
  TM model, 88, 173, 217
  XML, *see* XML

XML, 26, 121, 149, 182, 264